Oral Health and Aging

Christie-Michele Hogue • Jorge G. Ruiz
Editors

Oral Health and Aging

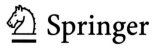
Springer

Editors
Christie-Michele Hogue
Department of Dental Services - VA
Healthcare System, Division of
Geriatrics and Gerontology, Emory
University School of Medicine
Atlanta, GA, USA

Jorge G. Ruiz
Geriatric Research, Education and Clinical
Center (GRECC)
Miami VA Healthcare System
Miami, FL, USA

Division of Geriatrics and
Palliative Care
University of Miami Miller School of
Medicine
Miami, FL, USA

ISBN 978-3-030-85992-3   ISBN 978-3-030-85993-0 (eBook)
https://doi.org/10.1007/978-3-030-85993-0

© The Editor(s) (if applicable) and The Author(s), under exclusive license to Springer Nature Switzerland AG 2022
This work is subject to copyright. All rights are solely and exclusively licensed by the Publisher, whether the whole or part of the material is concerned, specifically the rights of translation, reprinting, reuse of illustrations, recitation, broadcasting, reproduction on microfilms or in any other physical way, and transmission or information storage and retrieval, electronic adaptation, computer software, or by similar or dissimilar methodology now known or hereafter developed.
The use of general descriptive names, registered names, trademarks, service marks, etc. in this publication does not imply, even in the absence of a specific statement, that such names are exempt from the relevant protective laws and regulations and therefore free for general use.
The publisher, the authors and the editors are safe to assume that the advice and information in this book are believed to be true and accurate at the date of publication. Neither the publisher nor the authors or the editors give a warranty, expressed or implied, with respect to the material contained herein or for any errors or omissions that may have been made. The publisher remains neutral with regard to jurisdictional claims in published maps and institutional affiliations.

This Springer imprint is published by the registered company Springer Nature Switzerland AG
The registered company address is: Gewerbestrasse 11, 6330 Cham, Switzerland

Contents

Age-Related Changes in Oral Health 1
Ezekiel Ijaopo and Christie-Michele Hogue

Epidemiology of Oral Health Conditions in the Older Population 13
W. Murray Thomson and Moira B. Smith

Nutrition and Oral Health 29
Rena Zelig, Samantha Honeywell, and Riva Touger-Decker

Swallowing, Dysphagia, and Aspiration Pneumonia 47
Atsuko Kurosu, Rebecca H. Affoo, Shauna Hachey,
and Nicole Rogus-Pulia

Xerostomia and Hyposalivation................................. 85
Rosa María López-Pintor, Lucía Ramírez Martínez-Acitores,
Julia Serrano Valle, José González-Serrano, Elisabeth Casañas,
Lorenzo de Arriba, and Gonzalo Hernández

Management of Periodontal Disease in Older Adults 109
Nadia Laniado, Liran Levin, and Ira Lamster

Management of Caries in Older Adults 131
Gerry McKenna, Martina Hayes, and Cristiane DaMata

Systemic Disease That Influences Oral Health..................... 145
Jaisri R. Thoppay and Akhilanand Chaurasia

The 3 Ds: Dementia, Delirium and Depression in Oral Health 161
Natasha Resendes, Iriana Hammel, and Christie-Michele Hogue

Oral Care in Long-Term Care Settings........................... 177
Ronald Ettinger and Leonardo Marchini

Oral Health of the Palliative and Hospice Patient 201
Valerie Hart, Dominique Tosi, and Khin Zaw

Ethical Considerations in Geriatric Dentistry 223
Carlos S. Smith

Health Disparities in Oral Health 239
Cherae M. Farmer-Dixon, Machelle Fleming Thompson,
and Joyce A. Barbour

Frailty and Oral Health 253
Jorge G. Ruiz and Christie-Michele Hogue

The Role of Oral Health Literacy and Shared Decision Making 263
Marlena Fernandez, Christie-Michele Hogue, and Jorge G. Ruiz

Barriers to Access to Dental Care 279
Janet Yellowitz

Index 287

Contributors

Rebecca H. Affoo, PhD, CCC-SLP, SLP-Reg, SLP(C) School of Communication Sciences and Disorders, Faculty of Health, Dalhousie University, Halifax, NS, Canada

Joyce A. Barbour, DDS, MBA Meharry Medical College, Nashville, TN, USA

Elisabeth Casañas, DDS, PhD Department of Dental Clinical Specialties, School of Dentistry, Complutense University, Madrid, Spain

Akhilanand Chaurasia, MDS Department of Oral Medicine and Radiology, Faculty of Dental Sciences, King George's Medical University, Lucknow, UP, India

Cristiane DaMata, BDS, MFD RCSI, MPH, PhD Cork University Dental School and Hospital, University College Cork, Cork, Ireland

Lorenzo de Arriba, DDS, MD, PhD Department of Dental Clinical Specialties, School of Dentistry, Complutense University, Madrid, Spain

Ronald L. Ettinger, BDS, MDS, DDSc, DDSc(hc) Department of Prosthodontics, College of Dentistry, University of Iowa, Iowa City, IA, USA

Cherae M. Farmer-Dixon, DDS, MSPH, MBA Meharry Medical College, Nashville, TN, USA

Marlena Fernandez, MD Miami VA Healthcare System, Geriatric Research, Education and Clinical Center (GRECC), Miami, FL, USA

José González-Serrano, DDS, PhD Department of Dental Clinical Specialties, School of Dentistry, Complutense University, Madrid, Spain

Shauna Hachey, MHS, RDH School of Dental Hygiene, Faculty of Dentistry, Dalhousie University, Halifax, NS, Canada

Iriana Hammel, MD Miami VA Healthcare System, Geriatric Research, Education and Clinical Center, Miami, FL, USA

Division of Geriatrics and Palliative Medicine, University of Miami Miller School of Medicine, Miami, FL, USA

Valerie Hart, MD University of Miami/Jackson Health System, Miami, FL, USA

Martina Hayes, BDS, MFDS RCSEd, PgDipTLHE, PhD Cork University Dental School and Hospital, University College Cork, Cork, Ireland

Gonzalo Hernández, DDS, MD, PhD Department of Dental Clinical Specialties, School of Dentistry, Complutense University, Madrid, Spain

Christie-Michele Hogue, DDS, AGSF Department of Dental Services - VA Healthcare System, Division of Geriatrics and Gerontology, Emory University School of Medicine, Atlanta, GA, USA

Samantha Honeywell, MS, RD, CNSC Department of Clinical and Preventive Nutrition Sciences, School of Health Professions, Rutgers, The State University of New Jersey, Newark, NJ, USA

Ezekiel Ijaopo, MD, MPH, MRCP-UK, DGM, MSc Combined Geriatric Medicine/Hospice and Palliative Medicine Fellow, University of Miami/Jackson Health System, Miami, FL, USA

Atsuko Kurosu, PhD Department of Medicine, School of Medicine and Public Health, University of Wisconsin–Madison, Madison, WI, USA

Ira Lamster, DDS MMSc School of Dental Medicine, Stony Brook University, Stony Brook, NY, USA

Nadia Laniado, DDS MPH MSc Department of Dentistry, Albert Einstein College of Medicine, Bronx, NY, USA

Liran Levin, DMD Faculty of Medicine and Dentistry, University of Alberta, Edmonton, AB, Canada

Rosa María López-Pintor, DDS, PhD Department of Dental Clinical Specialties, School of Dentistry, Complutense University, Madrid, Spain

Leonardo Marchini, DDS, MSD, PhD Department of Preventive and Community Dentistry, College of Dentistry, University of Iowa, Iowa City, IA, USA

Lucía Ramírez Martínez-Acitores, DDS Department of Dental Clinical Specialties, School of Dentistry, Complutense University, Madrid, Spain

Gerry McKenna, BDS,PhD,FDS(Rest Dent)RSCEd,FHEA Centre for Public Health, Queen's University Belfast, Belfast, Northern Ireland, UK

Natasha Resendes, MD Miami VA Healthcare System, Geriatric Research, Education and Clinical Center (GRECC), Miami, FL, USA

Department of Medical Education, University of Miami Miller School of Medicine, Miami, FL, USA

Nicole Rogus-Pulia, PhD, CCC-SLP Division of Geriatrics and Gerontology, Department of Medicine, School of Medicine and Public Health, University of Wisconsin–Madison, Madison, WI, USA

Swallowing and Salivary Bioscience Laboratory, Geriatric Research Education and Clinical Center (GRECC), William S. Middleton Memorial Veterans Hospital, Madison, WI, USA

Jorge G. Ruiz, MD Miami VA Healthcare System, Geriatric Research, Education and Clinical Center (GRECC), Miami, FL, USA

Division of Geriatrics and Palliative Medicine, University of Miami Miller School of Medicine, Miami, FL, USA

Carlos S. Smith, DDS, MDiv, FACD Department of Dental Public Health and Policy, VCU School of Dentistry, Richmond, VA, USA

Moira B. Smith, BDS, PhD, PGDipSci DPH Department of Public Health, University of Otago, Wellington, New Zealand

Machelle Fleming Thompson, RDH, BS, MSPH Meharry Medical College, Nashville, TN, USA

W. Murray Thomson, PhD Sir John Walsh Research Institute, Faculty of Dentistry, The University of Otago, Dunedin, New Zealand

Jaisri R. Thoppay, DDS, MBA, MS Center for Integrative Oral Health, Winter Park, FL, USA

Dominique Tosi, MD Miami VA Healthcare System, Geriatric Research, Education and Clinical Center (GRECC), Miami, FL, USA

Department of Medical Education, University of Miami Miller School of Medicine, Miami, FL, USA

Riva Touger-Decker, PhD, RD,CDN, FADA Rutgers School of Dental Medicine, Newark, NJ, USA

Julia Serrano Valle, DDS, PhD Department of Dental Clinical Specialties, School of Dentistry, Complutense University, Madrid, Spain

Janet Yellowitz, DMD, MPH, FASGD, DABSCD University of Maryland School of Dentistry, Baltimore, MD, USA

Khin Zaw, MD Palliative Medicine Program, Miami VA Healthcare System, Miami, FL, USA

Division of Geriatrics and Palliative Medicine, University of Miami Miller School of Medicine, Miami, FL, USA

Rena Zelig, DCN, RDN, CDCES, CSG Department of Clinical and Preventive Nutrition Sciences, School of Health Professions, Rutgers, The State University of New Jersey, Newark, NJ, USA

Age-Related Changes in Oral Health

Ezekiel Ijaopo and Christie-Michele Hogue

This chapter reviews common age-related changes in oral health that affect the structures and functions of the oral cavity and how they may predispose older adults to the development of a variety of oral pathologies. We will address some of the limitations and challenges in the study of age-related changes in oral health. Clinicians and investigators often overlook age-related changes in oral health due to the wrong perception that these problems are inconsequential or non-life-threatening. Further evidence of this oversight is in the limited number of cross-sectional, longitudinal studies and randomized controlled trials that have been conducted. When available, existing studies have included relatively small sample sizes or shorter follow-up periods. Another consideration when discussing age-related changes is that oral conditions may not necessarily reflect the effects of the aging but rather the effects of chronic diseases, lifestyle, environmental, and social determinants. These factors may negatively impact oral health by accelerating the effects of aging on the oral cavity.

E. Ijaopo
Combined Geriatric Medicine/Hospice and Palliative Medicine Fellow, University of Miami/Jackson Health System, Miami, FL, USA

C.-M. Hogue (✉)
Department of Dental Services - VA Healthcare System, Division of Geriatrics and Gerontology, Emory University School of Medicine, Atlanta, GA, USA
e-mail: christie.michele.hogue@emory.edu

© The Author(s), under exclusive license to Springer Nature Switzerland AG 2022
C.-M. Hogue, J. G. Ruiz (eds.), *Oral Health and Aging*,
https://doi.org/10.1007/978-3-030-85993-0_1

1 Age-Related Changes in Oral Structures and Function

The development of oral structures is a complex process that began during the embryonic stage. The main structures in the oral cavity include the lips, soft and hard palates, oral mucous membranes, teeth, gingiva, tongue, salivary glands, and bones of the upper (maxilla) and lower (mandible) jaws. These structures provide a framework that supports the oral cavity and play critical roles in the physiologic processes of tasting, speaking, chewing, (mastication), and swallowing (deglutition) which will impact the process of digestion and articulation. Table 1 summarizes the main age-related changes in the structures and functions of the oral cavity.

2 Oral Mucous Membranes

The oral mucosa becomes smooth and dry with aging. Several studies [1, 3] have described age-related changes in the oral mucosa that include the thinning of the oral epithelium which results from reduction in the thickness of epithelial ridges and a decrease in salivary secretion. Arteriosclerotic changes with progressive obliteration of the capillaries and a reduction of cell metabolism are the main causes of oral mucosa changes with aging. The connective tissue of the oral mucosa also becomes atrophic with loss of elasticity. Similarly, nerves and end organs in the oral mucosa may also be affected by age, thus leading to a gradual loss of sensitivity to thermal, chemical, and mechanical stimuli [3].

As stated earlier, environmental factors may contribute to some of the observed changes in the oral cavity. Evidence shows that exposure of the lining of the oral mucosa to a variety of environmental factors may resemble many of the changes attributed to aging. While few age-related structural changes occur in the surface epithelia, there is mixed evidence regarding age-related changes in epithelial thickness, rates of tissue turnover, and metabolic activity [25]. Indeed, it can be challenging to differentiate normal aging changes in the oral mucosa from the variable effects of lifestyle, genetics, and environmental factors on these oral structures.

An observational study that included 38 cadavers from Japanese adults ranging in age from 62 to 98 years investigated age-related changes in the buccal mucous membranes. Serial sections of the buccal mucous membrane in the vicinity of the anguli oris were observed under a light microscope. The investigators identified five age-related changes: (1) a significant decrease in the thickness of the buccal mucous membrane; (2) a disappearance of the functional arrangement of collagenous and elastic fibers in the lamina propria and submucous membrane, accompanied by prominent fibrosis; (3) a reduction in the number and distribution of blood vessels in the mucous membrane; (4) fat infiltration and fibrosis of the small salivary glands; and (5) a decrease in the thickness of the tunica muscularis [2]. Limitations of this study are the cross-sectional nature of the data and the technical limitations of postmortem examinations which may limit the interpretation of age-related changes.

Table 1 Age-related changes in the structure and function of the oral cavity

Oral cavity structures and functions	Changes with aging	Predispose to oral pathologies
Structure		
Oral mucous membranes	↑ epithelial thinning [1] ↑ atrophy of connective tissue [2] ↑ dry, thin, and smooth oral mucosal surfaces [1, 3] ↓ thickness of epithelial ridges [3] ↓ elasticity [1, 2]	Oral cancers Oral candidiasis Oral lichen planus Chronic aphthous stomatitis Oral hairy leukoplakia Pemphigus vulgaris
Teeth	↑ enamel hardness and brittleness [4] ↑ wearing of occlusal surface [1, 5] ↓ thickness of mantle dentine and globular dentine [6] ↑ cemental irregularities [7] ↑ secondary dentine deposition/calcification [4]	Dental caries Tooth loss Chewing dysfunction
Periodontium	↓ fibroblast density of periodontal ligament tissue [8] ↓ quality and quantity of collagen [9] ↑ alveolar bone resorption [10] ↑ thinning of gingival epithelium [7] ↓ vascularity and mitotic activity [9] ↓ keratinization of gingival epithelium [7] ↑ resorption and apposition of cementum [7]	Gingivitis Chronic periodontitis Periodontitis as a manifestation of systemic diseases Necrotizing periodontal diseases Periodontal abscess
Salivary glands	↑ replacement of parenchyma by fibrous and/or adipose tissue [7, 11, 12] ↓ acinar volume (acinar atrophy) [11, 13] ↓ salivary secretions [12]	Xerostomia Swallowing disorders Sialolithiasis Sialadenitis Tumors Sjogren's syndrome
Tongue	↓ filiform papillae [1] ↓ thickness of epithelium [14] ↓ epithelium of lingual mucosa [15] ↓ lingual muscle diameter [14] ↑ lingual gland acinar atrophy [14]	Glossitis Geographic tongue Fissured tongue Taste dysfunctions Oral candidiasis Oral cancers
Function		
Masticatory function	↓ thickness of the masseter muscle [16, 17] ↓ masticatory performance [18] → functional feeding skills [19]	Chewing dysfunction
Swallowing function	↑ (prolonged) initiation of swallowing [20] ↓ maximal tongue strength [21, 22] ↓ tongue motor function and tongue pressure [23] ↑ rigidity of the esophageal wall [24] ↓ esophageal contractility [24]	Swallowing dysfunction

3 Teeth

With increasing age, the teeth show wearing of the enamel, chipping and fracture lines, and thinning of the enamel that may cause stain of the dentin, leading to a darker appearance of the teeth. The pulp chamber and canals become reduced in size due to the deposition of secondary dentin [4]. Other studies have reported the wearing away of the occlusal surface and proximal contour of the enamel, making the teeth more vulnerable to damage and decay [1, 5]. Other changes include the appearance of a small, polished facet on the cusp tip or ridge or a slight flattening of the incisal edges. In addition, there is a reduction in the cuspal height with inclination and flattening of the proximal contour of the enamel. The shortening of the length of the dental arch may be due to reduction in the mesiodistal diameters of the teeth through proximal attrition [1, 26]. Tooth loss appears to be one of the main reasons why older people have difficulty with chewing. One study aimed to determine the age-related changes in pulp cell density, pulp area, and dentinal thickness with age. Incisors (50), canines (39), premolars (51), and molars (7) extracted from 60 patients, aged 10–59 years, were analyzed histomorphometrically for cell density (presence of odontoblasts, subodontoblasts, and pulp core fibroblasts) and dentinal thickness. The analyses revealed that with increasing age, dentinal thickness increases in both the crown and root aspects of the teeth, while the density of odontoblasts, subodontoblasts, and pulp fibroblasts decreases. However, the degree of age-related changes in the teeth appeared to be asymmetrical: the decreases in the root were more pronounced than those in the crown [6].

3.1 Edentulism

Edentulism, is the permanent absence of natural teeth in the dental arch. Edentulism, or the complete loss of teeth, represents a debilitating and irreversible condition and is the final outcome of a multifactorial process encompassing patient-related and environmental factors [27]. Data from the National Health and Nutrition Examination Survey (NHANES) (2005 through 2008) were used to estimate dentate status and prevalence of untreated dental disease by age (50–64 years, 65–74 years, and ≥75 years). The investigators gathered information on persons' reports of fair or poor general health, chronic disease status, race/ethnicity (non-Hispanic Whites, non-Hispanic Blacks, and Hispanics), and income levels. In this cohort of older adults, tooth loss was highest among persons aged 75 years and older. When compared with persons aged 50–64 years, persons aged 75 years and older were three times more likely to be edentulous (32% vs 10%), and, among the dentate, persons aged ≥75 years had four fewer teeth on average (18 vs 22). A significant number of older adults had untreated dental disease. Individuals aged ≥75 years were nearly 50% more likely to have untreated root caries than persons aged 50–64 years (16% vs 11%) [28]. Another survey study conducted among 308 older adults >65 years old living in large rural communities of Colorado, USA, examined factors associated with tooth loss. This study demonstrated that rural residents of racial and ethnic minority groups along with people who had levels of education below high school had fewer teeth than their urban peers and were at higher risk of becoming edentulous at older ages [29]. A more recent study, based again on data from NHANES, analyzed data obtained from 1999–2004 and 2009–2014. It revealed a lower incidence of age-related tooth loss in adults aged 50 years and older in the 2009–2014 cohort as compared with the earlier 1999–2004 cohort (11% vs 17%) indicating an improvement in the oral health status of older individuals over time. However, this decrease was not observed among poor and disadvantaged groups. Complete tooth retention improved from 14% to 21% between 1999–2004 and 2009–2014 for persons aged 50 years and older. The improvements in teeth retention were mostly attributed to better public health measures in the last decade including exposure to fluoride and better preventive practices [30]. This evidence suggests that social determinants of health including poor lifestyle choices, access to appropriate dental care, poverty, and lack of education [31, 32] may work in association with age-related changes in the teeth to cause edentulism in older adults.

4 Salivary Glands

Salivary glands have many roles in the oral cavity. In addition to producing and secreting digestive fluids, salivary glands are responsible for producing the saliva that lubricates the mouth, protects the teeth against bacteria, makes foods moist, and aids in the digestion of food by helping with the formation of the alimentary bolus in preparation for the process of swallowing. There are three main pairs of salivary glands: parotid, submandibular, and sublingual. Salivary glands undergo degenerative changes with normal aging, including a reduced number of acini and infiltration of fatty and fibrous tissue that may contribute to reductions in salivary secretion [11–13]. However, there is mixed evidence on whether salivary flow rate declines with aging. While some authors have described reduced levels of salivary flow rates with aging, including an increase in the ionic concentrations of saliva [11, 12], others report that salivary flow rates are unchanged with aging [13].

One observational study examined salivary flow rates and saliva composition in healthy individuals ranging in age from 18 to 89 years. Saliva samples were collected in unstimulated conditions followed by sialometrical and sialochemical analyses. The study showed three main findings:

(a) Older people have significantly reduced and altered salivary secretion as compared with younger people. Although the salivary concentrations of some chemicals increased with aging, the total values of most salivary components decreased.
(b) Over one half of the older individuals reported idiopathic oral sensorial complaints (OSCs) including taste disturbances, burning mouth syndrome, or xerostomia.

(c) Older individuals reporting OSCs were more likely to use prescription drugs, highlighting again the difficulties in studying age-related changes.

The authors concluded that a reduction in salivary function and alteration in salivary composition are mostly age-related [33]. More longitudinal studies are needed that investigate age-related alterations in salivary gland morphology and function and on whether or not salivary flow rate decreases with increasing age. For a more in-depth discussion on xerostomia, please refer to the chapter "Xerostomia and Hyposalivation".

5 Tongue-Lip Motor Function (TLMF)

The tongue-lip motor function is an essential component of the innate oral-motor skills underpinning the ability to move the muscles of the facial structures, namely, the mouth, jaw, tongue, and lips. This function is fundamental for speech and feeding skills, such as sucking, biting, swallowing, and chewing. TLMF achieves this functionality by controlling muscle tone, strength, coordination, and range of motion. In older adults with missing teeth, the tongue may also play an important role in compensating for alterations in masticatory function [34]. An experimental study conducted on animals investigated age-related changes in the intrinsic lingual muscle fibers. The main age-related findings were a decreased in the number of rapid-contracting muscle fibers and an increased in the proportion of slow-contracting muscle fibers. The authors reported that shifts in muscle composition from faster to slower myosin heavy chain (MyHC) fiber types may contribute to age-related changes in swallowing duration. The decreasing muscle fiber size in transverse and verticalis muscles may add to reductions in the maximum isometric tongue pressure found in older individuals [35].

One study explored the relationship between tongue motor skills and masticatory performance in dentate older adults and denture wearers. Investigators examined 30 healthy, normal adults with teeth, 10 normal older adults with teeth, and 20 edentulous adults wearing complete dentures that were constructed following similar methods and materials. They assessed tongue motor skills via an ultrasound system and used a sieving method to evaluate masticatory performance. The study showed age-related decreases in tongue motor skills and masticatory performance [18]. Although the outcome from this study revealed that tongue-lip motor function deteriorates with increasing age, other studies have argued that these skills are not age-dependent. One longitudinal study investigated whether functional oral-motor skills change with age by measuring the functional feeding skills and oral praxis abilities of 79 healthy adults aged 60–97 years who were followed up for up to four decades. The investigators administered the Modified Functional Feeding Assessment (FFAm) subscale of the Multidisciplinary Feeding Profile (MFP) and the Oral Praxis Subtest (OPS) of the Southern California Sensory Integration Test. The results showed that older people maintained functional feeding skills throughout the four decades of the study. Individuals in their 70s and 80s experienced difficulties with a variety of food textures including soft, hard, fibrous, and tough skins [19]. It is, however, important to exercise caution when interpreting these results as several factors could have influenced the findings. The investigators measured random portions of muscle fibers from each muscle cross section rather than including all fibers within that particular muscle. Analyzing the complete muscle cross sections may have improved the accuracy and perhaps provided different data. Two other studies examined the maximal tongue strength during swallowing and chewing in healthy adults. The first study enrolled 51 dentate adults with a mean age of 25 years. The investigators evaluated tongue and lip functions by measuring the maximum tongue pressure and oral diadochokinesis with a multiple sieving method using peanuts to evaluate chewing ability [36]. The second study assessed 80 healthy young (aged 20–39 years) and older adults (aged ≥65 years) recruited from the community. They used the Iowa Oral Performance Instrument to measure maximal tongue strength and tongue strength during swallowing [22]. The first study showed that chewing ability was significantly correlated with maximum tongue pressure. The second study revealed that compared to older adults, the maximal tongue strength was significantly higher in the younger adult age group.

Although the evidence from these studies is still inconclusive on how age-related changes in tongue-lip motor function affect swallowing and masticatory functions, there is consistent evidence that tongue motor function, tongue pressure, and maximal tongue strength decrease with aging.

6 Oral Microbiome

Oral microbes are essential components of the oral cavity. The term "microbiome" represents the ecological community of symbiotic, commensal, and pathogenic microorganisms that closely share our body space. Although they are often ignored, they play crucial roles as determinants of health and disease [37]. In fact, after the gut, the oral cavity has the second largest and diverse microbiota providing a habitat for over 700 species of bacteria, fungi, viruses, and protozoa. The oral microbiome is essential to maintaining oral and systemic health [38]. Aging changes including the chronic state of low-grade inflammation or "inflammaging" may interact with the oral microbiota of older adults increasing the susceptibility of older adults to several infectious and degenerative disease processes [39].

The oropharyngeal microbiome of older people may promote the growth of several microorganisms including enterobacteria, pseudomonads, staphylococci, and yeasts that in older individuals with weakened immunity or deteriorated general health may become opportunistic pathogens [40]. Whether through the influence of the natural aging process or facilitated by the effects of disease, the bionomics of the oral cavity are likely to change, leading to alterations in the makeup of the oral microbiome. A survey study examined the relationship between the oral and gut microbiota. The findings demonstrated higher similarity between the microbiota of the gut and the subgingival plaque in older adults than in younger individuals [41]. A Japanese study investigated changes in the gut microbiota composition of age groups ranging from newborns to centenarians. They found a higher proportion of *Bacteroidetes* and *Proteobacteria* species in individuals older than 70 years. The authors postulated that nutrients in the gut might play an important role in changing the gut microbiota composition with age [42]. In addition to aging, the oral and gut microbiota may be affected by changes in dietary habits, lifestyle, immunologic reactivity, exposure to certain medications (i.e., antibiotics, proton pump inhibitors), and the increased incidence of chronic multimorbidity in the older adult population which can potentially contribute to dysbiosis of the oral microbiome which in turn may predispose older adults to oral and systemic pathologies [43–46].

Research into the role of the oral microbiome in aging and disease is rapidly evolving. Studies using diverse research techniques, lack of standardization, and small sample sizes have produced findings that are often inconsistent. Future research with larger sample sizes along with improved techniques and standardization are needed to generate more consistent results.

7 Masticatory Function

The ability to chew food particles ensures an adequate nutritional status critical for oral health and quality of life [47–50]. Optimal chewing ability will be highly dependent on the number of functional teeth, number of missing teeth, and whether the individual uses dental prostheses. The chewing ability of an individual will have direct and indirect impact on general health and may serve as an indicator of the overall oral health of an individual [51].

A cross-sectional study investigated the relationship between aging and tooth loss on the quantity and quality of masseter muscle among 112 participants, aged 20–90 years old, who were cognitively intact and independent in their activities of daily living. The study excluded participants with a lack of molar occlusal support, diseases that could affect muscle function, and presence of temporomandibular disorders. The investigators used ultrasound to measure masseter muscle thickness (MMT), an indicator of muscle quantity, and masseter muscle echo intensity (MMEI), a measure of muscle quality. Findings revealed that aging was associated with lower quantity and quality of the masseter muscle [17]. While preservation of natural dentition or prosthetic treatment may be effective at maintaining masseter muscle function in females, males may require resistance exercise training to maintain the same level of function. In another cross-sectional study, 547 community-dwelling older persons (246 men and 301 women, mean age 73.8 ± 6.2 years) underwent a comprehensive annual geriatric health examination. Their chewing ability was evaluated by masseter muscle tension palpation, differences of masseter muscle thickness measured with ultrasound, occlusal force, self-reported chewing ability, and number of remaining and functional teeth. The study showed that masseter muscle thickness and occlusal force were significantly different between males and females [52]. Another study found that masseter muscle thickness in dentate older adults at rest and during contraction was significantly higher than that found in edentulous older individuals [53]. By aiding chewing ability, masseter muscle thickness may represent an indicator of good oral health-related quality of life.

Although it has been argued that feeding skills are usually unaffected with normal aging, available evidence shows a decreased thickness of the masseter muscle and an increased acinar atrophy of lingual glands with normal aging. In addition, the prolonged initiation of swallowing and decreased masticatory performance reported with age may predispose older adults to swallowing and chewing dysfunction. These age-related changes may cause detrimental effects on the dietary habits of older individuals by limiting the intake of foods rich in vitamins, minerals, fiber, and protein while increasing the consumption of sugary and easy-to-chew, less nutritious foods [54–56]. These dietary habits may in turn contribute to nutritional deficiencies, ultimately increasing the risk for malnutrition and poor quality of life in older adults [57]. For a more in-depth discussion on these topics, please refer to chapters "Nutrition and Oral Health" and "Swallowing, Dysphagia, and Aspiration Pneumonia".

8   Conclusions

Available evidence revealed that age-related structural and functional changes in the oral cavity occur with normal aging in older people. The structural changes range from increased epithelial thinning of the oral mucosa membranes; dry, thin, and smooth oral mucosal surfaces; increased enamel hardness and brittleness; wearing of occlusal surface; and cemental irregularities. Similarly, the periodontium undergoes increased resorption and apposition of cementum and increased thinning of gingival epithelium along with decreased keratinization. With aging, salivary glands also experience more replacement of parenchyma by fibrous and/or adipose tissue and decreased acinar volume along with decreased saliva production. However, available studies are inconclusive on whether the salivary flow rate decreases with normal aging. Decreased thickness of the masseter muscle and increased acinar atrophy of lingual glands with normal aging affect masticatory function and result in altered perception of food taste, respectively. These age-related changes may predispose older individuals to malnutrition, disease, and poor quality of life.

References

1. Khare A, Thahriani A, Chauhan AS, Khare A. Age changes in oral tissues. Heal Talk. July–August 2015, 2015 ed. p. 41–50.
2. Akimoto K. Observations on the structural changes according to aging of oral mucous membrane in the elderly--structure of buccal mucous membrane in the vicinity of angulus oris. Kokubyo Gakkai zasshi. J Stomatol Soc Jpn. 2004;71(2):80–94.

3. Breustedt A. Age-induced changes in the oral mucosa and their therapeutic consequences. Int Dent J. 1983;33(3):272–80.
4. Lamster IB, Asadourian L, Del Carmen T, Friedman PK. The aging mouth: differentiating normal aging from disease. Periodontology 2000. 2016;72(1):96–107.
5. Sulyanto R. Effects of aging on the mouth and teeth: MERCK MANUAL consumer version; 2020 [updated Feb. 2020; cited 2021]. Available from: https://www.merckmanuals.com/home/mouth-and-dental-disorders/biology-of-the-mouth-and-teeth/effects-of-aging-on-the-mouth-and-teeth.
6. Murray PE, Stanley HR, Matthews JB, Sloan AJ, Smith AJ. Age-related odontometric changes of human teeth. Oral Surg Oral Med Oral Pathol Oral Radiol Endod. 2002;93(4):474–82.
7. Huttner EA, Machado DC, De Oliveira RB, Antunes AGF, Hebling E. Effects of human aging on periodontal tissues. Spec Care Dentist. 2009;29(4):149–55.
8. Krieger E, Hornikel S, Wehrbein H. Age-related changes of fibroblast density in the human periodontal ligament. Head Face Med. 2013;9(1):1–4.
9. Lim WH, Liu B, Mah SJ, Chen S, Helms JA. The molecular and cellular effects of ageing on the periodontal ligament. J Clin Periodontol. 2014;41(10):935–42.
10. Arai K, Tanaka S, Yamamoto-Sawamura T, Sone K, Miyaishi O, Sumi Y. Aging changes in the periodontal bone of F344/N rat. Arch Gerontol Geriatr. 2005;40(3):225–9.
11. Razak PA, Richard KJ, Thankachan RP, Hafiz KA, Kumar KN, Sameer K. Geriatric oral health: a review article. J Int Oral Health: JIOH. 2014;6(6):110.
12. Xu F, Laguna L, Sarkar A. Aging-related changes in quantity and quality of saliva: where do we stand in our understanding? J Texture Stud. 2019;50(1):27–35.
13. Vissink A, Spijkervet FKL, Amerongen AVN. Aging and saliva: a review of the literature. Spec Care Dentist. 1996;16(3):95–103.
14. Nakayama M. Histological study on aging changes in the human tongue. Nippon Jibiinkoka Gakkai Kaiho. 1991;94(4):541–55.
15. Sasaki M. Histomorphometric analysis of age-related changes in epithelial thickness and Langerhans cell density of the human tongue. Tohoku J Exp Med. 1994;173(3):321–36.
16. Watanabe Y, Hirano H, Arai H, Morishita S, Ohara Y, Edahiro A, et al. Relationship between frailty and oral function in community-dwelling elderly adults. J Am Geriatr Soc. 2017;65(1):66–76.
17. Yamaguchi K, Hara K, Nakagawa K, Namiki C, Ariya C, Yoshimi K, et al. Association of aging and tooth loss with masseter muscle characteristics: an ultrasonographic study. Clin Oral Investig. 2020:1–8.
18. Koshino H, Hirai T, Ishijima T, Ikeda Y. Tongue motor skills and masticatory performance in adult dentates, elderly dentates, and complete denture wearers. J Prosthet Dent. 1997;77(2):147–52.
19. Fucile S, Wright PM, Chan I, Yee S, Langlais M-E, Gisel EG. Functional oral-motor skills: do they change with age? Dysphagia. 1998;13(4):195–201.
20. Hiramatsu T, Kataoka H, Osaki M, Hagino H. Effect of aging on oral and swallowing function after meal consumption. Clin Interv Aging. 2015;10:229.
21. Crow HC, Ship JA. Tongue strength and endurance in different aged individuals. J Gerontol Ser A Biol Med Sci. 1996;51(5):M247–M50.
22. Park J-S, Oh D-H, Chang M. Comparison of maximal tongue strength and tongue strength used during swallowing in relation to age in healthy adults. J Phys Ther Sci. 2016;28(2):442–5.
23. Iyota K, Mizutani S, Oku S, Asao M, Futatsuki T, Inoue R, et al. A cross-sectional study of age-related changes in oral function in healthy Japanese individuals. Int J Environ Res Public Health. 2020;17(4):1376.
24. Jungheim M, Schwemmle C, Miller S, Kühn D, Ptok M. Swallowing and dysphagia in the elderly. HNO. 2014;62(9):644–51.
25. Hill MW. The influence of aging on skin and oral mucosa 1. Gerodontology. 1984;3(1):35–45.
26. Bishara SE, Jakobsen JR, Treder JE, Stasl MJ. Changes in the maxillary and mandibular tooth size-arch length relationship from early adolescence to early adulthood: a longitudinal study. Am J Orthod Dentofac Orthop. 1989;95(1):46–59.

27. Emami E, de Souza RF, Kabawat M, Feine JS. The impact of edentulism on oral and general health. Int J Dent. 2013;2013:498305.
28. Griffin SO, Jones JA, Brunson D, Griffin PM, Bailey WD. Burden of oral disease among older adults and implications for public health priorities. Am J Public Health. 2012;102(3):411–8.
29. Tiwari T, Scarbro S, Bryant LL, Puma J. Factors associated with tooth loss in older adults in rural Colorado. J Community Health. 2016;41(3):476–81.
30. Dye BA, Weatherspoon DJ, Mitnik GL. Tooth loss among older adults according to poverty status in the United States from 1999 through 2004 and 2009 through 2014. J Am Dent Assoc. 2019;150(1):9–23.e3.
31. Gaio EJ, Haas AN, Carrard VC, Oppermann RV, Albandar J, Susin C. Oral health status in elders from South Brazil: a population-based study. Gerodontology. 2012;29(3):214–23.
32. Moon J-H, Heo S-J, Jung J-H. Factors influencing self-rated oral health in elderly people residing in the community: results from the Korea community health survey, 2016. Osong Public Health Res Perspect. 2020;11(4):245.
33. Nagler RM, Hershkovich O. Age-related changes in unstimulated salivary function and composition and its relations to medications and oral sensorial complaints. Aging Clin Exp Res. 2005;17(5):358–66.
34. Kikutani T, Tamura F, Nishiwaki K, Kodama M, Suda M, Fukui T, et al. Oral motor function and masticatory performance in the community-dwelling elderly. Odontology. 2009;97(1):38–42.
35. Cullins MJ, Connor NP. Alterations of intrinsic tongue muscle properties with aging. Muscle Nerve. 2017;56(6):E119–E25.
36. Yamada A, Kanazawa M, Komagamine Y, Minakuchi S. Association between tongue and lip functions and masticatory performance in young dentate adults. J Oral Rehabil. 2015;42(11):833–9.
37. Kilian M, Chapple I, Hannig M, Marsh P, Meuric V, Pedersen A, et al. The oral microbiome–an update for oral healthcare professionals. Br Dent J. 2016;221(10):657–66.
38. Deo PN, Deshmukh R. Oral microbiome: unveiling the fundamentals. J Oral Maxillofac Pathol: JOMFP. 2019;23(1):122.
39. Zapata HJ, Quagliarello VJ. The microbiota and microbiome in aging: potential implications in health and age-related diseases. J Am Geriatr Soc. 2015;63(4):776–81.
40. Belibasakis GN. Microbiological changes of the ageing oral cavity. Arch Oral Biol. 2018;96:230–2.
41. Iwauchi M, Horigome A, Ishikawa K, Mikuni A, Nakano M, Xiao JZ, et al. Relationship between oral and gut microbiota in elderly people. Immun Inflammation Dis. 2019;7(3):229–36.
42. Odamaki T, Kato K, Sugahara H, Hashikura N, Takahashi S, Xiao J-Z, et al. Age-related changes in gut microbiota composition from newborn to centenarian: a cross-sectional study. BMC Microbiol. 2016;16(1):1–12.
43. Conlon MA, Bird AR. The impact of diet and lifestyle on gut microbiota and human health. Nutrients. 2015;7(1):17–44.
44. Cullen CM, Aneja KK, Beyhan S, Cho CE, Woloszynek S, Convertino M, et al. Emerging priorities for microbiome research. Front Microbiol. 2020;11:136.
45. Imhann F, Vich Vila A, Bonder MJ, Lopez Manosalva AG, Koonen DP, Fu J, et al. The influence of proton pump inhibitors and other commonly used medication on the gut microbiota. Gut Microbes. 2017;8(4):351–8.
46. Jackson MA, Goodrich JK, Maxan M-E, Freedberg DE, Abrams JA, Poole AC, et al. Proton pump inhibitors alter the composition of the gut microbiota. Gut. 2016;65(5):749–56.
47. Lee IC, Yang YH, Ho PS, Lee IC. Chewing ability, nutritional status and quality of life. J Oral Rehabil. 2014;41(2):79–86.
48. Motokawa K, Mikami Y, Shirobe M, Edahiro A, Ohara Y, Iwasaki M, et al. Relationship between chewing ability and nutritional status in Japanese older adults: a cross-sectional Study. Int J Environ Res Public Health. 2021;18(3):1216.
49. Samnieng P, Ueno M, Shinada K, Zaitsu T, Wright FAC, Kawaguchi Y. Oral health status and chewing ability is related to mini-nutritional assessment results in an older adult population in Thailand. J Nutr Gerontol Geriatr. 2011;30(3):291–304.

50. Tada A, Miura H. Association of mastication and factors affecting masticatory function with obesity in adults: a systematic review. BMC Oral Health. 2018;18(1):1–8.
51. Brennan DS, Spencer AJ, Roberts-Thomson KF. Tooth loss, chewing ability and quality of life. Qual Life Res. 2008;17(2):227–35.
52. Ohara Y, Hirano H, Watanabe Y, Edahiro A, Sato E, Shinkai S, et al. Masseter muscle tension and chewing ability in older persons. Geriatr Gerontol Int. 2013;13(2):372–7.
53. Mayil M, Keser G, Demir A, Pekiner FN. Assessment of masseter muscle appearance and thickness in edentulous and dentate patients by ultrasonography. Open Dent J. 2018;12:723.
54. Kossioni AE. The association of poor oral health parameters with malnutrition in older adults: a review considering the potential implications for cognitive impairment. Nutrients. 2018;10(11):1709.
55. Sahyoun NR, Lin C-L, Krall E. Nutritional status of the older adult is associated with dentition status. J Am Diet Assoc. 2003;103(1):61–6.
56. Sheiham A, Steele J. Does the condition of the mouth and teeth affect the ability to eat certain foods, nutrient and dietary intake and nutritional status amongst older people? Public Health Nutr. 2001;4(3):797–803.
57. Ijaopo E, Ijaopo R. A review of oral health in older adults: key to improving nutrition and quality of life. OBM Geriatr. 2018;2:1.

Epidemiology of Oral Health Conditions in the Older Population

W. Murray Thomson and Moira B. Smith

Oral epidemiological research makes inferences about oral health and ill-health in the source population from measurements conducted on representative samples. The purpose of this chapter is to provide an overview of what is currently known of the epidemiology of oral health and disease in older people using data from epidemiological studies.

1 Thinking About Old Age and Oral Health

Old age is more than just a chronological concept; the age at which a person is considered "old" is arbitrary and varies globally. While 65 years has traditionally been the accepted threshold for old age in most Western societies, the greater longevity accrued in recent decades means that it is an administrative threshold (enabling access to retirement benefits and other services) more than a chronological or social one. Low- and middle-income countries have relatively younger populations, and so their threshold for old age is typically 60 years; it is also the age used when considering the global older population.

It is important to bear in mind that older people have not appeared de novo. They have been shaped by their journey along the life course, having been subjected to age effects (maturation and then senescence), period effects

---

W. M. Thomson (✉)
Sir John Walsh Research Institute, Faculty of Dentistry,
The University of Otago, Dunedin, New Zealand
e-mail: murray.thomson@otago.ac.nz

M. B. Smith
Department of Public Health, University of Otago, Wellington, New Zealand

© The Author(s), under exclusive license to Springer Nature Switzerland AG 2022
C.-M. Hogue, J. G. Ruiz (eds.), *Oral Health and Aging*,
https://doi.org/10.1007/978-3-030-85993-0_2

(exposures occurring at particular times), and cohort effects (generation-specific characteristics). Ettinger summarized these well: "Elderly (sic) individuals are a complex combination and expression of their individual genetic predispositions, lifestyles, socialization and environments, all of which affect their health beliefs and, consequently, their health behavior. To understand an individual, one must evaluate the social, cultural, economic and chronologically specific cohort experiences which have shaped his/her life" [1]. Older people comprise the most heterogenous of any of the life stage groups (childhood, adolescence, adulthood, and old age), and we cannot lump all older people together and make generalizations about their oral health. Recognizing this diversity and to more accurately reflect the changes that typically occur as people age, the older population may be divided into the subgroups of "young-old" (65–74), "middle-old" or "old" (75–84), and "oldest-old" (85+) [2].

How might this work in practice? Consider, for example, a situation where we are interpreting findings from an oral health survey of people aged 65 years and older that we conducted in 2020. We recorded their dentition and periodontal status. Our sample ranges in age from 65 to 95 years. For reporting purposes, we have categorized age into the four age groups of 65–74, 75–84, 85–94, and 95+ years. Comparisons of dentition status across those age groups will show noteworthy and not entirely unpredictable differences in tooth loss and Decayed, Missing, or Filled Teeth (DMFT) scores. After all, both tooth loss and dental caries are chronic, cumulative conditions which increase in severity as we age. However, what we cannot do is state with any confidence that the accumulated disease experience observed in the oldest age group would be what we would observe in the youngest age group if we were to replicate the survey in three decades' time. This is because of differences arising from the abovementioned period and cohort effects.

Figure 1 illustrates the challenges. Those who were 95 in 2020 would have been 45 in 1970; by contrast, those aged 65 years in 2020 were only 15 in 1970. Their behaviors, beliefs, and norms would have been very different, as would their life trajectories over the subsequent decades. The same applies to their exposures, whether adverse or beneficial. For example, fluoride toothpaste, widely credited for the most precipitous fall in dental caries experienced in recent decades, was introduced in the early 1970s. While those aged 65 years in 2020 would have spent three quarters of their lives exposed to it, their 95-year-old counterparts would have used it for only half of their lives, and that would be reflected in their DMFT scores (as well as in their cumulative tooth loss). Such differences are depicted in Table 1, which presents nationally representative data from a survey of older New Zealanders, conducted in 2012 [3]. While the date of the survey differs from 2020, the differences are marked enough to illustrate the principle well. The observed differences between the oldest group and those aged 65–74 years are generational in nature, yet we tend to aggregate them together, considering those aged 65 years or more as "older people."

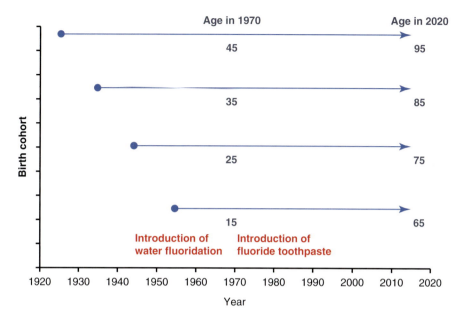

Fig. 1 Cohort differences in respect to dental caries among older adults

Table 1 Age group differences in dentition status in 2012 among older New Zealanders[a] (brackets contain 95% CI)

	Age group (years)			
	65–74	75–84	85–94	95+
% dentate	42.9 (36.8, 49.2)	41.8 (37.8, 45.8)	36.0 (32.2, 40.0)	29.9 (23.5, 37.1)
Mean no. of teeth	19.6 (18.2, 21.0)	16.9 (16.0, 17.7)	15.1 (14.3, 15.9)	14.9 (12.7, 17.2)
Mean DMFT	21.6 (20.4, 22.9)	23.6 (22.9, 24.2)	25.3 (24.7, 25.8)	25.0 (23.4, 26.6)
Mean DT	2.1 (1.6, 2.7)	2.0 (1.6, 2.3)	2.4 (2.0, 2.9)	1.9 (1.1, 2.7)
Mean MT	12.2 (11.0, 13.4)	14.9 (14.1, 15.8)	16.7 (15.9, 17.5)	17.0 (14.8, 19.3)
Mean FT	7.3 (5.9, 8.7)	6.7 (5.9, 7.5)	6.1 (5.4, 6.9)	6.0 (4.2, 7.9)

Abbreviations: *DMFT* Decayed, Missing, or Filled Teeth, *DT* decayed teeth, *MT* missing teeth, *FT* filled teeth
[a]Source of data: see CBG Health Research Ltd [3]

2 Sociodemographic Changes

Rising life expectancy and falling birth rates have meant that, in almost all countries, populations comprise more older people, and a greater share of older people, than ever before. What is more, almost all societies are aging at unprecedented rates [4, 5]. By 2050, the proportion of the global population aged over 60 years is projected to more than double, rising from 1 billion in 2019 to 2.1 billion. In some regions, such as North America and Europe, almost one in four people will be "older" [5]. Longer life expectancies also mean that populations will comprise a substantial proportion of "oldest-old" people. In many countries, that age category is the fastest growing of all older age groups. The number of people aged 85 years or older is expected to triple in the period from 2019 to 2050, to make up almost one quarter of all older people. Rates of aging also vary regionally. While the older populations in many industrialized countries, most notably Japan, have been aging for some time, the most rapid shifts in population distribution are projected to occur in developing countries, in which four in five of the world's older people will live [5].

Population aging presents health, social, and economic systems with myriad challenges in meeting older people's complex dental and medical needs, in protecting and promoting their health and well-being, and in reducing the years lived with disability and poor quality of life. While Western societies have had some time to consider how to address these challenges, low- and middle-income countries' rapid acceleration of aging, and a lack of capacity and resources to cope with these changes, means that they are less well-prepared to respond and face imminent and substantial pressures [6]. It is thought that the health, social, and economic implications—for individuals and society alike—of the demographic changes are so substantial that population aging will be a hallmark of the twenty-first century [5]. Consequently, there has been a burgeoning of gerontological research aimed at understanding the demographic, geographic, sociocultural, and political influences on the associated dental and medical phenomena.

3 Health Differences by Gender, Ethnicity, and Socioeconomic Position

Marked differences by gender among older populations are evident [7, 8]. Most notably, women live approximately 5 years longer than men, the gap being greater among countries with higher levels of development [5, 9]. Unsurprisingly, then, women make up more than half of older populations and an even larger share of the oldest-old subgrouping [5]. However, the gender longevity gap appears to be narrowing (especially in more developed countries), a consequence of a reduction in gender differences in tobacco and alcohol consumption. While men's rates of tobacco and alcohol consumption have typically been higher than women, they are now falling; women's uptake of tobacco and alcohol also occurred later than men. Improvements in the treatment of cardiovascular disease, which is more prevalent in men than women, have further contributed to the convergence of men's and women's life expectancies [8, 10].

Aside from living longer, women are disadvantaged in almost all other aspects of health [7]. In many societies, women (of all ages) do not have the same access as men to several key determinants of health, including education, paid employment and other economic opportunities, and health services. Not only do the consequences of such inequities and disadvantage accumulate through the life course and persist into older age but they also exist and have an impact in old age. In some countries, sources of social support and income for older people, such as pensions and care assistance, may be inadequate or non-existent; these situations especially impact women. Consequently, many older women (especially those in low- and middle-income countries) live in or close to poverty, and typically have poorer health and health-related quality of life, and live longer with disability than men [7, 11]. Older women also live with greater levels of dependency than men, and fewer can live independently [12]. Disparities in health and social support between older men and women, particularly those living in developing countries, are exacerbated by prevailing gender-related cultural norms, such as women's lack of financial autonomy, capacity to own property, and the realization of other rights and freedoms [7].

Ethnic differences in health and well-being among older populations are also evident. Indigenous older people and those in "minority" ethnic groups typically have poorer access to health services, social supports, income, and other key determinants of health than non-indigenous and majority ethnic groups. They also experience racial prejudice and discrimination. In turn, their health and well-being are poorer; they have higher prevalence of chronic conditions, multimorbidity, levels of disability, and lower life expectancy and poorer quality of life than their non-indigenous peers and those of majority ethnicities [13–15]. Addressing these disparities is critical in maintaining and improving the health and well-being of future older generations, given that the proportion and absolute numbers of these groups among most populations are expected to rise [4, 16].

Similarly, the prevalence rates for chronic diseases, multimorbidity, cognitive decline, and disability are higher among older adults living in more deprived areas than in those living in wealthier neighborhoods [8, 17, 18]. Deprivation also accelerates decline in older people [17]; those living in the least deprived areas live up to 10 years longer than their counterparts in poorer areas [8]. For a more in-depth discussion on the topic of health disparities, please refer to the chapter "Health Disparities in Oral Health".

4 Chronic Conditions, Multimorbidity, and Disability

Globally, the prevalence of non-communicable diseases—and deaths resulting from them—is overtaking that of communicable diseases. A substantial proportion of the global burden of chronic disease is attributable to those aged over 60 years [19, 20], and the slow progression and long duration of chronic conditions, combined with greater life expectancy, means that older people are disproportionately burdened by mental, neurological, and musculoskeletal disorders, diabetes, cardiovascular and chronic respiratory diseases, and cancer [21]. What is more, multimorbidity—the co-occurrence of two or more chronic conditions—is high among older people; over half to almost all older people have multiple chronic conditions [22, 23]. The number of conditions a person has increases with age and greater deprivation [22–24], and multimorbidity prevalence is higher among women than men. Other limitations associated with older age include compromised vision, poorer nutrition, more falls and other accidents, hearing loss, and speaking difficulties (the latter two make communication more challenging).

For the older person, chronic conditions (and multimorbidity) are associated with greater risk of disability, poorer quality of life, and greater rate of hospitalizations, use of health and social services, and mortality [22–24]. There is also the likelihood of greater dependency on others for functioning, ranging from support to undertake activities of daily living (such as housework and shopping) through to assistance with self-care or full personal care. For societies, these lead to greater use of health and social services and, in turn, substantive burdens on social and health resources [21, 24]. Given that older people are expected to live longer with chronic conditions and disability, it is thought that the costs associated with their long-term care needs will be substantial and exceed those directly associated with health care [21].

5 Dementia

One of the unforeseen features of greater longevity has been considerable growth in the incidence of dementia. Approximately 5–8% of those over 60 worldwide have dementia, with Alzheimer's diseases accounting for approximately two-thirds of all cases [25]. Concurrent with projections of population aging, the number of people with dementia is expected to rise rapidly, from 50 million in 2019 to 152 million in 2050, the majority living in low- and middle-income countries [23]. Although not a normal part of aging, dementia incidence rises sharply from age 75 [25].

Dementia is characterized by cognitive decline and loss of independence in daily functioning and is a leading cause of disability and dependency among older people. The consequences of dementia are profound, are wide-ranging, and are both direct and indirect, not only for the person with the disease but also for their caregivers and family members. Dementia also has substantial societal social and economic impacts; addressing dementia costs low- and middle-income countries 0.2% of GDP, while it accounts for 1.4% of the GDP in high-income countries [25]. For a more in-depth discussion on the topic of dementia, please refer to chapter "The 3 Ds: Dementia, Delirium and Depression in Oral Health".

6 Frailty

Frailty is a clinically recognizable state of greater vulnerability, resulting from age-associated declines in physiologic reserve and function across multiple organ systems, such that the ability to cope with everyday or acute stressors is compromised. It is commonly associated with aging [26]. Its prevalence is high among older people, higher among women than men, and increases with age [27]. While it is distinct from multimorbidity, it shares features with chronic conditions and similarly increases the risk of disability, hospitalization, and death. Of those aged over 50 years, 12–24% are frail and a further half are prefrail [28]. For a more in-depth discussion on the topic of frailty, please refer to the chapter "Frailty and Oral Health".

7 Ageism

Population aging places considerable burdens on social and health-care systems and communities [21]. Assumptions that all older people are frail, disabled, and dependent, and therefore a burden on society and families, prevail, and ageism and discrimination against older people exist. Consequently, in many societies, older people are an often overlooked and excluded population group whose needs and rights are not sufficiently addressed.

There are differences in the rate at—and level to—which people decline as they age. Some decline rapidly and substantially, while others remain cognitively and physically intact throughout life, and older people are important members of society. Many continue to contribute to (and are active agents in) communities and societal development. Not only do they have extensive and valuable life experience, skills, and knowledge but they also participate politically and socially, and some continue in paid work, thus also making important economic contributions. Many older people (particularly women) engage in informal, unpaid work, volunteering for community organizations, and caring for grandchildren or an aging spouse.

8 Active Aging

To address the needs and rights of older people and advance their health and well-being, in recent decades, global [29] and national [30] strategies have been developed that aim to promote active aging, "the process of optimizing opportunities for health, participation and security in order to enhance quality of life as people age" [29]. Emphasis is placed on the implementation of actions that support older people's independence and autonomy and to ensure that people remain unencumbered by ill health, poor quality of life, and disability as they age.

Where older people live is a key feature of active aging, determined by cultural, economic, political, and health factors. As populations become more urbanized, family structures and functions also change. Generations of families are now more likely to be living separately, with older relatives being cared for less and less by their family. In Western societies in particular, older people are encouraged to "age in place," that is, to remain in their own homes for as long as possible as they age. Aging in place has benefits for the older person's quality of life and social connectedness, and it can reduce care-related costs for health systems [31]. Despite older people spending 2.5–3 years, on average, with considerable care needs, the majority will continue to live in the community in their own homes [12], possibly with support for their care, either from family members or more increasingly from support workers. Nevertheless, some older people will require more intensive support provided in residential care facilities, the rate of use depending on countries' attitudes to the care of older people, economic resources, and supply of such facilities [32]. Approximately 5% of the older population reside in aged residential care facilities [33], for 2 years, on average [32], although up to half of the older population are likely to use such facilities for care at some point in the late stages of their life [34]. As the number of older people aging in place rises, those entering aged care facilities are predominantly the oldest-old, those with the greatest cognitive decline, the very frail, and those with the most complex care needs [34–37].

9 The Common Oral Conditions Affecting Older People

The most common oral conditions among older people are tooth loss, dental caries, periodontitis, dry mouth, and oral mucosal lesions [38–40]. Those are chronic noncommunicable conditions which increase in severity with age because of their cumulative nature, and all can compromise older people's quality of life.

9.1 Tooth Loss

Almost all older people have lost at least one tooth on their journey through life, and most of that tooth loss has occurred because of dental caries or periodontitis [41]. Before thinking about the occurrence of tooth loss, however, it is useful to make a distinction between edentulism (the state of having had all the natural teeth removed) and the more common incremental loss of teeth (but short of the full dentition) which tends to occur throughout life. People who are edentulous have at some stage made the decision (or had it made for them) to undergo complete removal of their remaining dentition. The decision to make that transition is as much a social one as it is a clinical one [42, 43], and there are marked inequities by socioeconomic position and accumulation of adversity through the life course [44, 45]. In industrialized countries, edentulism prevalence has fallen markedly over the past few decades.

Regarded as an undesirable, "biographically disruptive" endpoint which perhaps reflects the collective failure of both self-care and the dental care system [46], the transition to edentulism can also mark the end of decades of misery and eating problems [47]. The influence of the dental system and prevailing social norms on tooth loss rates in older people was underlined in findings from a comparison of oral status in older people in a Western society (New Zealand) and one rooted in the Confucian tradition (China), whereby tooth retention among the latter was considerably greater, not only in their lower edentulism prevalence but also in a higher proportion with a functional dentition and in the higher mean number of teeth present among dentate individuals [48]. The authors pointed out that those dissimilarities represent differences in not only access to—and use of—dental care but also sociocultural differences in norms and values.

Incremental tooth loss is now far more common than edentulism, among adults of all ages. The most important reason for it is dental caries, with trauma and periodontitis making minor contributions, although the latter becomes more important with increasing age [41, 49]. There appears to be no readily identifiable life stage at which the bulk of tooth loss takes place, although, given the chronic, cumulative nature of its main cause, it would be expected that perhaps the tooth loss increment rate might stay reasonably constant with age, and this has been confirmed by several reports from prospective cohort studies of older people [47, 50]. Its less predictable nature means that incremental tooth loss can pose more of a prosthodontic challenge, given that its sequelae can include the drifting or over-eruption of the remaining teeth. Most descriptions of tooth loss among older adults have focused on indicators such as the edentulous proportion, the mean number of restored and missing teeth, and the proportion with a functional dentition (usually defined as having 21 or more remaining teeth [51]). While those indicators remain useful, they lack the detail required for a more nuanced understanding of the remaining dentition. Recently published estimates from a national survey of dependent older adults in New Zealand have shown that their residual dentitions vary considerably, and having a complete dentition is rare [52]. Those residual dentition patterns come about through influences which range from the pathological through to the societal; what is observed in old age is the outcome of a lifetime's steady accumulation of adverse and beneficial exposures.

9.2 Dental Caries

It is now well-recognized that dental caries is a disease that continues through life and that, other than the greater susceptibility of the deciduous dentition (due to its lower mineralization), the typical annual caries increment is constant through life, at about one new surface per year in the average person [53]. That holds in old age, where coronal caries continues to predominate [54, 55]. However, where the caries increment has been shown to increase considerably is after admission to aged residential care, where it is more than double that observed among community-dwelling older people, and more than twice as high again among those with dementia [56].

There is no shortage of anecdotal reports from clinicians of dentitions deteriorating rapidly in such circumstances. For a more in-depth discussion on the topic of caries, please refer to the chapter "Management of Caries in Older Adults".

9.3 Periodontitis

Most dentate older people show evidence of periodontitis, with moderate levels of attachment loss apparent in most [57]. While a substantial minority have more advanced attachment loss [58], relatively few sites are affected. The attachment loss manifests mainly as gingival recession. A complicating factor when considering periodontitis in older people is that their experience of incremental tooth loss means that the remaining dentition is the "healthy survivors," and so their lifetime periodontitis experience is likely to be underestimated from a contemporary clinical dental examination. This makes the interpretation of periodontal epidemiological data on older people particularly difficult. For a more in-depth discussion on the topic of periodontal disease, please refer to the chapter "Management of Periodontal Disease in Older Adults".

9.4 Dry Mouth

The term "dry mouth" covers both salivary gland hypofunction (SGH) and xerostomia. With the former, someone has low salivary flow, while the latter involves the subjective sensation of dry mouth. The degree of concordance between the two aspects of dry mouth remains unclear, and it is likely that much of the occurrence of xerostomia may be due to differences in saliva quality rather than quantity [59]. Not only is dry mouth common but its prevalence is highest among older people, with more than one in five affected [60].

People who have Sjögren's syndrome (1% of the population) or who have undergone radiotherapy for head/neck cancer (0.1% of the population) can suffer from severe chronic dry mouth, but medications are by far the most important risk factor for chronic dry mouth, responsible for more than 95% of cases [59]. Older people take a lot of medications: polypharmacy is common [60]. Determining the effects of medications on salivary flow and subjective dry mouth is challenging because not only may a particular drug exert its effect at more than one step in the salivary secretion pathway but the strength of that effect is determined by dose, duration, metabolism, and the concurrent effects of other drugs which are being taken [60]. Epidemiological investigations of associations between medications and dry mouth have found many drugs to be risk factors, but those most consistently identified as such have been antidepressants, diuretics, anti-anginal, bronchodilators, and antihistamines. Polypharmacy continues to complicate such investigations, but people taking many different medications have higher rates of dry mouth, regardless of the actual preparations being taken.

Dry mouth has been shown to affect sufferers' quality of life [61], and they also have higher rates of dental caries [62]. Managing dry mouth remains a difficult and challenging process, mostly empirical in nature. For a more in-depth discussion on the topic of dry mouth, please refer to the chapter "Xerostomia and Hyposalivation".

9.5   Oral Mucosal Lesions

While lesions of the oral mucosa are common among older people, population-based estimates are scarce. In the USA, the most recent estimates come from the third NHANES study (conducted from 1988 to 1994), where one or more oral mucosal lesions were observed in 39.4% of 60–69-year-olds and 42.6% of those aged 70 years or older [63]. More recent estimates come from New Zealand's 2009 national oral health survey [64], where one-third of those aged 65 years or older had at least one oral mucosal lesion. Almost all of those were relatively harmless, arising from local trauma or chronic infection (such as denture stomatitis). Given its catastrophic personal implications, oral cancer should always be considered, of course, given that most cases of oral cancer are diagnosed in older people.

The terms "oral precancer" and "oral cancer" cover several oral mucosal lesions. The former term is generally applied to lesions such as leukoplakia, lichen planus, and erythroplakia; these are acknowledged to have malignant transformation potential. Erythroplakia is very rare but is the most sinister of those, invariably featuring dysplastic epithelium. The term "oral cancer" most commonly refers to oral squamous cell carcinoma [65]. It is a condition for which the death-registration ratio is comparable to those of breast cancer and cervical cancer and exceeds that of melanoma [66]. Tobacco use (whether smoked, chewed, or rinsed as a "tuibur" solution [67]) is the most well-known risk factor. It also has a synergistic effect with heavy alcohol use [68]. Human papilloma virus (HPV) has also been implicated in the occurrence of oropharyngeal cancer, particularly among younger adults [69], but it will be intriguing to observe what happens as that population enters old age.

10   Conclusions

Most countries are faced with the challenge of older people with more teeth. Such an unprecedented situation is challenging for health systems which (for the most part) are not ready for it. Epidemiological investigations of older people's oral health provide essential information for understanding the nature and extent of that challenge. A life course perspective is essential to interpreting and understanding the data.

References

1. Ettinger RL. Cohort differences among aging populations: a challenge for the dental profession. Spec Care Dent. 1993;13:19–26.
2. von Humboldt S, Leal I. The old and the oldest-old: do they have different perspectives on adjustment to aging? Int J Gerontol. 2015;9(3):156–60.
3. CBG Health Research Ltd. Our older people's oral health: key findings of the 2012 New Zealand older people's oral health survey. Auckland: CBG Health Research Ltd; 2015.
4. Vespa J, Armstrong D, Medina L. Demographic turning points for the United States: population projections for 2020 to 2060. USA: US Census Bureau; 2018. Contract No.: P25-1144.
5. United Nations. Department of Economic and Social Affairs Population Division. World population ageing 2019: highlights. New York: United Nations; 2019. Report No.: ST/ESA/SER.A/430.
6. Sudharsanan N, Bloom DE. The demography of aging in low- and middle-income countries: chronological versus functional perspectives. In: National Academies of Sciences Engineering, and Medicine; Division of Behavioral and Social Sciences and Education; Committee on Population, Majmundar MK, Hayward MD, editors. Future directions for the demography of aging: proceedings of a workshop. Washington, DC: National Acadamies Press; 2018.
7. Carmel S. Health and well-being in late life: gender differences worldwide. Front Med (Lausanne). 2019;6:218.
8. Mayhew L, Harper G, Villegas A. Inequalities matter - an investigation into the impact of deprivation on demographic inequalities in adults. London: Cass Business School; 2018.
9. GBD 2017 Disease and Injury Incidence and Prevalence Collaborators. Global, regional, and national age–sex-specific mortality and life expectancy, 1950–2017: a systematic analysis for the Global Burden of Disease Study 2017. Lancet. 2018;392(10159):1684–735.
10. Kolip P, Lange C. Gender inequality and the gender gap in life expectancy in the European Union. Eur J Pub Health. 2018;28(5):869–72.
11. Lee KH, Xu H, Wu B. Gender differences in quality of life among community-dwelling older adults in low- and middle-income countries: results from the Study on global AGEing and adult health (SAGE). BMC Public Health. 2020;20(1):114.
12. Kingston A, Wohland P, Wittenberg R, Robinson L, Brayne C, Matthews FE, et al. Is late-life dependency increasing or not? A comparison of the Cognitive Function and Ageing Studies (CFAS). Lancet. 2017;390(10103):1676–84.
13. Ng JH, Bierman AS, Elliott MN, Wilson RL, Xia C, Scholle SH. Beyond black and white: race/ethnicity and health status among older adults. Am J Manag Care. 2014;20(3):239–48.
14. Evandrou M, Falkingham J, Feng Z, Vlachantoni A. Ethnic inequalities in limiting health and self-reported health in later life revisited. J Epidemiol Community Health. 2016;70(7):653–62.
15. Moriarty JO, Butt J. Inequalities in quality of life among older people from different ethnic groups. Ageing Soc. 2004;24(5):729–53.
16. Coleman D. Projections of the ethnic minority populations of the United Kingdom 2006–2056. Popul Dev Rev. 2010;36(3):441–86.
17. Steptoe A, Zaninotto P. Lower socioeconomic status and the acceleration of aging: an outcome-wide analysis. Proc Natl Acad Sci. 2020;117(26):14911–7.
18. Shahar S, Vanoh D, Mat Ludin AF, Singh DKA, Hamid TA. Factors associated with poor socioeconomic status among Malaysian older adults: an analysis according to urban and rural settings. BMC Public Health. 2019;19(4):549.
19. GBD 2017 Disease and Injury Incidence and Prevalence Collaborators. Global, regional, and national age-sex-specific mortality for 282 causes of death in 195 countries and territories, 1980–2017: a systematic analysis for the Global Burden of Disease Study 2017. Lancet. 2018;392(10159):1736–88.
20. GBD 2017 Disease and Injury Incidence and Prevalence Collaborators. Global, regional, and national incidence, prevalence, and years lived with disability for 354 diseases and injuries

for 195 countries and territories, 1990–2017: a systematic analysis for the Global Burden of Disease Study 2017. Lancet. 2018;392(10159):1789–858.
21. Prince MJ, Wu F, Guo Y, Gutierrez Robledo LM, O'Donnell M, Sullivan R, et al. The burden of disease in older people and implications for health policy and practice. Lancet. 2015;385(9967):549–62.
22. Marengoni A, Angleman S, Melis R, Mangialasche F, Karp A, Garmen A, et al. Aging with multimorbidity: a systematic review of the literature. Ageing Res Rev. 2011;10(4):430–9.
23. Ofori-Asenso R, Chin K, Curtis A, Zomer E, Zoungas S, Liew D. Recent patterns of multimorbidity among older adults in high-income countries. Popul Health Manag. 2019;22(2):127–37.
24. McPhail SM. Multimorbidity in chronic disease: impact on health care resources and costs. Risk Manag Healthc Policy. 2016;9:143–56.
25. Langa KM. Cognitive Aging, dementia, and the future of an aging population. In: National Academies of Sciences Engineering, and Medicine; Division of Behavioral and Social Sciences and Education; Committee on Population, Majmundar MK, Hayward MD, editors. Future directions for the demography of aging: proceedings of a workshop. Washington, DC: National Acadamies Press; 2018.
26. Clegg A, Young J, Iliffe S, Rikkert MO, Rockwood K. Frailty in elderly people. Lancet. 2013;381(9868):752–62.
27. Fried LP, Tangen CM, Walston J, Newman AB, Hirsch C, Gottdiener J, et al. Frailty in older adults: evidence for a phenotype. J Gerontol A Biol Sci Med Sci. 2001;56(3):M146–M57.
28. O'Caoimh R, Sezgin D, O'Donovan MR, Molloy DW, Clegg A, Rockwood K, et al. Prevalence of frailty in 62 countries across the world: a systematic review and meta-analysis of population-level studies. Age Ageing. 2020;50(1):96–104.
29. World Health Organization. Active ageing: a policy framework. Geneva: World Health Organization; 2002. Report No.: WHO/NMH/NPH/02.8.
30. Associate Minister of Health. Healthy ageing strategy. Wellington: Ministry of Health; 2016.
31. Horner B, Boldy DP. The benefit and burden of "ageing-in-place" in an aged care community. Aust Health Rev. 2008;32(2):356–65.
32. Ribbe MW, Ljunggren G, Steel K, Topinková E, Hawes C, Ikegami N, et al. Nursing homes in 10 nations: a comparison between countries and settings. Age Ageing. 1997;26(Suppl 2):3–12.
33. Broad JB, Ashton T, Lumley T, Connolly MJ. Reports of the proportion of older people living in long-term care: a cautionary tale from New Zealand. Aust N Z J Public Health. 2013;37(3):264–71.
34. Broad JB, Ashton T, Gott M, McLeod H, Davis PB, Connolly MJ. Likelihood of residential aged care use in later life: a simple approach to estimation with international comparison. Aust N Z J Public Health. 2015;39(4):374–9.
35. Khadka J, Lang C, Ratcliffe J, Corlis M, Wesselingh S, Whitehead C, et al. Trends in the utilisation of aged care services in Australia, 2008–2016. BMC Geriatr. 2019;19(1):213.
36. Gordon AL, Franklin M, Bradshaw L, Logan P, Elliott R, Gladman JR. Health status of UK care home residents: a cohort study. Age Ageing. 2014;43(1):97–103.
37. Broad JB, Gott M, Kim H, Boyd M, Chen H, Connolly MJ. Where do people die? An international comparison of the percentage of deaths occurring in hospital and residential aged care settings in 45 populations, using published and available statistics. Int J Public Health. 2013;58(2):257–67.
38. Sussex PV, Thomson WM, Fitzgerald RP. Understanding the "epidemic" of complete tooth loss among older New Zealanders. Gerodontology. 2010;27(2):85–95.
39. Persson GR. Dental geriatrics and periodontitis. Periodontol 2000. 2017;74(1):102–5.
40. Jamieson LM, Thomson WM. Xerostomia: its prevalence and associations in the adult Australian population. Aust Dent J. 2020;65(Suppl 1):S67–70.
41. Phipps KR, Stevens VJ. Relative contribution of caries and periodontal disease in adult tooth loss for an HMO dental population. J Public Health Dent. 1995;55(4):250–2.
42. Sanders AE, Slade GD, Carter KD, Stewart JF. Trends in prevalence of complete tooth loss among Australians, 1979–2002. Aust N Z J Public Health. 2004;28(6):549–54.

43. Gibson BJ, Sussex PV, Fitzgerald RP, Thomson WM. Complete tooth loss as status passage. Sociol Health Illn. 2017;39(3):412–27.
44. Fantin R, Delpierre C, Kelly-Irving M, Barboza SC. Early socio-economic conditions and severe tooth loss in middle-aged Costa Ricans. Community Dent Oral Epidemiol. 2018;46(6):555–62.
45. Lee H. A life course approach to total tooth loss: testing the sensitive period, accumulation, and social mobility models in the Health and Retirement Study. Community Dent Oral Epidemiol. 2019;47(4):333–9.
46. Rousseau N, Steele JG, May C, Exley C. "Your whole life is lived through your teeth": biographical disruption and experiences of tooth loss and replacement. Sociol Health Illn. 2014;36(3):462–76.
47. Thomson WM. Epidemiology of oral health conditions in older people. Gerodontology. 2014;31(Suppl 1):9–16.
48. He S, Thomson WM. An oral epidemiological comparison of Chinese and New Zealand adults in two key age groups. Community Dent Oral Epidemiol. 2018;46(2):154–60.
49. Haworth S, Shungin D, Kwak SY, Kim H-Y, West NX, et al. Tooth loss is a complex measure of oral disease: determinants and methodological considerations. Community Dent Oral Epidemiol. 2018;46(6):555–62.
50. Silva Junior MF, Batista MJ, de Sousa MDLR. Risk factors for tooth loss in adults: a population-based prospective cohort study. PLoS One. 2019;14(7): e0219240.
51. Nuttall N, Steele JG, Nunn J, et al. A guide to the UK adult dental health survey 1998. London: British Dental Association; 2001.
52. Hyland N, Smith MB, Gribben B, Thomson WM. The residual dentition among New Zealanders in aged residential care. Gerodontology. 2019;36(3):216–22.
53. Broadbent JM, Foster Page LA, Thomson WM, Poulton R. Permanent dentition caries through the first half of life. Br Dent J. 2013;215(7):E12.
54. Thomson WM. Dental caries experience in older people over time: what can the large cohort studies tell us? Br Dent J. 2004;196(2):89–92.
55. Griffin SO, Griffin PM, Swann JL, Zlobin N. Estimating rates of new root caries in older adults. J Dent Res. 2004;83(8):634–8.
56. Chalmers JM, Carter KD, Spencer AJ. Caries incidence and increments in Adelaide nursing home residents. Spec Care Dent. 2005;25(2):96–105.
57. Locker D, Slade GD, Murray H. Epidemiology of periodontal disease among older adults: a review. Periodontol 2000. 1998;16:16–33.
58. Eke PI, Wei L, Borgnakke WS, Thornton-Evans G, Zhang X, Lu H, McGuire LC, Genco RJ. Periodontitis prevalence in adults >65 years of age, in the USA. Periodontol 2000. 2016;72(1):76–95.
59. Villa A, Wolff A, Narayana N, Dawes C, Aframian D, Lynge Pedersen AM, Vissink A, Aliko A, Sia YW, Joshi RK, et al. World Workshop on Oral Medicine VI: a systematic review of medication-induced salivary gland dysfunction: prevalence, diagnosis, and treatment. Clin Oral Invest. 2016;22(5):365–82.
60. Ferguson CA, Thomson WM, Kerse NM, Peri K, Gribben B. Medication taking in a national sample of dependent older people. Res Soc Adm Pharm. 2020;16:299–307.
61. Benn AML, Broadbent JM, Thomson WM. Occurrence and impact of xerostomia among dentate adult New Zealanders: findings from a national survey. Aust Dent J. 2015;60(3):362–7.
62. Thomson WM, Spencer AJ, Slade GD, Chalmers JM. Is medication a risk factor for dental caries among older people? Evidence from a longitudinal study in South Australia. Community Dent Oral Epidemiol. 2002;30(3):224–32.
63. Shulman JD, Beach MM, Rivera-Hidalgo F. The prevalence of oral mucosal lesions in U.S. adults: data from the Third National Health and Nutrition Examination Survey, 1988–1994. J Am Dent Assoc. 2004;135(9):1279–86.
64. Ministry of Health. Our oral health: key findings of the 2009 New Zealand oral health survey. Wellington: New Zealand Ministry of Health; 2010.

65. Glick M, Johnson NW. Oral and oropharyngeal cancer: what are the next steps? J Am Dent Assoc. 2011;142(8):892–4.
66. Johnson NW, Warnakulasuriya KA. Epidemiology and aetiology of oral cancer in the United Kingdom. Community Dent Health. 1993;10(Suppl 1):13–29.
67. Madathil SA, Nachimuthu SK, Zodinouii D, Muthukumaran RB, Lalmuanpuii R, Nicolau B. Tuibur: tobacco in a bottle – commercial production of tobacco smoke aqueous concentrate in Mizoram, Northeast India. Addiction. 2018;113:577–80.
68. Tanaka TI, Alawi F. Human papilloma virus and oropharyngeal cancer. Dent Clin N Am. 2018;62(1):111–20.
69. Chaturvedi AK. Epidemiology and clinical aspects of HPV in head and neck cancers. Head and Neck Pathology 2012;6:S16–S24.

Nutrition and Oral Health

Rena Zelig, Samantha Honeywell, and Riva Touger-Decker

There are synergistic and multifaceted associations between diet, nutrition, and oral health. As the "gateway to the gastrointestinal tract," a healthy functioning mouth is essential for individuals to eat and drink. Diet can directly impact oral soft and hard tissues, and, conversely, the integrity of the mouth can affect biting, chewing, and swallowing. If the impact is prolonged, the risk for micronutrient deficiencies and malnutrition increases, potentially increasing the risk for compromised systemic health. Soft tissue integrity can be negatively impacted by nutrient deficiencies, infection(s), surgery, and medication(s). Changes to soft or hard tissue including tooth loss with or without replacement can negatively impact food, fluid intake, nutritional status, and in turn can further compromise oral health.

Screening to detect factors influencing the ability to consume a healthy diet and risk for micronutrient deficiencies and malnutrition as well as factors influencing the ability to consume foods and fluids can help identify older adults needing intervention early and prevent or mitigate the severity of problems. The primary aims of this chapter are to describe nutrition risk factors within the context of validated approaches to nutrition risk screening of older adults; describe associations between diet, nutrition, and tooth loss and dentures; and address interventions to improve the functional ability to eat in the face of tooth loss and replacement. The other chapters of this text cover additional topics that can also influence nutritional status including chapter "Age-Related Changes in Oral Health", and as such, they are not covered herein. Similarly, content covered in the chapters on dysphagia (chapter "Swallowing, Dysphagia, and Aspiration Pneumonia"), hyposalivation (chapter "Xerostomia and

---

R. Zelig (✉) · S. Honeywell
Department of Clinical and Preventive Nutrition Sciences, School of Health Professions, Rutgers, The State University of New Jersey, Newark, NJ, USA
e-mail: zeligre@shp.rutgers.edu

R. Touger-Decker
Rutgers School of Dental Medicine, Newark, NJ, USA

© The Author(s), under exclusive license to Springer Nature Switzerland AG 2022
C.-M. Hogue, J. G. Ruiz (eds.), *Oral Health and Aging*,
https://doi.org/10.1007/978-3-030-85993-0_3

Hyposalivation"), oral, infectious, and systemic diseases (chapter "Systemic Disease That Influence Oral Health"), alterations in mental status (chapter "The 3 Ds: Dementia, Delirium and Depression in Oral Health"); and long-term care settings (chapter "Oral Care in Long-Term Care Settings"), includes factors that impact diet and nutritional status. While there are no screening tools that are specific to predict the impact on nutritional status due to oral disease, infections, and altered soft or hard tissue function or integrity, clinicians should consider the location(s) of the problem, whether it is acute or chronic, and patient self-reported and clinician anticipated impact on food and fluid consumption in determining risk for problems with diet that require patient education and/or referral. If such factors are not addressed in a timely and comprehensive manner, changes in diet may ultimately negatively impact nutritional status and risk for malnutrition.

1 Nutrition Risk Factors and Screening Tools Used with Older Adults

Nutrition risk factors are any factors that elevate the chances of getting a disease or having a certain outcome or condition [1]. For the purposes of this chapter, nutrition and oral health risk factors will refer to any factor that may increase an older adult's risk for difficulty eating or drinking which can lead to inadequate nutrient intake, micronutrient deficiencies, or malnutrition. There are nutrition risk screening tools for older adults [2–8]; however, the integrity or function of the oral cavity as a risk factor is only addressed to a small extent in the Mini Nutritional Assessment (MNA) [2, 3]. Common nutrition screening factors are addressed in the next section. Consideration of factors affecting the integrity and function (mandibular opening, biting, chewing, swallowing, lip seal) of the mouth (including pain, saliva, soft tissue, nerves, muscles, joints, teeth) that may in turn affect food and fluid consumption is important both in regard to provider examination and patient self-report as part of comprehensive care [9]. The findings can be integrated with any of the nutrition screening tools addressed herein to determine interventions to maximize patient response to treatment and systemic health.

1.1 Weight Status and Change

Unintentional weight change, either loss or gain, may reflect a change in appetite or ability to eat and/or drink, alterations in energy needs due to a systemic issue, an eating disorder, or food insecurity. With unintentional weight loss, losses in both fat and muscle mass may occur. Body compositional changes seen in aging include loss of muscle mass and an increase in body fat mass. This process may be expedited in the face of decreased mobility either due to voluntary or involuntary causes [10].

Asking patients about their weight history is valuable to establish a basis for comparison. Both actual and usual weights are used to calculate percent weight change [(Actual − Usual)/Usual × 100]. A 5–10% unintentional weight loss in 3–6 months is considered a risk factor for malnutrition according to the Malnutrition Universal Screening Tool (MUST) [5], while the Mini Nutritional Assessment (MNA) [2, 3] considers a 3 kilograms or more loss of weight in the preceding 3 months a risk factor for malnutrition. Unintentional weight gain can reflect a change in health status, diet, or a decline in physical activity. If the gain is due to excess fluid accumulation, such as in edema or ascites, prompt medical attention is needed to determine the cause and treat the fluid excess.

Evaluation of weight and weight change over time is inexpensive, noninvasive, and rapid. Body mass index (BMI) reflects weight in proportion to height; it does not differentiate between fat and muscle mass. Hence, even a person with no weight change may have a shift in the proportion of muscle and fat mass that will not be reflected in the BMI. Weight status classifications are based on BMI [underweight, normal, overweight, obesity (class I or II), and extreme obesity (class III)] and can be used to identify risk for cardiometabolic diseases as well as mortality. BMI can be calculated using applications from the National Institutes of Health and the Centers for Disease Control and Prevention (http://www.nhlbi.nih.gov/guidelines/obesity/BMI/bmicalc.htm, and https://www.cdc.gov/healthyweight/assessing/index.html).

1.2 Medical, Surgical, and Dental History

Patient history of acute or chronic diseases provides insights into factors that may influence oral integrity and subsequently oral intake. Oral manifestations of diabetes including increased risk of oral infectious diseases, burning tongue, xerostomia, and compromised wound healing can negatively affect appetite, eating ability, and intake [11, 12]. Infections can impact glycemic control and ultimately nutritional status.

Other systemic diseases not specific to older adults that can affect nutritional status and diet include autoimmune diseases such as Crohn's disease, rheumatoid arthritis, Sjögren's syndrome, systemic lupus erythematosus, scleroderma, and pemphigus vulgaris. In these diseases, both functional and sensory abilities may be altered either by virtue of the impact of the disease on muscle and joint pain or function, sensory impacts due to oral lesions or altered cranial nerve function, or the medications used to treat the systemic conditions. Xerostomia and hyposalivation which may be due to medications or Sjögren's syndrome increase the risk for oral infectious diseases and mucosal injury. Joint pain such as in the temporomandibular joint can limit mandibular opening and the ability to bite and chew. While these factors may not be included specifically in nutrition risk screening or assessment tools, they are essential for health professionals to consider.

Most cancers can affect nutritional status as well as the integrity of the oral cavity. In particular, upper gastrointestinal (GI) cancers from the mouth through the esophagus can impact nutrition via the disease itself causing altered energy and nutrient needs, location, and extent of surgeries and treatments. Radiation to the mouth can alter sensory and functional abilities and may, depending on the extent, cause hyposalivation and xerostomia. Chemotherapies can cause oral infections including stomatitis, along with anorexia, nausea, and vomiting. Surgical resections depending on the location, extent, and any need for oral devices such as a palatal obturator can have short- and long-term impacts on eating and drinking ability.

1.3 Oral Risk Factors

The integrity and function (mandibular opening, biting, chewing, swallowing, lip seal) of the mouth (including pain, saliva, soft tissue, nerves, muscles, joints, teeth) are not addressed in the majority of nutrition screening tools. However, failure to consider these factors as part of the assessment of the older adult, in terms of both physical examination and patient interview, can impact the plan of care and may result in missing contributing causal factors to risk for or presence of malnutrition. Readers are urged to consider the impact of material covered in other sections and chapters as part of their nutrition screening.

1.4 Dietary Intake

Changes in dietary intake of foods and fluids merit consideration as part of nutrition screening. Simple questions about whether food intake has changed or declined due to appetite, masticatory or swallowing problems, or gastrointestinal disorders and, if so, the extent and timeframe of the decline or change help to identify the severity of the problem. In some circumstances, the clinician may choose to further assess dietary intake to determine eating patterns, energy and nutrient intake, and diet quality. Diet assessment methods commonly used include dietary recalls and food frequencies. With any approach, there is the potential for over- and underreporting of error [13].

Dietary recalls refer to asking the patient to "recall" everything they consumed (foods and fluids) either on a typical day or the preceding 24 hours. With this approach, one documents the pattern, specific food(s) and fluid(s), and portion sizes. Dietary recall data can be analyzed using a nutrient analysis web application to determine total energy intake, macro- and micronutrients, and food groups. In contrast, food frequency questionnaires (FFQs) assess patient consumption of foods and fluids over a period of time such as a week, a month, or a year [14]. Validated FFQs exist and are typically used in epidemiological studies. The use of FFQs in clinical settings is limited as they may not reflect short-term changes in intake or eating and drinking patterns. There are other approaches to dietary intake assessment; the National Cancer Institute *Dietary Assessment Primer* [14] provides greater detail on these approaches.

1.5 Nutrition Screening and Assessment Tools

Nutrition screening refers to the identification of patient characteristics that are associated with nutritional problems [15]. It is intended to identify whether further comprehensive nutrition assessment should be conducted prior to intervention. Validated tools for nutrition assessment and screening specific to older adults which can be used in a variety of settings include the Mini Nutritional Assessment in the complete and short forms (MNA, MNA-SF) and the self-administered version (Self-MNA), the Malnutrition Screening Tool (MST), the Malnutrition Universal Screening Tool (MUST), and the Nutritional Risk Screening 2002 (NRS 2002). These tools are compared in Table 1. The choice of the tool to use is dependent on the intent (screening or diagnosis), population (some tools have only been validated in specific countries), care setting, time, and user.

The MNA family of tools originated with the validation of the MNA in 1994 in its full and complete form [16]. The MNA forms are specific to adults aged 65 years and older in any care setting. The original 18-item MNA (https://www.mna-elderly.com/forms/MNA_english.pdf) is intended as a nutrition assessment tool; it addresses food intake, BMI, weight loss, diet, activities of daily living, mobility, psychological stress or acute disease, neuropsychological problems, medications, presence of decubiti, and mid-arm and calf circumferences. Of note, the change in food intake question specifically asks whether the change is due to difficulty chewing or swallowing, appetite loss, or digestive problems. It is intended to be used by healthcare professionals to determine if patients have normal nutritional status or are at risk of or have malnutrition.

The MNA Short-Form (MNA-SF) (https://www.mna-elderly.com/forms/mini/mna_mini_english.pdf) was validated in 2001 [17] and 2009 [3] against the original

Table 1 Validated nutrition screening and assessment tools [2–8]

	MNA	MNA-SF	MST	MUST	NRS 2002
Unintentional weight loss	X	X	X	X	X
Change in intake due to oral function and appetite	X	X	X (only appetite)		X
Acute disease	X	X		X	
Cognition	X	X			
Mobility	X	X			
BMI or calf circumference	X	X		X	X
Medications	X				
Decubiti	X				
Mode of feeding	X				
Mid-arm circumference	X				
Specific to older adults	X	X			X has a correction score

BMI body mass index, *MNA* Mini Nutritional Assessment, *MNA-SF* Mini Nutritional Assessment Short-Form, *MST* Malnutrition Screening Tool, *MUST* Malnutrition Universal Screening Tool, *NRS 2002* Nutrition Risk Screening 2002

MNA. It is designed as a nutritional status screening tool for use by any healthcare professional to determine the risk of malnutrition in older adults. The two validation studies reflect its original validation [17] with BMI, and then in 2009, the validation included the use of calf circumference as an alternative to BMI when it is not available [3]. The six items include the same questions as the original MNA in regard to intake, unintentional weight loss, mobility, psychological stress/acute disease, neuropsychological problems, and BMI (or calf circumference).

The 2013 validated Self-MNA (https://www.mnaelderly.com/forms/Self_MNA_English_Imperial.pdf) can be used by older adults to self-assess their risk for malnutrition [18]. The Self-MNA asks for self-assessment of decline in food intake (but does not evaluate the specific cause of the decline), weight loss, mobility status, stress or severe illness, dementia, and BMI. The tool is limited by its self-evaluative nature and whether a person can self-identify as having dementia or experiencing the other symptoms evaluated.

The Malnutrition Screening Tool (MST), like the MNA Short-Form, was validated with adults in acute, rehabilitation, and long-term care settings, including inpatients with cancer in ambulatory care settings [4, 6]. It is designed for use by healthcare professionals as well as consumers to identify the risk for malnutrition. It asks about weight loss (intentional or unintentional and extent) and change in appetite.

The Malnutrition Universal Screening Tool (MUST) was validated in community, long-term care, and acute care settings in Australia, the United Kingdom, and the European Union with adults to identify risk for malnutrition [5, 7]. It can be used by any healthcare professional and includes the evaluation of BMI, unintentional weight loss over the previous 3–6 months, and acute illness with or without lack of intake in the preceding 5 days. Without an accurate weight or self-reported weight, a recalled weight can be used. If height measurement is not feasible, knee height may be used.

The Nutritional Risk Screening 2002 (NRS 2002) was validated in Denmark for use with hospitalized patients to identify risk for malnutrition [8]. It includes a correction factor in the scoring system for patients who are 70 years of age or older. The use of the tool is limited to adults in acute care settings; it classifies patients as having "undernutrition" to varying extents based on the presence of an unintentional weight loss, change in intake, and BMI.

2 Associations Between Tooth Loss and Replacement, Diet, and Nutritional Status in Older Adults

Tooth loss, with or without replacement with dentures, can lead to compromised oral function and changes in biting, chewing, and swallowing ability [19]. The quantity and distribution of the remaining teeth and the type, fit, and location of dentures all influence masticatory ability, food choices, diet quality, and nutritional status [19–24]. Associations between these factors reported in the research are heterogeneous due to variability in the methods used to assess diet, nutritional status, tooth loss, and denture type(s). Tada et al. found that those who are missing all or some of their natural teeth are more likely to have impaired ability to bite and chew compared with those who are fully dentate [20]. Having fewer natural teeth and poorer occlusion and mastication are associated with poorer food diversity and diet quality, as well as lower intakes of energy, vegetables, fruits, fiber, protein, dairy, carbohydrates, fat (especially polyunsaturated fatty acids), and micronutrients including vitamins A, C, D, E, K, beta carotene, thiamine, riboflavin, niacin, B6, folate, B12, pantothenic acid, calcium, sodium, potassium, phosphorus, magnesium, iron, zinc, selenium, and copper [24–42].

Likewise, denture type and pattern may also impact nutrient intake; however, research findings vary in part due to the types of tools used to assess intake and denture type and pattern [43]. Individuals with implant-supported dentures (ISD) consume more vegetables, B12 and animal proteins, fiber, calcium, and iron and have less difficulty masticating raw, hard, and fibrous foods as compared to those who wear other types of dentures [44–47]. However, other researchers have not demonstrated significant differences in food and nutrient intake based on denture type [26, 48, 49]. Individuals with ill-fitting dentures, or those who remove their dentures while eating, are more likely to have poorer diet quality and avoid more foods than those who consistently wear their dentures for eating [26, 50–52]. A simple yet often overlooked question with patients is whether they use their dentures for eating.

Aside from changes in overall quantity of nutrient intake, difficulty biting and chewing can lead to the selection of softer foods that require less masticatory effort and that may be richer in carbohydrate and calories in place of nutrient-dense foods that may be harder to chew [33, 38, 53]. Such changes in diet can ultimately result in changes in weight and nutritional status [28, 29, 38, 54, 55]. Older adults with poorer occlusion and compromised masticatory ability are significantly more likely to be both underweight or have lower BMI values [54–60] and to be overweight/obese or have higher BMI values [28, 54, 56, 61–63], when compared to those with more teeth and better occlusion, placing them at higher risk of malnutrition. Longitudinal studies have found that complete edentulism is a significant risk factor for both weight loss [64] and gain [53].

However, others have not found significant associations between tooth loss and changes in weight or weight status [38, 65, 66] or replacement with dental prostheses and changes in weight or weight status [46, 54, 67, 68] which contributes to the lack of definitive findings. The variation in these findings may be due in part to the heterogeneity in study design and populations. Regardless, screening for changes in nutrient intake and weight status that may occur in association with tooth loss and replacement can help prevent malnutrition [69].

The MNA is the most commonly used nutrition screening tool reported in research that assesses the associations between tooth loss, replacement, and malnutrition risk [70–80]. However, this body of research is heterogeneous in that the studies measure dental status differently, which make the results somewhat difficult to compare. When the nutritional status of participants with complete edentulism has been compared to participants with partial edentulism, most studies have found significant positive associations between complete edentulism and increased risk of malnutrition [71–74].

Associations between functional dentition [81, 82] and the risk of malnutrition have also been documented. Those without functional dentition are at a higher risk of malnutrition than those with functional dentition [70, 80]. Others have only reported trends [79] or found significant findings but only in unadjusted models for this association [76]. Yet other research findings do not support significant differences in nutritional status based on the number of remaining teeth or occlusal status [75, 77, 78]. While the findings of these individual studies are heterogeneous, Zelig et al. completed a meta-analysis and found that older adults who were fully edentulous or lacked functional dentition were 21% more likely to be at risk of or have malnutrition than older adults who were partially dentate or with functional dentition [21].

Older adults with removable partial or full dentures are at greater risk of malnutrition than those with complete posterior occlusion [83] or implant-supported dentures [44]. Some have found that the replacement of missing teeth with dentures can improve nutritional status [84–87]. However, replacement of older dentures with newer complete dentures has not been shown to significantly improve MNA scores and reduce malnutrition risk [68, 88]. Dentures do not provide the same masticatory ability as natural teeth. Changes in eating behaviors and dietary patterns take time, education, and adjustment and may be difficult to attain.

Ikebe et al. found that adults in the poorest quintile of masticatory ability were approximately two times more likely to be underweight and those in the lowest quintile of occlusal force were almost two times more likely to be overweight [55]. These findings shed some light on the heterogeneity of this body of research and suggest that in relation to their effect on nutritional status, functional ability (masticatory and occlusal force) may be equally or more important than morphology (number of teeth and presence and type of dentures). Thus, rehabilitation to improve oral function and masticatory ability combined with education and interventions to improve nutritional status are warranted for older adults with tooth loss.

3 Dietary Interventions for Older Adults With Tooth Loss With or Without Dentures

Older adults experience both adaptive and maladaptive behaviors as they adjust to tooth loss and replacement [89–92]. Individuals with tooth loss may take more time to eat, chew food longer, and chew on the side of the mouth that has better occlusion. Intervention to minimize risk for declines in the intake of energy or nutrient and maximize adaptive behaviors can also help individuals consume a healthy dietary pattern and enjoy a better quality of life.

Simply telling patients to "eat soft foods" is insufficient as it is open to interpretation and some soft foods like white bread readily absorb saliva and form a bolus and are hard to swallow. In contrast, cooked, cut, or chopped foods may be easier to bite and chew initially, and thus the degree of "softness" may be better stated "as tolerated." Advising patients to use their knives and forks as "teeth" and to cut foods to minimize biting and chewing is also useful.

According to the World Health Organization (WHO), consuming a healthy diet throughout the lifespan is essential for preventing malnutrition and chronic disease [93, 94]. A healthy diet emphasizes vegetables, fruits, legumes, nuts, and whole grains and includes low-fat dairy products and lean protein sources like fish and poultry [93–96]. Preference is given to unsaturated fat sources, such as olive, canola, sunflower, or soybean oils, as well as fish, nuts, and avocados. Intake of sugar, sweets, sugar-sweetened beverages, trans and saturated fats including red meats and tropical oils, sodium, and processed foods is discouraged [93–96]. Within this framework, clinicians can guide patients toward adaptation of healthier dietary choices based on personal and cultural food preferences, food availability, and budgetary constraints to reduce the potential for maladaptive behaviors [93, 94].

Maladaptive behaviors include the avoidance of difficult to chew foods, like raw vegetables and fruits, hard or fibrous nuts, grains, and meat products, and increased consumption of foods that are higher in fat (i.e., mayonnaise), sugar (i.e., ice cream), or other carbohydrate sources (i.e., mashed potatoes) [89–92]. Approaches to replace maladaptive with adaptive behaviors have been developed for older adults with tooth loss and with dentures [89–92].

4 Guidance for Healthcare Providers and Older Adults with Tooth Loss

Zelig et al. found that older adults with tooth loss employed adaptive strategies to compensate for chewing difficulty [89]. These included modifications in food texture selection and cooking methods, such as choosing foods that are naturally easier to bite and chew, like overripe fruits, and cooking foods until they acquire a softer consistency. Other compensatory strategies include chopping, mashing, peeling, shredding, and grinding foods or adding fats and gravies to make foods softer, moister, and easier to chew. Table 2 provides tips for oral health and other healthcare providers to use with older adults experiencing tooth loss to help them eat better and enhance their eating experience.

5 Guidance for Healthcare Providers and Older Adults with Dentures

Replacement of missing teeth with removable partial or full dentures (RPD, FD) also impacts the eating experience. While dentures replace teeth, functional ability to bite and chew foods varies depending on many factors including type(s) of

Table 2 Guidance for eating healthier with tooth loss [89]

Tips to improve fruit and vegetable intake
Choose softer fruits and vegetables like bananas or avocados
Peel or remove hard-to-chew skin
Cut or chop into bite-sized pieces
Cook to a softer consistency
Blend or puree into a smoothie or a cold soup
Buy canned (without added salt or sugar) or frozen as needed
Tips to improve whole grain intake
Choose cooled whole grains like oatmeal, brown rice, quinoa, or couscous
Cut bagels and rolls into smaller pieces
Cook pasta and rice until soft
Allow cereals to soften in milk or other liquid
Toast lightly and add a spread like butter or cream cheese
Have sips of fluids while eating to add moisture
Tips to improve protein intake
Choose easy-to-eat and drink, protein-rich foods like ground meat or poultry, fish or seafood, eggs, cooked beans, tofu, or dairy products like cottage cheese, cow or other dairy or non-dairy alternative milks, yogurts, and cheese
Remove hard-to-chew skin
Cook foods that will shred or flake easily like fish, shredded or pulled beef, chicken, or pork, or vegetable protein alternatives
Cook to a softer consistency or until tender; try a slow cooker
Add sauces and gravies to moisten
Use a knife and fork or mini-food chopper to cut foods into bite-sized pieces
Tips to become more comfortable eating around others
Share eating challenges with family and friends so you can enjoy eating with them
Plan meals with family and friends where everyone can eat the same thing
When going to a party or event, eat first or bring something you can eat just in case there are no foods you can tolerate
Leave yourself enough time to eat
Go to restaurants where the menu includes foods you can eat, and don't be afraid to ask how foods are prepared, and specify how you would like them cooked

dentures, location (maxillary or mandibular), age, and fit [19, 43]. Ideally, denture fit and stability should be evaluated while observing a patient eating. Observation of mandibular movement while attempting to bite and chew foods permits the examiner to check for movement, noise, and function of the denture(s) as well as food pocketing. Adults with dentures should be asked if they use them for eating, and, if not, they should be questioned on why in order to determine potential causes and solutions. Consideration of patient complaints of difficulty biting, chewing, and swallowing with or without dentures is critical. This information can be used for the dental and diet treatment plans.

Dietary guidelines for those wearing dentures recommend that individuals start slow and progress gradually, *as tolerated* [97]. At least initially, it is best to avoid dry foods that fall apart in the mouth like rice, muffins, and nuts. On the day of and initially 1–3 days following insertion, some patients may need to eat easy-to-masticate items. This helps minimize the need to bite or chew while maintaining nutrient quality of food along with sensory qualities like taste and smell. Chopping and cooking a variety of vegetables to make a vegetable soup, mashing them to the consistency of mashed potatoes, or cooking any vegetables until they are fork-tender allows for consumption of a greater variety of vegetables to enhance flavor and increase the nutrient value.

Cut-up and peeled raw soft fruits and vegetables, grains, and protein products should come next, followed by progression to raw, whole items, *as tolerated*. Using a knife and fork to cut food into bite-sized pieces so that the teeth don't have to do the work can help. Trying to chew foods at corners of the mouth can take the pressure off the front teeth which are generally used to bite. Fluids should also be encouraged to help moisten food.

Adjusting to dentures takes time. A progressive diet plan can ease the adjustment and allow the patients to consume foods they enjoy and that are healthy. Hard, crunchy, and tough foods like crusty breads, tough stringy meats (e.g., steaks, ribs), nuts, and seeds may be challenging, and soft, sticky foods like white bread and some soft rolls may be very difficult. Similarly, peanut and other nut butters can be difficult to manage with dentures. Chewing gum is generally discouraged [97].

Individuals who wear dentures also benefit from modification of food choices and consistencies, in addition to instruction on how to improve denture stability and function while eating [91, 92]. Table 3 provides a guide for oral health and other healthcare providers for use with older adults who wear dentures to help them eat better and enhance their eating experience.

6 Conclusions

A healthy mouth is a key component to being able to consume a healthy diet. Changes to soft and hard tissues and cranial nerves that affect oral sensations and movement have the potential to affect food and fluid choices and nutrient and energy intake and ultimately increase the risk for malnutrition. The extent to which the risk for malnutrition occurs may be mitigated by early identification of risk factors, followed by the provision of appropriate interventions. An interprofessional team including medical, oral health, and diet and nutrition professionals working together to provide screening and appropriate referrals between professions can promote optimal patient-centered care.

Nutrition screening and identification of factors that affect the ability to eat and drink can be identified early as part of the initial patient evaluation by oral healthcare professionals. Dietitians can integrate oral screening into their physical examination as part of nutrition assessment. Diet education may be provided by a dentist or hygienist, physician, physician assistant, nurse, or a credentialed dietitian, depending on the setting. In settings without a credentialed dietitian, a referral can be provided to one for medical nutrition therapy. A synergistic approach to patient care by all members of the interprofessional team can help to maximize oral, systemic, and nutritional health as well as quality of life.

Table 3 Guidance for eating following denture provision [91, 92, 97]

Tips for diet progression following provision of new dentures:
Day #1: May need to eat chopped, minced, pureed, or blenderized foods; smoothies, soups, puddings
Days #2–3: Choose soft or cut-up foods as tolerated
Animal and vegetable protein sources: cook until soft[a], cut into small pieces, moisten with gravy or sauces
Dairy and non-dairy alternatives: milk, yogurt, spreads, cheeses, hot/cold cereal with milk, smoothies
Fruits and vegetables: soups, smoothies; peel and cook until mashable or fork-tender as tolerated
Grains: mashed potatoes, oatmeal, cream of wheat, pastas
Days #4–5: Progress to raw cut-up foods as tolerated
Peel and cut or chop raw fruits and vegetables
Use a knife and fork to cut food into bite-sized pieces
Foods to avoid (at least initially)
Dry foods that fall apart in the mouth like rice, quinoa, grains, biscuits, crackers, and muffins
Hard, crunchy, tough-to-chew foods like crusty breads, stringy meats, nuts, and seeds
Soft, sticky foods like white bread and soft rolls and nut butters
Foods that may get stuck like seeds and pulp or other foods that break into small pieces
Chewing gum and hard candies
Other tips for eating well with dentures[b]
Cut food using a knife and fork and take small bites
Chew foods at corners of the mouth to take the pressure off the front teeth
Balance the bite force on both sides of the mouth
Fluids should also be encouraged to help moisten food
Choose softer[a] foods as tolerated
Cook foods to a softer[a] consistency
Modify the way the food is prepared and consumed
Practice good oral hygiene after meals and snacks
Troubleshooting pain or discomfort and denture instability
Use fixatives as needed under the guidance of an oral healthcare professional
Follow up with a dentist for denture adjustment as needed

[a]The narrative describes how to interpret the word "soft"
[b]See Table 2 for further discussion of appropriate food modifications for patients with tooth loss and replacement

References

1. US National Library of Medicine MedlinePlus Medical Encyclopedia. Heart disease – risk factors [updated 6/25/2020]. Available from: https://medlineplus.gov/ency/patientinstructions/000106.htm.
2. Vellas B, Guigoz Y, Garry PJ, Nourhashemi F, Bennahum D, Lauque S, et al. The Mini Nutritional Assessment (MNA) and its use in grading the nutritional state of elderly patients. Nutrition. 1999;15(2):116–22.
3. Kaiser MJ, Bauer JM, Ramsch C, Uter W, Guigoz Y, Cederholm T, et al. Validation of the Mini Nutritional Assessment short-form (MNA-SF): a practical tool for identification of nutritional status. J Nutr Health Aging. 2009;13(9):782–8.

4. Ferguson M, Capra S, Bauer J, Banks M. Development of a valid and reliable malnutrition screening tool for adult acute hospital patients. Nutrition. 1999;15(6):458–64.
5. BAPEN Malnutrition Advisory Group. The 'MUST' report. Nutritional screening of adults: a multidisciplinary responsibility. Development and use of the 'Malnutrition Universal Screening Tool' ('MUST') for adults; 2003.
6. Skipper A, Coltman A, Tomesko J, Charney P, Porcari J, Piemonte TA, et al. Adult malnutrition (undernutrition) screening: an evidence analysis center systematic review. J Acad Nutr Diet. 2020;120(4):669–708.
7. Stratton RJ, Hackston A, Longmore D, Dixon R, Price S, Stroud M, et al. Malnutrition in hospital outpatients and inpatients: prevalence, concurrent validity and ease of use of the 'malnutrition universal screening tool' ('MUST') for adults. Br J Nutr. 2004;92(5):799–808.
8. Kondrup J, Rasmussen HH, Hamberg O, Stanga Z. Ad Hoc ESPEN Working Group. Nutritional risk screening (NRS 2002): a new method based on an analysis of controlled clinical trials. Clin Nutr. 2003;22(3):321–36.
9. O'Keeffe M, Kelly M, O'Herlihy E, O'Toole PW, Kearney PM, Timmons S, et al. Potentially modifiable determinants of malnutrition in older adults: a systematic review. Clin Nutr. 2019;38(6):2477–98.
10. Shaw KA, Srikanth VK, Fryer JL, Blizzard L, Dwyer T, Venn AJ. Dual energy X-ray absorptiometry body composition and aging in a population-based older cohort. Int J Obes. 2007;31(2):279–84.
11. Lalla E, Kunzel C, Burkett S, Cheng B, Lamster IB. Identification of unrecognized diabetes and pre-diabetes in a dental setting. J Dent Res. 2011;90(7):855–60.
12. Barasch A, Safford MM, Qvist V, Palmore R, Gesko D, Gilbert GH, et al. Random blood glucose testing in dental practice: a community-based feasibility study from The Dental Practice-Based Research Network. J Am Dent Assoc. 2012;143(3):262–9.
13. Beaton GH. Approaches to analysis of dietary data: relationship between planned analyses and choice of methodology. Am J Clin Nutr. 1994;59(1 Suppl):253S–61S.
14. National Cancer Institute. Food frequency questionnaire at a glance. Available from: https://dietassessmentprimer.cancer.gov/profiles/questionnaire/index.html.
15. American Dietetic Association. Identifying patients at risk: ADA's definition for nutrition screening and nutrition assessment. J Am Diet Assoc. 1994;94(8):838–9.
16. Guigoz Y, Vellas B, Garry PJ. Mini Nutritional Assessment: a practical assessment tool for grading nutritional state of elderly patients. Facts Res Gerontol. 1994:15–59.
17. Rubenstein LZ, Harker JO, Salva A, Guigoz Y, Vellas B. Screening for undernutrition in geriatric practice: developing the short-form mini-nutritional assessment (MNA-SF). J Gerontol A Biol Sci Med Sci. 2001;56(6):M366–72.
18. Huhmann MB, Perez V, Alexander DD, Thomas DR. A self-completed nutrition screening tool for community-dwelling older adults with high reliability: a comparison study. J Nutr Health Aging. 2013;17(4):339–44.
19. Kiesswetter E, Poggiogalle E, Migliaccio S, Donini LM, Sulmont-Rosse C, Feart C, et al. Functional determinants of dietary intake in community-dwelling older adults: a DEDIPAC (DEterminants of DIet and Physical ACtivity) systematic literature review. Public Health Nutr. 2018;21(10):1886–903.
20. Tada A, Miura H. Systematic review of the association of mastication with food and nutrient intake in the independent elderly. Arch Gerontol Geriatr. 2014;59(3):497–505.
21. Zelig R, Goldstein S, Touger-Decker R, Firestone E, Golden A, Johnson Z, et al. Tooth loss and nutritional status in older adults: a systematic review and meta-analysis. JDR Clin Trans Res. 2020:2380084420981016.
22. Kazemi S, Savabi G, Khazaei S, Savabi O, Esmaillzadeh A, Keshteli AH, et al. Association between food intake and oral health in elderly: SEPAHAN systematic review no. 8. Dent Res J. 2011;8(Suppl 1):S15–20.
23. Okamoto N, Amano N, Nakamura T, Yanagi M. Relationship between tooth loss, low masticatory ability, and nutritional indices in the elderly: a cross-sectional study. BMC Oral Health. 2019;19(1):110.

24. Inomata C, Ikebe K, Kagawa R, Okubo H, Sasaki S, Okada T, et al. Significance of occlusal force for dietary fibre and vitamin intakes in independently living 70-year-old Japanese: from SONIC study. J Dent. 2014;42(5):556–64.
25. Bailey RL, Ledikwe JH, Smiciklas-Wright H, Mitchell DC, Jensen GL. Persistent oral health problems associated with comorbidity and impaired diet quality in older adults. J Am Diet Assoc. 2004;104(8):1273–6.
26. Marshall TA, Warren JJ, Hand JS, Xie XJ, Stumbo PJ. Oral health, nutrient intake and dietary quality in the very old. J Am Dent Assoc. 2002;133(10):1369–79.
27. Zhu Y, Hollis JH. Tooth loss and its association with dietary intake and diet quality in American adults. J Dent. 2014;42(11):1428–35.
28. Sahyoun NR, Lin CL, Krall E. Nutritional status of the older adult is associated with dentition status. J Am Diet Assoc. 2003;103(1):61–6.
29. Sheiham A, Steele J. Does the condition of the mouth and teeth affect the ability to eat certain foods, nutrient and dietary intake and nutritional status amongst older people? Public Health Nutr. 2001;4(3):797–803.
30. Marcenes W, Steele JG, Sheiham A, Walls AW. The relationship between dental status, food selection, nutrient intake, nutritional status, and body mass index in older people. Cad Saude Publica. 2003;19(3):809–16.
31. Kwon SH, Park HR, Lee YM, Kwon SY, Kim OS, Kim HY, et al. Difference in food and nutrient intakes in Korean elderly people according to chewing difficulty: using data from the Korea National Health and Nutrition Examination Survey 2013 (6th). Nutr Res Pract. 2017;11(2):139–46.
32. de Andrade FB, de Franca Caldas Jr A, Kitoko PM. Relationship between oral health, nutrient intake and nutritional status in a sample of Brazilian elderly people. Gerodontology. 2009;26(1):40–5.
33. Osterberg T, Tsuga K, Rothenberg E, Carlsson GE, Steen B. Masticatory ability in 80-year-old subjects and its relation to intake of energy, nutrients and food items. Gerodontology. 2002;19(2):95–101.
34. Kagawa R, Ikebe K, Inomata C, Okada T, Takeshita H, Kurushima Y, et al. Effect of dental status and masticatory ability on decreased frequency of fruit and vegetable intake in elderly Japanese subjects. Int J Prosthodont. 2012;25(4):368–75.
35. Kimura Y, Ogawa H, Yoshihara A, Yamaga T, Takiguchi T, Wada T, et al. Evaluation of chewing ability and its relationship with activities of daily living, depression, cognitive status and food intake in the community-dwelling elderly. Geriatr Gerontol Int. 2013;13(3):718–25.
36. Iwasaki M, Taylor GW, Manz MC, Yoshihara A, Sato M, Muramatsu K, et al. Oral health status: relationship to nutrient and food intake among 80-year-old Japanese adults. Community Dent Oral Epidemiol. 2014;42(5):441–50.
37. Iwasaki M, Yoshihara A, Ogawa H, Sato M, Muramatsu K, Watanabe R, et al. Longitudinal association of dentition status with dietary intake in Japanese adults aged 75 to 80 years. J Oral Rehabil. 2016;43(10):737–44.
38. Yoshida M, Kikutani T, Yoshikawa M, Tsuga K, Kimura M, Akagawa Y. Correlation between dental and nutritional status in community-dwelling elderly Japanese. Geriatr Gerontol Int. 2011;11(3):315–9.
39. Brennan DS, Singh KA, Liu P, Spencer A. Fruit and vegetable consumption among older adults by tooth loss and socio-economic status. Aust Dent J. 2010;55(2):143–9.
40. Ervin RB, Dye BA. The effect of functional dentition on Healthy Eating Index scores and nutrient intakes in a nationally representative sample of older adults. J Public Health Dent. 2009;69(4):207–16.
41. Yoshihara A, Watanabe R, Nishimuta M, Hanada N, Miyazaki H. The relationship between dietary intake and the number of teeth in elderly Japanese subjects. Gerodontology. 2005;22(4):211–8.
42. Kim JM, Stewart R, Prince M, Kim SW, Yang SJ, Shin IS, et al. Dental health, nutritional status and recent-onset dementia in a Korean community population. Int J Geriatr Psychiatry. 2007;22(9):850–5.

43. Sanchez-Ayala A, Lagravere MO, Goncalves TM, Lucena SC, Barbosa CM. Nutritional effects of implant therapy in edentulous patients--a systematic review. Implant Dent. 2010;19(3):196–207.
44. Tsai AC, Chang TL. Association of dental prosthetic condition with food consumption and the risk of malnutrition and follow-up 4-year mortality risk in elderly Taiwanese. J Nutr Health Aging. 2011;15(4):265–70.
45. Goncalves TM, Campos CH, Garcia RC. Effects of implant-based prostheses on mastication, nutritional intake, and oral health-related quality of life in partially edentulous patients: a paired clinical trial. Int J Oral Maxillofac Implants. 2015;30(2):391–6.
46. Morais JA, Heydecke G, Pawliuk J, Lund JP, Feine JS. The effects of mandibular two-implant overdentures on nutrition in elderly edentulous individuals. J Dent Res. 2003;82(1):53–8.
47. Tajbakhsh S, Rubenstein JE, Faine MP, Mancl LA, Raigrodski AJ. Selection patterns of dietary foods in edentulous participants rehabilitated with maxillary complete dentures opposed by mandibular implant-supported prostheses: a multicenter longitudinal assessment. J Prosthet Dent. 2013;110(4):252–8.
48. Liedberg BN, Norlen P, Owall B, Stoltze K. Masticatory and nutritional aspects on fixed and removable partial dentures. Clin Oral Investig. 2004;8(1):11–7.
49. Liedberg B, Stoltze K, Norlen P, Owall B. 'Inadequate' dietary habits and mastication in elderly men. Gerodontology. 2007;24(1):41–6.
50. Sahyoun NR, Krall E. Low dietary quality among older adults with self-perceived ill-fitting dentures. J Am Diet Assoc. 2003;103(11):1494–9.
51. Lin YC, Chen JH, Lee HE, Yang NP, Chou TM. The association of chewing ability and diet in elderly complete denture patients. Int J Prosthodont. 2010;23(2):127–8.
52. Savoca MR, Arcury TA, Leng X, Chen H, Bell RA, Anderson AM, et al. Impact of denture usage patterns on dietary quality and food avoidance among older adults. J Nutr Gerontol Geriatr. 2011;30(1):86–102.
53. Lee JS, Weyant RJ, Corby P, Kritchevsky SB, Harris TB, Rooks R, et al. Edentulism and nutritional status in a biracial sample of well-functioning, community-dwelling elderly: the health, aging, and body composition study. Am J Cin Nutr. 2004;79(2):295–302.
54. Musacchio E, Perissinotto E, Binotto P, Sartori L, Silva-Netto F, Zambon S, Manzato E, Corti MC, Baggio G, Crepaldi G. Tooth loss in the elderly and its association with nutritional status, socio-economic and lifestyle factors. Acta Odontol Scand. 2007;65(2):78–86.
55. Ikebe K, Matsuda KI, Morii K, Nokubi T, Ettinger RL. The relationship between oral function and body mass index among independently living older Japanese people. Int J Prosthodont. 2006;19(6):539–46.
56. Sheiham A, Steele JG, Marcenes W, Finch S, Walls AW. The relationship between oral health status and Body Mass Index among older people: a national survey of older people in Great Britain. Br Dent J. 2002;192(12):703–6.
57. Ostberg AL, Nyholm M, Gullberg B, Rastam L, Lindblad U. Tooth loss and obesity in a defined Swedish population. Scand J Public Health. 2009;37(4):427–33.
58. Hashimoto M, Yamanaka K, Shimosato Y, Ozawa A, Takigawa T, Hidaka S, Sakai T, Noguchi T. Oral condition and health status of elderly 8020 achievers in Aichi Prefecture. Bull Tokyo Dent Coll. 2006;47(2):37–43.
59. Soini H, Routasala P, Lagstrom H. Nutritional status in cognitively intact older people receiving home care services--a pilot study. J Nutr Health Aging. 2005;9(4):249–53.
60. Adiatman M, Ueno M, Ohnuki M, Hakuta C, Shinada K, Kawaguchi Y. Functional tooth units and nutritional status of older people in care homes in Indonesia. Gerodontology. 2013;30(4):262–9.
61. Andreas Zenthofer A, Rammelsberg P, Cabrera T, Hassel A. Prosthetic rehabilitation of edentulism prevents malnutrition in nursing home residents. Int J Prosthodont. 2015;28(2):198–200.
62. Ando A, Ohsawa M, Yaegashi Y, Sakata K, Tanno K, Onoda T, et al. Factors related to tooth loss among community-dwelling middle-aged and elderly Japanese men. J Epidemiol. 2013;23(4):301–6.

63. Osterberg T, Dey DK, Sundh V, Carlsson GE, Jansson JO, Mellstrom D. Edentulism associated with obesity: a study of four national surveys of 16 416 Swedes aged 55–84 years. Acta Odontol Scand. 2010;68(6):360–7.
64. Ritchie CS, Joshipura K, Silliman RA, Miller B, Douglas CW. Oral health problems and significant weight loss among community-dwelling older adults. J Gerontol A Biol Sci Med Sci. 2000;55(7):M366–71.
65. Hanioka T, Ojima M, Tanaka K, Aoyama H. Association of total tooth loss with smoking, drinking alcohol and nutrition in elderly Japanese: analysis of national database. Gerodontology. 2007;24(2):87–92.
66. Syrjala AMH, Ylostalo P, Hartikainen S, Sulkava R, Knuuttila M. Number of teeth and selected cardiovascular risk factors among elderly people. Gerodontology. 2010;27(3):189–92.
67. Awad MA, Morais JA, Wollin S, Khalil A, Gray-Donald K, Feine JS. Implant overdentures and nutrition: a randomized controlled trial. J Dent Res. 2012;91(1):39–46.
68. Muller F, Duvernay E, Loup A, Vazquez L, Herrmann FR, Schimmel M. Implant-supported mandibular overdentures in very old adults: a randomized controlled trial. J Dent Res. 2013;92(12 Suppl):154S–60S.
69. Guigoz Y, Vellas B. Nutritional assessment in older adults: MNA(R) 25 years of a screening tool and a reference standard for care and research; what next? J Nutr Health Aging. 2021;25(4):528–83.
70. Lopez-Jornet P, Saura-Perez M, Llevat-Espinosa N. Effect of oral health dental state and risk of malnutrition in elderly people. Geriatr Gerontol Int. 2013;13(1):43–9.
71. Starr JM, Hall RJ, Macintyre S, Deary IJ, Whalley LJ. Predictors and correlates of edentulism in the healthy old people in Edinburgh (HOPE) study. Gerodontology. 2008;25(4):199–204.
72. Gil-Montoya JA, Subira C, Ramon JM, Gonzalez-Moles MA. Oral health-related quality of life and nutritional status. J Public Health Dent. 2008;68(2):88–93.
73. Krzyminska-Siemaszko R, Chudek J, Suwalska A, Lewandowicz M, Mossakowska M, Kroll-Balcerzak R, et al. Health status correlates of malnutrition in the polish elderly population – results of the Polsenior Study. Eur Rev Med Pharmacol Sci. 2016;20(21):4565–73.
74. Saarela RK, Lindroos E, Soini H, Hiltunen K, Muurinen S, Suominen MH, et al. Dentition, nutritional status and adequacy of dietary intake among older residents in assisted living facilities. Gerodontology. 2016;33(2):225–32.
75. Furuta M, Takeuchi K, Adachi M, Kinoshita T, Eshima N, Akifusa S, et al. Tooth loss, swallowing dysfunction and mortality in Japanese older adults receiving home care services. Geriatr Gerontol Int. 2018;18(6):873–80.
76. Furuta M, Komiya-Nonaka M, Akifusa S, Shimazaki Y, Adachi M, Kinoshita T, et al. Interrelationship of oral health status, swallowing function, nutritional status, and cognitive ability with activities of daily living in Japanese elderly people receiving home care services due to physical disabilities. Community Dent Oral Epidemiol. 2013;41(2):173–81.
77. Soini H, Routasalo P, Lagstrom H. Nutritional status in cognitively intact older people receiving home care services--a pilot study. J Nutr Health Aging. 2005;9(4):249–53.
78. Soini H, Routasalo P, Lauri S, Ainamo A. Oral and nutritional status in frail elderly. Spec Care Dentist. 2003;23(6):209–15.
79. Zelig R, Byham-Gray L, Singer SR, Hoskin ER, Fleisch Marcus A, Verdino G, et al. Dentition and malnutrition risk in community dwelling older adults. J Aging Res Clin Pract. 2018;7:107–14.
80. Kikutani T, Yoshida M, Enoki H, Yamashita Y, Akifusa S, Shimazaki Y, et al. Relationship between nutrition status and dental occlusion in community-dwelling frail elderly people. Geriatr Gerontol Int. 2013;13(1):50–4.
81. Dye BA, Weatherspoon DJ, Lopez MG. Tooth loss among older adults according to poverty status in the United States from 1999 through 2004 and 2009 through 2014. J Am Dent Assoc. 2019;150(1):9–23 e3.
82. Walls AW, Steele JG. The relationship between oral health and nutrition in older people. Mech Ageing Dev. 2004;125(12):853–7.

83. Cousson PY, Bessadet M, Nicolas E, Veyrune JL, Lesourd B, Lassauzay C. Nutritional status, dietary intake and oral quality of life in elderly complete denture wearers. Gerodontology. 2012;29(2):e685–92.
84. Su Y, Yuki M, Hirayama K, Sato M, Han T. Denture wearing and malnutrition risk among community-dwelling older adults. Nutrients. 2020;12(1):151.
85. Wallace S, Samietz S, Abbas M, McKenna G, Woodside JV, Schimmel M. Impact of prosthodontic rehabilitation on the masticatory performance of partially dentate older patients: can it predict nutritional state? Results from a RCT. J Dent. 2018;68:66–71.
86. McKenna G, Allen PF, O'Mahony D, Cronin M, DaMata C, Woods N. Impact of tooth replacement on the nutritional status of partially dentate elders. Clin Oral Investig. 2015;19(8):1991–8.
87. McKenna G, Allen PF, Flynn A, O'Mahony D, DaMata C, Cronin M, et al. Impact of tooth replacement strategies on the nutritional status of partially-dentate elders. Gerodontology. 2012;29(2):e883–90.
88. Allen PF. Association between diet, social resources and oral health related quality of life in edentulous patients. J Oral Rehabil. 2005;32(9):623–8.
89. Zelig R, Jones VM, Touger-Decker R, Hoskin ER, Singer SR, Byham-Gray L, et al. The eating experience: adaptive and maladaptive strategies of older adults with tooth loss. JDR Clin Trans Res. 2019;4(3):217–28.
90. Hyland R, Ellis J, Thomason M, El-Feky A, Moynihan P. A qualitative study on patient perspectives of how conventional and implant-supported dentures affect eating. J Dent. 2009;37(9):718–23.
91. Al-Sultani H, Thomason JM, Field J, Breckons M, Moynihan P. Co-design of patient-centred advice about eating with complete dentures (poster presentation). London: International Association for Dental Research; 2018.
92. Al-Sultani H, Moynihan P, Holmes R, Thomason JM, Field J, Breckons M. Patient's opinions on advice about eating with complete dentures (poster presentation). Continental European and Scandinavian divisions meeting; 2017; Vienna, Austria.
93. World Health Organization. Healthy diet 2020 [updated April 29, 2020]. Available from: https://www.who.int/news-room/fact-sheets/detail/healthy-diet.
94. U.S. Department of Health and Human Services and U.S. Department of Agriculture. 2020–2025 dietary guidelines for Americans. 9th Edition. 2020. Available from: https://www.dietaryguidelines.gov/sites/default/files/2020-12/Dietary_Guidelines_for_Americans_2020-2025.pdf.
95. Van Horn L, Carson JA, Appel LJ, Burke LE, Economos C, Karmally W, et al. Recommended dietary pattern to achieve adherence to the American Heart Association/American College of Cardiology (AHA/ACC) guidelines: a scientific statement from the American Heart Association. Circulation. 2016;134(22):e505–e29.
96. US Preventive Services Taskforce, Krist AH, Davidson KW, Mangione CM, Barry MJ, Cabana M, et al. Behavioral counseling interventions to promote a healthy diet and physical activity for cardiovascular disease prevention in adults with cardiovascular risk factors: US Preventive Services Task Force recommendation statement. JAMA: J Am Med Assoc. 2020;324(20):2069–75.
97. Mobley CC, Dounis G. Dietary guidance for people wearing removable prostheses. J Am Dent Assoc. 2013;144(2):e11–5.

Swallowing, Dysphagia, and Aspiration Pneumonia

Atsuko Kurosu, Rebecca H. Affoo, Shauna Hachey, and Nicole Rogus-Pulia

Abbreviations

BOHSE	Brief Oral Health Status Examination
CN	Cranial nerve
DHI	Dysphagia Handicap Index
DIGEST	Dynamic Imaging Grade of Swallowing Toxicity
EAT-10	Eating Assessment Tool-10
FESS	Fiberoptic endoscopic evaluation of swallowing
GOHAI	Geriatric Oral Health Assessment Index
GUSS	Gugging Swallowing Screen
IDDSI	International Dysphagia Diet Standardization Initiative
LTC	Long-term care
MBSImP	Modified Barium Swallow Impairment Profile

A. Kurosu (✉)
Department of Medicine, School of Medicine and Public Health, University of Wisconsin–Madison, Madison, WI, USA
e-mail: akurosu@wisc.edu

R. H. Affoo
School of Communication Sciences and Disorders, Faculty of Health, Dalhousie University, Halifax, NS, Canada

S. Hachey
School of Dental Hygiene, Faculty of Dentistry, Dalhousie University, Halifax, NS, Canada

N. Rogus-Pulia
Division of Geriatrics and Gerontology, Department of Medicine, School of Medicine and Public Health, University of Wisconsin–Madison, Madison, WI, USA

Swallowing and Salivary Bioscience Laboratory, Geriatric Research Education and Clinical Center (GRECC), William S. Middleton Memorial Veterans Hospital, Madison, WI, USA

MBSS	Modified barium swallow study
MPS	Mucosal-Plaque Index
OHAT	Oral Health Assessment Tool
OHrQoL	Oral health-related quality of life
PEM	Protein-energy malnutrition
ROAG	Revised Oral Assessment Guide
SLP	Speech-language pathologist
SLS	Sodium lauryl sulfate-free
SSQ	Sydney Swallowing Questionnaire
THROAT	The Holistic and Reliable Oral Assessment Tool
TOR-BSST	Toronto Bedside Swallowing Screening Test
UES	Upper esophageal sphincter
VFS	Videofluoroscopic swallowing study
VFSS	Videofluoroscopic examination of swallow

1 What Is Swallowing?

1.1 Swallowing Definition

Swallowing is defined as the process of moving material through the oral cavity, pharynx, and esophagus and into the stomach through a series of muscular actions [1]. Swallowing is an overly complex neuromuscular act which requires motor and sensory coordination as well as organized interaction of cortical, subcortical, brain stem, and peripheral systems [2, 3]. Despite this, healthy individuals swallow an average of 500 times a day [4]. There are two types of swallowing: volitional and spontaneous [2]. Volitional swallowing is initiated under a conscious and awake condition such as during mealtimes with an intention to swallow [2]. Spontaneous swallowing is thought to be an involuntary mechanism that facilitates clearance of secretions from the mouth and pharynx and supports oral health and airway protection [4–8]. Spontaneous swallowing occurs unconsciously or without intention such as during sleeping or between mealtimes and is initiated when the salivary volume reaches a critical threshold [2, 7, 9].

Previous work has identified that as the volume of saliva increases in the oral cavity, humans will respond by spontaneously swallowing more frequently. Studies exploring resting swallowing frequency in healthy adults have identified a highly variable rate of 24–61 swallows/hour [9]. It is not clear if this variability is influenced by the volume of saliva secreted into the oral cavity or if there are other factors that may contribute. Reduction in the rate of spontaneous swallowing has been associated with increased pharyngeal secretions which increase the risk of chest infection in health compromised individuals [4–8].

2 Swallow Physiology

2.1 Liquid Swallowing: Four Sequence Model of Swallowing

Swallow physiology is divided into four sequential phases: (1) oral preparatory phase, (2) oral phase, (3) pharyngeal phase, and (4) esophageal phase [1, 10–12]. These phases are not discrete from one another but rather often overlap.

2.1.1 Oral Preparatory Phase of Swallowing

During the oral preparatory phase, liquid is taken into the oral cavity, and it is held on the tongue surface against the hard palate. The liquid is coated by and integrated with saliva to form a lubricated mass, which is referred to as a "bolus," that has suitable size and consistency for swallowing [10–14]. To prevent the loss of a portion of the bolus, the oral cavity is sealed anteriorly by the upper and lower lips and posteriorly by the contact of the dorsum of the tongue and the soft palate [1, 12, 15, 16].

2.1.2 Oral Phase of Swallowing

The oral phase of swallowing is initiated after the bolus is adequately formed [16]. During the oral phase, the bolus is held between the elevating and retracting tongue and the hard palate and propelled posteriorly via sequential contact of the tongue against the hard palate from front to back [10]. The oral phase ends when the tail of the bolus fully enters the oropharyngeal region.

2.1.3 Pharyngeal Phase of Swallowing

When the head of the bolus passes any point between the anterior faucial arches and the point where the base of the tongue crosses the ramus of the mandible, the pharyngeal swallow is triggered [1, 10, 17]. Sequential neuromuscular events occur once the pharyngeal swallow is initiated [1, 10, 15, 17]. The velum is moved superiorly and posteriorly to contact the posterior and lateral wall of the pharynx to close off the nasopharynx. This prevents materials from entering the nasal cavity. The hyoid bone is pulled superiorly and anteriorly by the suprahyoid muscles [16]. Simultaneously, the larynx is moved toward the hyoid bone by the thyrohyoid muscle. The anterior and superior displacement of the hyolaryngeal complex contributes to closure of the airway [1, 10, 17]. The airway is closed at three levels: (1) the true vocal folds; (2) the laryngeal entrance including the false vocal folds, the arytenoid cartilages tilting forward to the epiglottic base, and thickening of the epiglottic base; and (3) the deflection of the epiglottis. Airway closure is critical for preventing materials from entering the airway. The anterior displacement of the hyolaryngeal complex, relaxation of the cricopharyngeal muscle, and intrabolus pressure contribute to the upper esophageal sphincter (UES) opening [18]. The opening of the UES allows the bolus to enter the esophagus [1, 15]. Then, the space between the base of the tongue and posterior pharyngeal wall sequentially collapses from the top to bottom to propel the bolus inferiorly when the bolus tail reaches the level of the base of the tongue.

2.1.4 Esophageal Phase of Swallowing

The esophageal phase of swallowing is initiated when the bolus enters the esophagus at the UES [1, 16]. When the bolus passes through the UES, the bolus is carried down to the stomach by a sequential peristaltic wave through the lower esophageal sphincter [1, 15].

2.2 Solid Food Swallowing: Process Model of Feeding

The process model of feeding divides swallow physiology into five stages: (1) stage I transport, (2) food processing, (3) stage II transport, (4) pharyngeal stage, and (5) esophageal stage [15, 19]. The pharyngeal and esophageal stages in this model are identical to those of the four- phase model for liquid swallowing.

2.2.1 Stage I Transport

After the solid food is placed in the oral cavity, the food is moved posteriorly to the post-canine region by the tongue. Then, the food is moved laterally to be placed onto the occlusal surface of the lower teeth for mastication [15, 19].

2.2.2 Food Processing

During food processing, the solid food is masticated and mixed with saliva until the food becomes suitable and safe for swallowing [15, 19, 20]. The properties of masticated bolus, such as particle size, bolus hardness, springiness, adhesiveness, and cohesiveness, may be used to determine when the bolus is ready for swallowing [20].

2.2.3 Stage II Transport

The masticated food is placed on the tongue surface, and it is propelled posteriorly. Then, the food is accumulated in the upper oropharynx and/or valleculae, which is referred to as "bolus aggregation," before it is propelled into the pharynx and beyond [15, 19]. This is also an example of overlap between the phases of swallowing given that the pharyngeal phase of the swallow may be initiated with a portion of the solid bolus that was adequately masticated while food processing with the rest of the solid bolus continues.

The purpose of mastication is to process food in the oral cavity into a bolus that can be transported through the oropharynx, swallowed safely, and then easily digested [21, 22]. During mastication, ingested food particles are mechanically reduced in size through the process of lingual particle selection as well as fragmentation between the occlusal surfaces of the teeth [23]. Factors such as total occlusal area, opposing occlusal contacts, bite force, number of teeth, and coordination between the movement of the jaw, tongue, and cheeks during manipulation of the food particles play an important role in effective mastication [22–24].

The secretion of saliva is critical for effective mastication, bolus formation, and bolus transport, and both the volume and composition of saliva contribute significantly to these functions [25]. The water in saliva is used to moisten the food particles, allowing the salivary amylase to access available starch and initiate chemical digestion [26]. Saliva contains mucins (primarily MUC5B and MUC7) that contribute to a slimy, viscoelastic coating of all surfaces in the oral cavity which is an important lubricant between opposing oral surfaces during mastication, swallowing, and speaking [27]. The salivary mucins bind masticated food into a coherent and slippery bolus that can easily be transported through the oropharynx [21]. The secretions rich in mucins can lubricate, stretch, and bond to one another to form tangled grids or webs known as spinnbarkeit that coat the epithelial surfaces of the mouth and pharynx. When food is mixed with the mucin-rich secretions, they serve to minimize shear stresses and potentially increase the extensional viscosity of the bolus allowing for less effort during mastication and improved pharyngeal transport with less post-swallow residue [28]. Even though mucins seem to play a critical role in mastication of solid food boluses, saliva secreted from the parotid glands during alimentation typically has the lowest concentrations of mucins and is also the least viscoelastic [27]. It has been hypothesized that parotid secretions may change the pH of saliva during bolus formation, which may consequently affect shear forces [29], but this process is not well understood, and it is unclear whether there is a threshold concentration of mucins or ideal viscoelasticity that results in optimal bolus formation and transport.

3 Swallowing Anatomy

3.1 Swallowing Musculature

Swallowing involves the precise coordination of more than 30 muscles in the face, oral cavity, pharynx, larynx, and esophagus [16]. Most of the muscles that participate in swallowing are striated muscles except for those in the middle and distal esophagus. The middle and distal esophagus are partially and completely comprised of smooth muscles [16]. Muscular movements during swallowing are controlled by the trigeminal (CN V), facial (CN VII), glossopharyngeal (CN IX), vagus (CN X), and hypoglossal (CN XII) nerves as well as the ansa cervicalis (C1–C3) and the pharyngeal plexus with fibers from the cranial division of accessory nerve (CN XI) [11, 16, 30]. The muscles involved during the oral phase include the muscles of the face, tongue (intrinsic and extrinsic tongue muscles), and mastication. The muscles involved during the pharyngeal phase include the muscles of the soft palate, pharyngeal musculature, hyoid (suprahyoid and infrahyoid), larynx, and upper esophagus [16, 31]. Figure 1 summarizes the muscles involved in swallowing.

3.2 Swallowing Neurophysiology

Swallowing requires the complex interaction of voluntary and involuntary neuronal networks including the cortical, subcortical, brain stem, and peripheral nervous system [2, 3]. There are sensory fibers that respond to temperature, touch, and pressure

Oral phase			Pharyngeal phase		
Group	Name	Innervation	Group	Name	Innervation
Face	Obicularis oris	Facial (CN VII)	Soft palate	Tensor veli palatini	Trigeminal (CN V)
	Buccinator	Facial (CN VII)		Levator veli palatini	Vagus nerve (CN X)
Tongue (Intrinsic)	Superior longitudinal	Hypoglossal (CN XII)		Musculus uvulae	Vagus nerve (CN X)
	Inferior longitudinal	Hypoglossal (CN XII)	Pharynx	Stylopharyngeus	Glossopharyngeal (IX)
	Transversus	Hypoglossal (CN XII)		Salpingopharyngeus	Vagus nerve (CN X)
	Verticalis	Hypoglossal (CN XII)		Palatopharyngeaus	Vagus nerve (CN X)
Tongue (Extrinsic)	Hyoglossus	Hypoglossal (CN XII)		Superior pharyngeal constrictor	Vagus nerve (CN X)
	Genioglossus	Hypoglossal (CN XII)		Middle pharyngeal constrictor	Vagus nerve (CN X)
	Styloglossus	Hypoglossal (CN XII)		Inferior pharyngeal constrictor	
	Palatoglossus	Vagus nerve (CN X)	Hyoid (Suprahyoid)	Geniohyoid	Hypoglossal (CN XII); Ansa cervicalis (C1-C2)
Mastication	Temporalis	Trigeminal (CN V)		Mylohyoid	Trigeminal (CN V)
	Masseter	Trigeminal (CN V)		Anterior belly of digastric	Trigeminal (CN V)
	Lateral pterygoid	Trigeminal (CN V)		Posterior belly of digastric	Facial (CN VII)
	Medial pterygoid	Trigeminal (CN V)		Styroid	Facial (CN VII)
			Hyoid (Infrahyoid)	Omohyoid	Ansa cervicalis (C1-C3)
				Thyrohyoid	Hypogiossal (CN XII); C1
				Sternohyoid	Ansa cervicalis (C1-C3)
				Sternohyoid	Ansa cervicalis (C1-C3)
			Larynx	Thyroartenoid	Vagus nerve (CN X)
				Transvers arytenoid	Vagus nerve (CN X)
				Lateral cricoarytenoid	Vagus nerve (CN X)
			Upper esophagus	Cricopharyngeaus	Vagus nerve (CN X)
				Inferior fibers of the inferior pharyngeal constrictor	Vagus nerve (CN X)
				Upper fibers of the esophagus	Vagus nerve (CN X)

Fig. 1 Musculature and innervation in the oral and pharyngeal phase of swallowing. (Adapted from Shaw and Martino [16])

as well as chemoreceptors or taste receptors in the oropharynx [32]. Sensory information is sent to the trigeminal nerve (CN V), facial nerve (CN VII), glossopharyngeal nerve (IX), and vagus nerve (CN X) and then transferred to various nuclei in the brain stem [32, 33]. The swallowing central pattern generator is located within the medulla oblongata in the brain stem [32, 33] and contains two swallow-related neuron groups which are the dorsal swallowing group within and around the nucleus tractus solitarius and the ventral swallowing group around the nucleus ambiguus [3, 33, 34].

Peripheral as well as supra-medullary inputs travel to the dorsal swallowing group. The dorsal swallowing group sends the motor signals to the ventral swallowing group and transmits the outputs to motor neuron pools [33, 34]. Studies with functional magnetic resonance imaging indicate multiple bilateral subcortical as well as cortical areas are activated during swallowing [35, 36]. The areas that are consistently active during swallowing include the primary sensory cortex, primary motor cortex, anterior cingulate cortex, and insular cortex [35, 36]. However, further studies are needed to clarify the supratentorial neural mechanisms of swallowing.

4 What Is Dysphagia?

4.1 Dysphagia Definition

Swallowing difficulty is called dysphagia. Dysphagia is characterized by any difficulty moving food, liquid, secretions, or medications from the mouth to the stomach [12, 37]. Dysphagia may result from any illnesses that cause neurological, anatomical, or physiological abnormalities or dysfunctions of swallow-related structures such as the oral cavity, larynx, pharynx, and esophagus [12, 38].

4.2 Prevalence of Dysphagia

The exact prevalence of dysphagia is unknown given that it varies widely in the literature [38]. This variability could be in part due to differences in the swallowing measures and definitions of dysphagia [39]. Additionally, the prevalence of dysphagia varies depending on the type and severity of the diseases that are causing dysphagia (e.g., dementia type and head and neck cancer stage and site) as well as treatment modalities for the diseases [39].

4.3 Signs and Symptoms of Dysphagia

Signs and symptoms of dysphagia include coughing, nasal regurgitation, choking of food, clearing throat, sensation of food sticking in the throat and/or chest, recurrent pneumonia, unexplained weight loss, and gurgly or wet voice [1, 14, 40, 41]. Patients with dysphagia may or may not self-report swallowing difficulties.

4.4 Types of Swallowing Impairments

Characteristics of swallowing impairments vary among patients. However, there are some typical swallowing impairment types that a patient may exhibit in each swallow phase [32].

4.4.1 Oral Phase Impairments

Weakness or dysfunction of the tongue, lips, and other muscles in the oral cavity and/or loss of or reduced oral sensation may result in swallowing impairments during the oral phase of swallowing. These impairments include reduced lip closure, absent or prolonged oral preparation, reduced tongue control, incomplete tongue-palate contact, difficulty chewing, reduced taste, and swallow apraxia [1, 14, 32]. Reduced lip closure may result in drooping or food falling from the oral cavity anteriorly [1, 42]. Reduced tongue control may result in premature loss of the bolus into the pharynx [41, 43].

4.4.2 Pharyngeal Phase Impairments

Swallowing impairments during the pharyngeal phase include delayed triggering of the pharyngeal swallow, absence of the pharyngeal response, reduced laryngeal closure, epiglottic dysfunction, reduced tongue base and posterior pharyngeal wall contact, reduced velopharyngeal closure, and reduced laryngopharyngeal sensation [12, 15, 32, 40, 41, 44]. Reduced velopharyngeal closure may result in nasal regurgitation. Delayed triggering of the pharyngeal swallow may result in penetration (entry of liquid or food into the airway above the true vocal folds) or aspiration (entry of liquid or food into the airway below the true vocal folds) *prior* to initiation of the pharyngeal phase of the swallow and associated airway closure [44]. Reduced laryngeal closure, hyolaryngeal excursion, and laryngopharyngeal sensation may lead to aspiration/penetration *during* or *at the height of* the pharyngeal phase of the swallow [32]. Reduced hyolaryngeal excursion and tongue base and posterior pharyngeal wall contact may result in pharyngeal residue (liquid or food left in the oropharynx after swallowing) that leads to penetration/aspiration *after* conclusion of the pharyngeal phase [41].

4.4.3 Esophageal Phase Impairments

Swallowing impairment during the esophageal phase will occur if patients have reduced upper esophageal sphincter (UES) opening, reduced duration of UES opening, and/or impaired esophageal peristalsis which may result in intraesophageal stasis and pharyngoesophageal reflux [1, 14, 32]. Zenker's diverticulum is an outpouching of mucosa at the level of UES [45, 46]. During swallowing, the diverticulum is filled with liquid or food, and then it is emptied after the swallow. The material in the diverticulum may enter the airway and cause aspiration *during* or *after* the swallow [46, 47]. Esophageal stricture is an abnormal narrowing of the esophagus that can be caused through neoplasm, fibrosis, or inflammation [48–50].

5 Risk Factors for Dysphagia

5.1 Risk Factors for Dysphagia in Older Adults

Older adults commonly experience normal age-related changes to swallowing anatomy and biomechanics, also known as "presbyphagia," that increase their susceptibility to dysphagia—increased time to initiate a swallow, reduced volume of the pharynx, reduced salivary secretion, and increasing rates of dental problems [51–62]. These changes are not considered pathological as many older adults are able to swallow safely, suggesting that functional reserve may allow older adults to compensate for age-related swallowing changes [63]. However, age has been identified as an independent risk factor for dysphagia in several studies including studies of community-dwelling older adults [64], as well as those in the hospital [65] or living in long-term care settings [66]. Age, therefore, is clearly an important factor related to dysphagia, and this may be due in part to the age-associated increase in the incidence of conditions and diseases that are known to be significant risk factors for developing dysphagia.

It is well-established that dysphagia is a symptom of many dysfunctions and disorders, including, but not limited to, stroke, Parkinson's disease, dementia, head and neck cancer, and brain injury [39]. Moreover, because the oropharynx is a shared pathway that supports ventilation as well as nutrition and hydration, diseases that impact the ventilatory system may also impact the process of deglutition. As such, dysphagia is a documented symptom of chronic respiratory diseases such as obstructive sleep apnea and chronic obstructive pulmonary disease [67, 68]. It is also commonly associated with laryngeal injury or deconditioning that may occur following endotracheal intubation and mechanical ventilation [69] and with the development of respiratory complications such as aspiration pneumonia that can further exacerbate existing respiratory disease [70].

Eating and swallowing requires an individual to address the meal, visually recognize food and drink, and respond with the appropriate motor movements that results in transportation of food and fluid to the mouth and then from the mouth to the stomach [37, 71, 72]. Given the important role that cognition plays in the process of eating and swallowing, it is not surprising that impaired cognitive function has been found to be a risk factor for dysphagia. Leder and group conducted a study with hospitalized participants and found that not being oriented to person, place, or time or being unable to follow single-step commands was associated with increased risk of aspiration [73]. Jo and group (2017) used a retrospective analysis of hospitalized patients and identified that cognitive status was an important predictor of dysphagia after a first-time stroke [74].

Furthermore, in a study of long-term care residents aged 60 years and older, Yatabe and colleagues (2018) identified that edentulous residents with higher Mini-Mental State Examination scores tended to have lower odds of dysphagia risk [75].

While the prevalence of dysphagia tends to increase with advancing age [65, 76], increased risk of adverse health outcomes, including dysphagia, may not necessarily be a consequence of aging. Some older adults are at greater risk of experiencing poor health outcomes compared with similar aged peers [77]. In a systematic review conducted by Madhavan and colleagues (2016), the authors identified significant risk factors for dysphagia, one of which was physical frailty [64]. Frailty, a condition marked by cumulative decline across several physiological systems [78], is generally measured in two different ways: as a specific physical syndrome [79] and as a deficit accumulation [80]. Evidence examining the relationship between dysphagia and physical frailty and frailty as deficit accumulation suggests that the two conditions may frequently co-occur [81–85], resulting in negative health outcomes [85]. The relationship between physical frailty and dysphagia may be driven by sarcopenia, or age-associated decreased muscle mass and function of the tongue [86]. The tongue plays a critical role in preparing the bolus to be swallowed and moving the bolus through the oral cavity and pharynx and into the esophagus [87]. Reduced tongue strength has been found to be an independent predictor of sarcopenic dysphagia in older hospitalized patients [88], it has been associated with aspiration in healthy, community-dwelling older adults [86], and with increased dysphagia risk and mealtime duration for individuals living in long-term care [89, 90]. Furthermore, a meta-analysis conducted by Zhao and colleagues (2018) revealed that individuals with sarcopenia are four times more likely to develop dysphagia [91]. Individuals with frailty due to their reduced functional reserve may no longer be able to compensate for age-related swallowing changes and may experience an acute, but potentially transient, reduction of swallowing safety and/or efficiency [92]. Even a transient dysphagia in these individuals has the potential for the negative sequelae associated with dysphagia to add to the burden of disease and worsen any existing frailty. It is critical to identify dysphagia and manage it appropriately to reduce these negative outcomes as well as others, including higher total costs, increased non-routine discharges (discharge to a short-term hospital, long-term care facility, or home health), more medical complications, and increased risk of inhospital mortality [85]. For a more in-depth discussion on the topic of frailty, please refer to the chapter "Frailty and Oral Health."

5.2 *Poor Oral Health as a Risk Factor for Dysphagia*

Due to the complexity and the multifactorial nature of oral health, the relationship between dysphagia and oral health has been hypothesized and explored in different ways. For example, the concepts of salivary [93–95] and oral function [96, 97], presence or absence of teeth [98], and oral hygiene [99] in relation to dysphagia have been discussed previously in the literature.

The oral cavity is the beginning of the digestive tract and contains numerous structures that function to deliver food and drink to the pharynx, including the teeth, orofacial muscles, lips, cheeks, and tongue. Missing teeth can decrease one's ability to masticate or chew [100], and tooth loss is also significantly associated with impaired water and saliva swallowing [98, 101].

Sarcopenia of the muscles of mastication may result in reduced bite force and jaw velocity and prolonged mastication duration, especially when eating tough foods such as meat. This may negatively impact nutritional status [53]. Dentures and tongue motor function have also been found to impact masticatory efficiency [102], which suggests that as tongue motor function declines with age, denture stability and retention may be compromised.

Other types of oral impairment have been identified as risk factors for dysphagia. Community-dwelling older adults may be two times more likely to self-report dysphagia if they have impaired oral function measured using a speech diadochokinesis task or the ability to repeat the /pa/ syllable as quickly as possible [97]. Reduced ability to complete diadochokinesis with the /pa/ syllable may be due to reduced lip force, which is associated with sarcopenic dysphagia in older hospitalized patients and may contribute to the downward turn of the lips and pooling of liquid at the labial commissures [88]. Impaired oral function may also impact functional oral intake.

Furuya and colleagues (2019) examined oral function in hospitalized patients with dysphagia and found that functional oral intake was significantly associated with level of consciousness, ability to independently complete activities of daily living, tongue coating, and posterior occlusal support [96]. Impaired oral hygiene has also been identified as a risk for dysphagia. Hida and colleagues (2021) examined oral cavity flora in community-dwelling older adults and identified that participants with colony-forming units of anaerobic *Prevotella* spp. were three times more likely to fail a water swallowing screening test [99].

5.3 *Dysphagia as Risk Factor for Poor Oral Health*

Older patients with dysphagia demonstrate poorer oral health than those without dysphagia. A study of 50 older patients with dysphagia revealed that this cohort had a higher prevalence of full edentulism, dental caries, gingivitis, and periodontitis compared to 15 older patients without dysphagia [103]. This same research group also conducted a study of 47 older patients with frailty (>70 years of age) in which they enrolled four groups: 17 patients with dysphagia and an acute episode of pneumonia, 14 patients with dysphagia and a history of pneumonia, 14 patients with dysphagia and no history of pneumonia, and 14 control participants without dysphagia [104]. Results showed that oral health was poor in all three groups (90% with periodontitis, 72% with caries). Total bacterial load was similar in all three groups. However, colonization of respiratory pathogens was significantly higher in the two groups of patients with dysphagia (93% in both groups) compared to the non-dysphagic control group (67%).

These findings highlight the ways in which swallowing function and various aspects of oral health may interact and influence one another. Regular and efficient swallowing supports a healthy microbiome by clearing food debris, detached cells, and microbial waste products. Saliva prevents dysbiosis through its antimicrobial components, pH buffering, and continuous refreshing. Salivary mucins induce bacterial aggregation preventing bacteria from attaching to the oral epithelial cell surface and promoting removal upon swallowing. Impaired swallowing biomechanics that result in more frequent and larger volume aspiration events in combination with a dysbiotic oral environment increase the risk of adverse health outcomes. In fact, a recent study revealed that, while poor oral health and dysphagia were both independently associated with mortality risk, those patients with both showed the highest mortality risk (2.6 times higher than those without either impairment) [105].

6 Consequences of Dysphagia

6.1 Pneumonia

Pneumonia is considered a major cause of morbidity and mortality globally for older adults and has been estimated to cause up to 1.1 million in-hospital deaths [106] and significant financial costs [107, 108] to patients and healthcare systems. Aspiration pneumonia is the third and fifth leading cause of infectious death in individuals aged >85 years and >65 years, respectively [109]. Bacterial pneumonia has been classified into several different types, and the categorization reflects differences in how the pneumonia was contracted and the pathogens responsible for the pneumonia [110–116] (Table 1).

6.2 Aspiration Pneumonia

Aspiration pneumonia is a lung infection that is acquired when bacteria-laden foreign materials, such as food/liquid, secretions, or regurgitated contents of the stomach or esophagus, enter the lungs, resulting in bacterial colonization [117]. In a meta-analysis conducted by van der Maarel-Wierink and colleagues, they found a positive correlation between dysphagia and aspiration pneumonia, which supports the common belief that dysphagia with aspiration is the essential predisposing element for the development of aspiration pneumonia [118]. However, Langmore and colleagues (1998) were the first to draw a connection between the condition of the oral cavity and the occurrence of aspiration pneumonia [119]. While dysphagia was

Table 1 Types of pneumonia

Pneumonia type	Description	Pathogen
Community-acquired pneumonia	Any pneumonia contracted outside the hospital	*Haemophilus influenzae, Streptococcus pneumoniae*
Hospital acquired pneumonia—nosocomial	Any pneumonia contracted by a patient in a hospital at least 48–72 hours after being admitted	*Staphylococcus aureus*
Hospital-acquired pneumonia—ventilator acquired	Any pneumonia contracted while on mechanical ventilation	*Pseudomonas aeruginosa, Staphylococcus aureus*
Healthcare-associated pneumonia	Any pneumonia contracted prior to hospital admission in patients with specific risk factors such as residing in long-term care, being immunocompromised, etc.	*Staphylococcus aureus*
Aspiration pneumonia	Any pneumonia contracted after bacteria-laden foreign materials, such as food/liquid, secretions, or regurgitated contents of the stomach or esophagus, enter the lungs, resulting in bacterial colonization	*Streptococcus pneumoniae, Staphylococcus aureus, Haemophilus influenzae*, and *Enterobacteriaceae* [117]

determined to be an important risk for aspiration pneumonia, it was not sufficient to cause pneumonia unless other risk factors were present. In that study, dependence for oral care and the number of decayed teeth were among the strongest predictors for pneumonia [120–122]. It is now accepted that there is a strong relationship between poor oral health and respiratory disease [123].

6.3 *Malnutrition and Dehydration*

Dysphagia is a risk factor for malnutrition in older adults [124–126]. A large secondary cross-sectional analysis of over 17,000 patients during hospitalization and in the nursing home setting revealed that those with dysphagia were at two times higher risk of malnutrition than those without dysphagia in the sample [127]. In one study examining patients with dysphagia (without tube feeding instigated), daily unsupported oral intake was found to be as low as 275 kcal (14.5% of estimated energy requirements) [128]. Protein-energy malnutrition (PEM) is a serious medical condition in which a person is not adequately receiving the correct amounts of protein/energy needed to sustain metabolic functions [129]. Individuals with dysphagia, especially those of advanced age, are at an increased risk for PEM and may experience a synergistic interaction between this nutritional vulnerability and reduced immune function that increases the chance for serious illness, including pneumonia onset [130]. The individual effects of poor oral health and dysphagia on food selection and nutrient intake may combine to exacerbate risk of malnutrition [131].

Similarly, individuals with dysphagia are at higher risk for dehydration. Patients with post-stroke dysphagia and modification of solid diets or on thickened liquids are significantly more likely to be dehydrated at discharge [132]. While thickened fluids and diet modification are often necessary for appropriate management of dysphagia, studies have shown that patients taking thickened liquids demonstrate decreased acceptance of the beverages [133]. One study of a group of patients post-stroke with comorbid dysphagia revealed that the intake of thickened fluids per day led to only 30% of the recommended 1500 mL/day [134].

6.4 Asphyxiation Risk

Asphyxiations of semisolid and solid foods are the cause of many deaths among older adults [135–137]. During 2007–2010 in the USA, 2214 deaths among persons aged >/= 65 years were attributed to choking on food [136]. These deaths were most associated with dementia (including Alzheimer's disease, Parkinson's disease, and pneumonitis) [136, 138]. Asphyxiation deaths can occur in all settings—hospital, nursing homes, at home, and in restaurants [139]. A maximum food sample size of 1.5 × 1.5 cm for hard and soft solid foods has been recommended by the International Dysphagia Diet Standardization Initiative (IDDSI) framework [140]. This particle size is small enough to pass completely into an adult trachea without obstructing it and has been shown to reduce the risk of asphyxiation [141, 142]. Issues related to inadequate oral health affecting masticatory efficiency, such as edentulism or low salivation, can increase the risk of asphyxiation due to poor bolus processing or breakdown to this necessary particle size [143].

6.5 Quality of Life for Oral Health and Swallowing

The ability to eat and swallow is critically important to maintaining the oral health-related quality of life of older adults. In a study conducted by Miura and colleagues (2010), they surveyed older adults and caregiver dyads and found that the most influential factors that impacted oral health-related quality of life (OHrQoL) were communication and dysphagia [144]. Dysphagia impacts OHrQoL in persons with neurodegenerative disease. In a study examining persons with Parkinson's disease, Barbe and colleagues (2016) found that many participants experienced xerostomia (49%), drooling (70%), and dysphagia (47%), and these symptoms significantly impacted oral health-related quality of life [145]. Dysphagia has also been found to mediate OHrQoL. Lu and group (2020) conducted a cross-sectional study of community-dwelling participants aged 65 years or older. They collected data on depression, dental status, oral dryness, masticatory performance, swallowing, physical function, and oral health-related quality of life and found that perceived oral dryness had the strongest direct negative effect on OHrQoL. Dysphagia and masticatory performance strongly mediated the effect of xerostomia on OHrQoL [146].

7 Evaluation of Swallowing

There are two main swallowing evaluations: clinical evaluation and instrumental evaluation [40]. Instrumental evaluation includes videofluoroscopic examination of swallow (VFSS) and fiberoptic endoscopic evaluation of swallowing (FESS) [40, 147].

7.1 Clinical Evaluation

The purpose of the clinical evaluation is to identify whether (1) patients are at a high risk of dysphagia and (2) referral for further instrumental swallowing evaluations [148]. There is no current standard protocol for the clinical evaluation. Typically, speech-language pathologists first conduct a thorough review of the patient's medical history from the medical chart. During the process, current and past medical issues that may cause dysphagia, current and past medications that may cause dysphagia and xerostomia (dry mouth), respiratory status including recent pneumonia episodes, history of intubation, mechanical ventilation and tracheostomy tube, cognitive functions, conscious level, and nutrition status are reviewed [1, 14, 40]. After the review, physical examination is conducted. Physical examination includes the oral anatomy examination, oral motor control examination, and oral sensitivity examination. During the oral anatomy examination, any abnormality of the lips, jaw, tongue, soft and hard palates, uvula, oral cavity, and neck is identified [1, 41, 149]. Dental and secretion status also is examined. For the oral motor examination, range, accuracy, and rate of the movement of the lips, jaw, tongue, and soft palate as well as laryngeal function (vocal quality) are assessed [1, 41, 150]. Muscular control of the head and trunk also is examined. The oral sensitivity examination includes the assessment of light touch of the face, lips, tongue, and palate to identify whether there are any areas with reduced sensitivity [1, 41, 150]. After completing the physical examination, the patient's swallowing function is evaluated. First, swallowing of saliva is observed. Then, liquid and/or food of various volumes and consistencies is administered to observe the swallowing functions including oral control of the bolus, elevations of the larynx, vocal quality after the swallow, and presence of coughing and choking during and after a swallow [1, 14, 40, 41]. When any signs and symptoms of dysphagia and/or any abnormality that may cause dysphagia are identified during the clinical evaluation, a referral for an in-depth comprehensive instrumental swallowing evaluation is made [1].

7.2 Screening Tests

There are several validated swallowing screening tests available to clinicians. Swallowing screening provides quick determination of (1) the likelihood of a patient having dysphagia; (2) need for referral for further swallowing evaluation; (3) safety of oral feeding for the purpose of nutrition, hydration, and medication; and (4) needs for referral to nutritional support and/or other medical services [151]. Swallowing screening protocols for adult patients include patient-reported outcome measures, water swallow tests, and solid food tests [152].

7.2.1 Patient-Reported Outcome Measures

Patient-reported outcomes are self-administered questionnaire-based screening tools. Some examples are the Eating Assessment Tool-10 (EAT-10) [153], the Sydney Swallowing Questionnaire (SSQ) [154], and the Dysphagia Handicap Index (DHI) [155]. The questionnaire-based patient-reported outcomes rely on patient's recall and cognitive ability. However, it is important to note that patients often underreport their dysphagia symptoms [152].

7.2.2 Water Swallow Tests

The water swallow test involves presentation of liquid boluses [152]. Water swallow test protocols include the Toronto Bedside Swallowing Screening Test (TOR-BSST) [156, 157], 3-Ounce Water Swallow Test [158, 159], Yale Swallow Screening Test [160], Barnes-Jewish Hospital Stroke Dysphagia Screen [161, 162], Gugging Swallowing Screen (GUSS) [161, 162], and Volume-Viscosity Test [163–166]. Most water swallow tests are pass/fail. The patient is asked to swallow liquid during the test. The volume administered for a water test varies depending on the protocol. Signs of dysphagia such as coughing, choking, clearing throat, voice quality change, breathlessness, and drooling and/or inability to complete the test indicate that a referral for instrumental swallowing evaluation is required.

7.2.3 Solid Food Test

A solid food test involves presentation of solid food. The Test of Masticating and Swallowing Solids (TOMASS) was developed to assess swallowing efficiency of solid food [167]. The TOMASS is composed of two short questionnaires regarding dental condition and mouth dryness and a solid swallowing test. The patient is asked to eat a commercially available cracker during the test.

7.3 Instrumental Swallow Evaluations

The goals for a comprehensive instrumental swallow evaluation are (1) to identify abnormalities in swallow anatomy and physiology that are causing swallowing difficulties and (2) to determine best swallow treatment strategies [1, 147]. Both videofluoroscopic examination of swallow (VFSS) and fiberoptic endoscopic evaluation of swallowing (FESS) are considered diagnostic standard assessment methods for evaluation of swallowing [147].

7.3.1 Videofluoroscopic Examination of Swallow (VFSS)

The videofluoroscopic examination of swallow (VFSS), also called the modified barium swallow study (MBSS) or videofluoroscopic swallowing study (VFS), is a dynamic radiographic procedure that can provide real time visualization of all phases of swallowing [1, 168, 169]. During VFSS, patients are asked to swallow barium of various volumes and viscosities, and the oropharyngeal region is radiographically visualized [32, 40]. While standard VFSS protocols have been proposed in the literature, heterogeneity may be observed among clinicians and facilities. The VFSS enables clinicians to examine bolus flow throughout all the phases of swallowing [1, 169]. It also allows clinicians to assess swallowing biomechanical functions that cause abnormal bolus flow and detect the presence, timing, and severity of aspiration and penetration [1]. VFSS does involve radiation exposure [168, 170]; however, the amount is minimal during the procedure [168, 170, 171]. Bedridden patients who cannot be transported to a fluoroscopy suite and are unable to maintain a seated position are ineligible for VFSS [172, 173].

There are standardized, validated tools for interpretation of swallowing function and outcomes on VFSS imaging. The severity of penetration and aspiration is quantifiable on VFSS by using the penetration-aspiration scale [174]. Also, the amount of residue is quantifiable using pixel-based measurements [175]. The Dynamic Imaging Grade of Swallowing Toxicity (DIGEST) is a validated scale that provides an overall rating of the function of the pharyngeal phase of swallowing [176]. The DIGEST first measures the swallowing safety (penetration and aspiration) and swallowing efficiency (estimation of the pharyngeal residue amount) through VFSS. Then, a single summary grade for the pharyngeal swallowing function is provided based on the swallowing safety and efficiency results [176, 177]. The Modified Barium Swallow Impairment Profile (MBSImP®) has 17 physiologic components to assess swallow physiology across the oral, pharyngeal, and esophageal phases [42].

7.3.2 Fiberoptic Endoscopic Evaluation of Swallowing (FEES)

Fiberoptic endoscopic evaluation of swallowing (FEES) involves insertion of a fiberoptic endoscope through the patient's nose into the oropharynx to obtain superior visual images of the larynx and hypopharynx, including the vocal folds [147]. FEES is portable and can be performed at bedside [172, 173, 178]. During a FEES examination, anatomical and physiological assessments of swallowing-related structural movements with liquid and solid boluses are conducted. Then, compensatory swallowing interventions (e.g., bolus modifications, postural changes, and behavioral changes) may be tested [172, 173, 178]. FEES does not involve radiation exposure [172]. FEES has higher sensitivity for detecting aspiration, penetration, and residue than VFSS [178]. However, FEES does not provide images of the oral cavity since an endoscope is placed transnasally [172]. Additionally, FEES does not visualize any swallow events that occur during the "white-out" period, when the pharynx collapses after the pharyngeal swallow is triggered [172]. Therefore, conclusions regarding swallowing impairment are based on the aspects of the swallow visualized before and after this period.

8 Prevention of Pneumonia

8.1 Daily Mouth Care for Individuals Intubated or with Dysphagia to Prevent Pneumonia

Daily mouth care for those who are experiencing impaired swallowing function is imperative to maintain oral health and OHrQoL [179, 180] and to reduce the risk of aspiration pneumonia [181]. The risk of aspiration pneumonia is reduced by minimizing bacterial colonization in the oral cavity and, in turn, minimizing bacteria in orogastric secretions. Bacterial colonization can occur on the teeth, tongue, fixed and removable prosthesis, and gingival and mucosal tissues. During intubation and mechanical ventilation, the endotracheal or tracheostomy tube is an additional structure for bacterial colonization [182, 183]. The following are daily mouth care considerations for individuals intubated or experiencing dysphagia post-extubation or for other reasons.

8.2 Daily Mouth Care Plans

Daily mouth care should be individualized and based on an oral health assessment [184]. Evidence suggests that following a step-by-step daily mouth care plan can reduce ventilator- associated or non-ventilator hospital-acquired pneumonia [185]. The following is an example of daily mouth care plan (Fig. 2).

8.3 Chlorhexidine

While once a standard of care, routine use of chlorhexidine gluconate in the oral cavity of mechanically ventilated patients has more recently come into question. Findings of a meta-analysis conclude that cardiac surgery patients whose oral care

Example

Oral Health Care Plan

Oral Health Assessment (OHA) Date: ____________ (OHA) Review Date: ____________

Oral Health Care Considerations

Problems: ☐ difficulty swallowing ☐ difficulty moving head ☐ difficulty opening mouth ☐ fear of being touched

Interventions: ☐ briding ☐ chaining ☐ hand over hand ☐ distraction (activity board/toy) ☐ rescue

☐ other ____________

Daily Activities of Oral Hygiene

	Morning	After Lunch	Night
Natural Teeth ☐ Yes ☐ No Cleaned by: ☐ Self ☐ Supervise ☐ i (Assist) Replace toothbrush (3 monthly) Date:	☐ clean teeth, gums, tongue	☐ rinse mouth with water ☐ antibacterial product (teeth & gums)	☐ clean teeth, gums, tongue
Denture ☐ Full ☐ Partial ☐ Upper ☐ Lower Inserted / removed by: ☐ Self ☐ Staff Cleaned by: ☐ Self ☐ Supervise ☐ Assist	☐ dean teeth, gums, tongue ☐ brush denture	☐ rinse mouth with water ☐ rinse denture ☐ antibacterial product (gums)	☐ clean teeth, gums, tongue ☐ brush denture with mild soap ☐ Leave dentures out overnight ☐ soak denture in cold water Disinfect dentures (weekly) Specify day:

Oral Hygiene Aids

☐ soft toothbrush ☐ modified toothbrush ☐ toothbrush grip ☐ denture brush ☐ spray bottle (labelled)

Oral Hygiene Care Products

☐ mild soap (denture) ____________ ☐ antibacterial product ____________ ☐ saliva substitute ____________

☐ lip moisturiser ____________ ☐ high fluoride (5000 ppm) toothpaste ____________

Additional Oral Care Instruction

☐ antifungal gel ____________ ☐ denture adhesive ____________

☐ interproximal brush ☐ tongue scraper ☐ normal saline mouth toilet

Comments

____

____

Check daily, document and report to RN if:

- bad breath
- bleeding gums
- lip blisters/sores/cracks
- tongue for any coating/change in colour
- sore mouth or gums
- mouth ulcer
- swelling of face/mouth
- broken / lost denture
- difficulty eating
- refusal of oral care
- denture not named
- excessive food left in mouth
- broken teeth

Signed RN: ____________ Date: ____________

18 | Oral Health Care Plan

Fig. 2 Example of an oral care plan. (Lewis and Fricker [221])

regime included chlorhexidine had significantly fewer respiratory tract infections, when compared with a placebo (95% CI, [0.41–0.77]). However, there was no significant difference in ventilator-associated pneumonia among non-cardiac surgical patients, with or without the use of chlorhexidine.

Furthermore, there is evidence to suggest that chlorhexidine does not reduce the risk of ventilator-associated pneumonia, regardless of concentration (0.12–2%) or preparation (liquid versus gel) [186]. In addition, chlorhexidine appears to be associated with increased mortality rate [186–188].

8.4 Suctioning

8.4.1 Oral Suctioning

Continuous suctioning of oral secretions during mechanical ventilation may reduce the risk of ventilator-associated pneumonia, duration of mechanical ventilation, and length of intensive care unit (ICU) admission, though research is limited. A pilot randomized controlled trial (RCT) study compared continuous suctioning using a saliva ejector with 100 mmHG of suction to routine care that did not include continuous suctioning. The saliva ejector was placed adjacent to the buccal mucosa. Statistically significant differences were found between the experimental group, who received continuous suctioning, and control groups in the rate of ventilator-associated pneumonia (3 (23.1%) vs 10 (83.3%), $p = 0.003$); number of days of mechanical ventilation (3.2 (SD 1.3) vs 5.9 (SD 2.8), $p = 0.009$); and number of days of ICU stay (4.8 (SD 1.6) vs 9.8 (SD 6.3), $p = 0.019$) [189].

8.4.2 Deep Suctioning

Deep suctioning of oropharyngeal secretions beyond the oral cavity is also recommended. Sole et al. (2011) used a repeated measures, single-group design to explore the frequency of deep suctioning among orally intubated adults. A 21-cm-deep suctioning catheter was used, and the patient's backrest was elevated to 30°. The catheter was inserted to the depth required to retrieve the secretions. Deep suctioning was required every 2–4 hours, depending on the volume of secretions. The group receiving deep suctioning had significantly shorter hospital length of stay [190]; however, more research is needed to explore the impact of deep suctioning on prevention of aspiration pneumonia.

8.4.3 Suction Toothbrushing

Evidence surrounding suction toothbrushes is also limited. The impact of a suction toothbrush as compared to a manual toothbrush on the incidence of aspiration pneumonia among dependent adults with dysphagia living in long-term care (LTC) has been explored in a pilot RCT. At the beginning of the study, participants received professional debridement, and the caregivers received training on daily mouth care. While statistically significant improvements in oral health were observed for all study participants between baseline and 1 month and the incidence of pneumonia for all study participants was significantly less compared to the general population within the LTC facility, no between-group differences were identified [191].

8.5 Toothbrushing

The best positioning for toothbrushing is sitting upright with the chin tucked downward and backward toward the chest. This helps to prevent aspiration and closure of the airway during swallowing. In the case of a stroke, the head should also be tilted toward the paralyzed side. If the person is unable to sit upright, toothbrushing can be performed with the person laying on their weaker side to allow for the oral secretions to flow out of the mouth. Suction, manual, or an electric toothbrush can be used, preferably with a small head and soft bristles [192–194].

8.6 Toothpaste

If a person is unable to expectorate voluntarily, a small pea-sized amount of fluoridated, nonfoaming (sodium lauryl sulfate-free [SLS]) toothpaste is recommended. After brushing, the remaining debris and excess moisture should be removed using a suction device or a moist thin face cloth or gauze to finger sweep in the buccal vestibule and the floor of the mouth. Rinsing the oral cavity after brushing is not recommended because the minimal amount of fluoridated toothpaste remaining is beneficial for caries prevention [192, 194].

8.7 Sample Protocol for Mechanically Ventilated Critically Ill Patients

A combination of oral hydration, lip moisturization, and toothbrushing is recommended for mechanically ventilated critically ill patients [195]. A non-petroleum, water-soluble lip moisturizer is preferred [193]. The proposed protocol for comprehensive oral care for mechanically ventilated critically ill patients is currently under investigation [196] (Table 2).

Table 2 Oral care bundle for mechanically ventilated critically ill patients

Comprehensive oral care Q12 hours	Equipment	Procedure
1. Oral assessment	• Flashlight • Tongue depressor • Gloves • Face shield	• Explain procedure to patient • Gently open mouth or use mouth prop • Inquire about mouth/throat pain (0–10 NRS) • Use CPOT tool to evaluate pain in non-verbal pt. • Treat pain prior to proceeding
2. Tooth brushing	• Yankauer • 12 or 14 French flexible catheter • Small soft-bristle or suction toothbrush • Sponge swabs • Sterile water • Gloves • Face shield	• Explain procedure to patient • Perform hand hygiene • Elevate HUB 30–45° as tolerated • Use oral prop to open mouth as needed • Oral suction with Yankauer or sterile flexible catheter to remove secretions that may migrate down airway • Moisten toothbrush with sterile water • Connect suction toothbrush to continuous suction if applicable • Brush accessible teeth and gums for 2 full minutes or 30 seconds per quadrant; brush in one continuous line LUQ > RUQ > RLQ > LLQ • Gently brush tongue
3. Mouth and lip moisturizer	• Swabs • Mouth moisturizer/saliva replacement or sterile water • Gloves • Face shield	• Explain procedure to patient • Use oral prop to open mouth as needed • Use 1–3 swabs to apply moisturizer to oral mucosa, tongue, and lips
4. Deep oral suctioning	• Yankauer or flexible catheter • Gloves • Face shield	• Explain procedure to patient • Use oral prop to open mouth as needed • Deep oropharyngeal suction (above the cuff) to remove pooled secretions
Maintenance oral care Q4 hours and PR	Equipment	Procedure
Mouth and lip moisturizer	• As above	• As above
Oral secretion removal	• As above	• As above

Dale et al. [196]

9 Prevention and Treatment of Dysphagia

9.1 Prevention and Treatment of Dysphagia in Older Adults

Dysphagia management approaches can be combined with oral care regimens to reduce the risk of pneumonia in older adults. Treatment for dysphagia can include surgical, pharmacologic, and behavioral interventions. Surgical interventions can be used to address a mechanical obstruction that is impeding bolus flow through the oral cavity or pharynx, such as tumor resection for patients with head and neck cancer or dilation for an esophageal stricture. Pharmacologic interventions may include medications to address the underlying medical condition that led to dysphagia (e.g., levodopa for Parkinson's disease) or a reduction or change in the dose of certain medications that can contribute to dysphagia (e.g., antipsychotics) in older patients, especially for those experiencing polypharmacy. Behavioral interventions for dysphagia are most commonly designed and implemented by speech-language pathologists (SLPs) who are typically the medical providers managing dysphagia. These SLP-led interventions can include compensatory approaches, eating and swallowing strategies, and rehabilitative interventions.

9.2 Compensatory Approaches to Dysphagia Management

These types of approaches to dysphagia management include dietary modifications, postural adjustments, and swallowing maneuvers that attempt to *bypass* or *compensate for* pathophysiologic changes in swallowing function. Dietary modifications may involve increasing the thickness of liquid or pureeing solid foods. The IDDSI framework has provided standardized definitions and clinically practical measurement approaches for the various dietary levels often prescribed to patients with dysphagia [140]. Thickened liquids are efficacious in reducing the incidence of airway invasion in certain groups of patients (post-stroke or with dementia) [197]; however, more research is needed in other patient populations, such as those with dysphagia following oncologic treatment for head and neck cancer [198]. However, studies have also suggested adverse outcomes of thickened liquid intake, including reduced fluid intake leading to dehydration [199]. Additionally, patients are often not adherent to this recommendation given the decreased palatability and thirst-quenching characteristics of thickened fluids. Modification to solid foods can assist with mastication, especially in older patients with missing dentition, and can also reduce the risk of asphyxiation.

Postural adjustments include a chin-down or chin-tuck posture, a head turn posture, or a head tilt posture. The chin-down posture has been shown to result in positioning of the base of the tongue closer to the posterior pharyngeal wall and to narrow the airway entrance [200]. The head turn posture is often recommended to patients with unilateral pharyngeal weakness in order to direct the flow of the bolus down the stronger side of the pharynx [201]. These two postures may be combined to improve clearance of the bolus through the pharynx [202].

Swallowing maneuvers also are often recommended as another way to compensate for impairments in swallowing physiology by altering the timing of select neuromuscular components of the pharyngeal phase [203]. These maneuvers include the effortful swallow, super supraglottic swallow, and Mendelsohn maneuver [203–206].

While these various compensatory approaches to dysphagia treatment can positively alter swallowing biomechanics, this must be evaluated and confirmed during an instrumental assessment for swallowing. The decision of which approach is most appropriate should be made by the SLP performing the assessment and will be based on the patient's specific swallowing impairments.

9.3 Rehabilitative Interventions for Dysphagia

In contrast to compensatory approaches to dysphagia treatment, rehabilitative interventions are intended to result in lasting change in swallowing physiology and result in improved function and outcomes. Beyond use of the maneuvers described above for immediate compensation of deficits during the swallow, these can also be used as an exercise protocol to improve strength and coordination. Other exercise protocols target various swallowing-related musculature, including the tongue, floor of the mouth, and pharyngeal muscles. The Shaker exercise consists of three 1-minute head lifts in the supine position with a 1-minute rest between lifts followed by 30 consecutive repetitions of head raisings in the same position [207, 208]. This exercise is performed twice per week for 6 weeks with the goal of increasing laryngeal elevation and upper esophageal opening [209]. Exercise regimens focused on increasing the strength of the oral tongue have been implemented. With a systematic, progressive protocol [210], these approaches have shown positive impact on swallowing biomechanics in older adults as well as patients with dysphagia [211–214]. These approaches may be facilitated by devices, like the Iowa Oral Performance Instrument® or the Tongueometer®. Expiratory muscle strength training (EMST) targets systematic exercise to increase maximum expiratory pressures and has been shown to improve respiratory function as well as swallowing function in patients with dysphagia [215–218].

9.4 Proactive Versus Reactive Approaches to Dysphagia Care

Despite evidence to support the use of rehabilitative approaches, dysphagia treatment frequently consists primarily of reactive approaches that include the compensatory techniques described previously. Reactive approaches also rely on clinical presence of dysphagia diagnosed through either bedside or instrumental assessment. For many patient populations including older adults with frailty or those with neurodegenerative disease or head and neck cancer, there is a shift to focusing on more proactive approaches to dysphagia management that are based on the concept of building functional physiologic reserve in swallowing-related muscles prior to onset of dysphagia [219]. Functional reserve refers to an organ's ability to fulfill its physiological activity when under stress which is the difference between its maximum capacity and the minimum activity necessary to function [220]. By shifting to more proactive approaches, rehabilitative interventions like those described previously can be implemented to build functional reserve in patients at risk for developing dysphagia [219]. Additionally, through earlier involvement in the patient's care trajectory, interprofessional management can include both SLPs and dental providers, thereby reducing risks associated with combined dysphagia and poor oral health. Even in light of a known dysphagia diagnosis, interventions like oral care protocols can optimize health and quality of life for patients living with swallowing difficulty.

10 Conclusions

Oral health and swallowing function are highly interrelated, and both are affected by the aging process as well as a variety of disease conditions. The presence of poor oral health along with dysphagia puts patients at increased risk for adverse health outcomes, including aspiration pneumonia. Interprofessional approaches to early evaluation and identification as well as proactive approaches to treatment that target both oral health and swallowing function will be most effective in positively impacting quality of life and overall health across vulnerable patient populations.

References

1. Logemann JA. Evaluation and treatment of swallowing disorders. 2nd ed. Austin: PRO-ED; 1998.
2. Ertekin C. Voluntary versus spontaneous swallowing in man. Dysphagia. 2011;26(2):183–92.
3. Miller AJ. The neurobiology of swallowing and dysphagia. Dev Disabil Res Rev. 2008;14(2):77–86.
4. Lear CS, Flanagan JB Jr, Moorrees CF. The frequency of deglutition in man. Arch Oral Biol. 1965;10:83–100.
5. Crary MA, Carnaby GD, Sia I, Khanna A, Waters M. Spontaneous swallowing frequency has potential to identify dysphagia in acute stroke. Stroke. 2013;44(12):3452–7.
6. Kapila YV, Dodds WJ, Helm JF, Hogan WJ. Relationship between swallow rate and salivary flow. Dig Dis Sci [Internet]. 1984;29(6):528–33. Available from: http://link.springer.com/10.1007/BF01296273
7. Rudney JD, Ji Z, Larson CJ. The prediction of saliva swallowing frequency in humans from estimates of salivary flow rate and the volume of saliva swallowed. Arch Oral Biol [Internet]. 1995;40(6):507–12. Available from: https://linkinghub.elsevier.com/retrieve/pii/0003996995000049
8. Shaker R, Ren J, Bardan E, Easterling C, Dua K, Xie P, et al. Pharyngoglottal closure reflex: characterization in healthy young, elderly and dysphagic patients with predeglutitive aspiration. Gerontology [Internet]. 2003;49(1):12–20. Available from: https://www.karger.com/Article/FullText/66504
9. Lagerlof F, Dawes C. The volume of saliva in the mouth before and after swallowing. J Dent Res [Internet]. 1984;63(5):618–21. Available from: http://journals.sagepub.com/doi/10.1177/00220345840630050201

10. Dodds WJ. The physiology of swallowing. Dysphagia [Internet]. 1989;3(4):171–8. Available from: http://link.springer.com/10.1007/BF02407219
11. Dodds WJ, Logemann JA, Stewart ET. Radiologic assessment of abnormal oral and pharyngeal phases of swallowing. Am J Roentgenol [Internet]. 1990;154(5):965–74. Available from: http://www.ajronline.org/doi/10.2214/ajr.154.5.2108570
12. Logemann JA. Swallowing disorders. Best Pract Res Clin Gastroenterol. 2007;21(4):563–73.
13. Hiiemae KM, Palmer JB. Tongue movements in feeding and speech. Crit Rev Oral Biol Med. 2003;14(6):413–29.
14. Logemann J. Treatment of oral and pharyngeal dysphagia. Phys Med Rehabil Clin N Am [Internet]. 2008;19(4):803–16. Available from: https://doi.org/10.1016/j.pmr.2008.06.003
15. Matsuo K, Palmer JB. Anatomy and physiology of feeding and swallowing: normal and abnormal. Phys Med Rehabil Clin N Am [Internet]. 2008;19(4):691–707. Available from: https://doi.org/10.1016/j.pmr.2008.06.001
16. Shaw SM, Martino R. The normal swallow: muscular and neurophysiological control. Otolaryngol Clin N Am. 2013;46(6):937–56.
17. Dodds WJ, Stewart ET, Logemann JA. Physiology and radiology of the normal oral and pharyngeal phases of swallowing. Am J Roentgenol [Internet]. 1990;154(5):953–63. Available from: http://www.ajronline.org/doi/10.2214/ajr.154.5.2108569
18. Kahrilas PJ. Upper esophageal sphincter function during antegrade and retrograde transit. Am J Med. 1997;103(5 A):56S–60S.
19. Matsuo K, Palmer JB. Coordination of mastication, swallowing and breathing. Jpn Dent Sci Rev. 2009;45(1):31–40.
20. Peyron MA, Gierczynski I, Hartmann C, Loret C, Dardevet D, Martin N, et al. Role of physical bolus properties as sensory inputs in the trigger of swallowing. PLoS One. 2011;6(6):e21167.
21. Pedersen AM, Bardow A, Jensen SB, Nauntofte B. Saliva and gastrointestinal functions of taste, mastication, swallowing and digestion. Oral Dis [Internet]. 2002;8(3):117–29. Available from: http://doi.wiley.com/10.1034/j.1601-0825.2002.02851.x
22. van der Bilt A, Engelen L, Pereira LJJ, van der Glas HWW, Abbink JHH. Oral physiology and mastication. Physiol Behav [Internet]. 2006;89(1):22–7. Available from: https://linkinghub.elsevier.com/retrieve/pii/S0031938406000382
23. Thexton AJ. Mastication and swallowing: an overview. Br Dent J [Internet]. 1992;173(6):197–206. Available from: https://doi.org/10.1038/sj.bdj.4808002
24. Hiiemae K, Thexton AJ, Crompton AW. Intra-oral food transport--a fundamental mechanism in feeding? In: Carlson DS, McNamara J, editors. Muscle adaptation in the craniofacial region, Craniofacial Growth Series, vol. 8. Ann Arbor: University of Michigan; 1978. p. 181–208.
25. Dawes C, Pedersen AML, Villa A, Ekström J, Proctor GB, Vissink A, et al. The functions of human saliva: a review sponsored by the World Workshop on Oral Medicine VI. Arch Oral Biol [Internet]. 2015;60(6):863–74. Available from: https://linkinghub.elsevier.com/retrieve/pii/S0003996915000692
26. Hoebler C, Karinthi A, Devaux M-F, Guillon F, Gallant DJG, Bouchet B, et al. Physical and chemical transformations of cereal food during oral digestion in human subjects. Br J Nutr [Internet]. 1998;80(5):429–36. Available from: https://www.cambridge.org/core/product/identifier/S0007114598001494/type/journal_article
27. Amerongen AN, Veerman E. Saliva the defender of the oral cavity. Oral Dis [Internet]. 2002;8(1):12–22. Available from: http://doi.wiley.com/10.1034/j.1601-0825.2002.1o816.x
28. Hadde EK, Cichero JAY, Zhao S, Chen W, Chen J. The importance of extensional rheology in bolus control during swallowing. Sci Rep [Internet]. 2019;9(1):16106. Available from: http://www.nature.com/articles/s41598-019-52269-4
29. Vijay A, Inui T, Dodds M, Proctor G, Carpenter G. Factors that influence the extensional rheological property of saliva. Singh B, editor. PLoS One [Internet]. 2015;10(8):e0135792. Available from: https://dx.plos.org/10.1371/journal.pone.0135792
30. Moore K, Dally A. Clinically oriented anatomy. 5th ed. Philadelphia: Lippincott Williams and Wilkins; 2006.

31. Sasegbon A, Hamdy S. The anatomy and physiology of normal and abnormal swallowing in oropharyngeal dysphagia. Neurogastroenterol Motil. 2017;29(11):1–15.
32. Malandraki G, Robbins J. Dysphagia. Handb Clin Neurol. 2013;110:255–71.
33. Jean A. Brain stem control of swallowing: neuronal network and cellular mechanisms. Physiol Rev. 2001;81(2):929–69.
34. Miller AJ. The search for the central swallowing pathway: the quest for clarity. Dysphagia. 1993;8(3):185–94.
35. Humbert IA, Robbins JA. Normal swallowing and functional magnetic resonance imaging: a systematic review. Dysphagia. 2007;22(3):266–75.
36. Malandraki G, Johnson S, Robbins J. Functional MRI of swallowing: from neurophysiology to neuroplasticity. Head Neck. 2011;33(Suppl 1 (0 1)):S14–20.
37. Rogus-Pulia N, Malandraki GA, Johnson S, Robbins J. Understanding dysphagia in dementia: the present and the future. Curr Phys Med Rehabil Rep [Internet]. 2015;3(1):86–97. Available from: http://link.springer.com/10.1007/s40141-015-0078-1
38. Carrau RL, Murry T, Howell R. Comprehensive management of swallowing disorders. Plural Publishing, Inc.; 2017.
39. Takizawa C, Gemmell E, Kenworthy J, Speyer R. A systematic review of the prevalence of oropharyngeal dysphagia in stroke, Parkinson's disease, Alzheimer's disease, head injury, and pneumonia. Dysphagia [Internet]. 2016;31(3):434–41. Available from: http://link.springer.com/10.1007/s00455-016-9695-9
40. Christmas C, Rogus-Pulia N. Swallowing disorders in the older population. J Am Geriatr Soc. 2019;67(12):2643–9.
41. Palmer JB, Drennan JC, Baba M. Evaluation and treatment of swallowing impairments. Am Fam Physician [Internet]. 2000;61(8):2453–62. Available from: http://www.ncbi.nlm.nih.gov/pubmed/10794585
42. Martin-Harris B, Brodsky MB, Michel Y, Castell DO, Schleicher M, Sandidge J, et al. MBS measurement tool for swallow impairment—MBSImp: establishing a standard. Dysphagia [Internet]. 2008;23(4):392–405. Available from: http://link.springer.com/10.1007/s00455-008-9185-9
43. Warnecke T, Labeit B, Schroeder J, Reckels A, Ahring S, Lapa S, et al. Neurogenic dysphagia: a systematic review and proposal of a classification system. Neurology. 2021;96(6):e876–89. https://doi.org/10.1212/WNL.0000000000011350.
44. Martin-Harris B, Brodsky MB, Michel Y, Lee F-S, Walters B. Delayed initiation of the pharyngeal swallow: normal variability in adult swallows. J Speech Lang Hear Res [Internet]. 2007;50(3):585–94. Available from: http://pubs.asha.org/doi/10.1044/1092-4388%282007%2F041%29
45. Cook I, Gabb M, Panagopoulos V, Jamieson G, Dodds W, Dent J, et al. Pharyngeal (Zenker's) diverticulum is a disorder of upper esophageal sphincter opening. Gastroenterology. 1992;103:1229–35.
46. Law R, Katzka DA, Baron TH. Zenker's diverticulum. Clin Gastroenterol Hepatol [Internet]. 2014;12(11):1773–82. Available from: https://doi.org/10.1016/j.cgh.2013.09.016
47. Ferreira LEVVC, Simmons DT, Baron TH. Zenker's diverticula: pathophysiology, clinical presentation, and flexible endoscopic management. Dis Esophagus. 2008;21(1):1–8.
48. Kruger D. Assessing esophageal dysphagia. J Am Acad Physician Assist. 2014;27(5):23–30.
49. Navaneethan U, Eubanks S. Approach to patients with esophageal dysphagia. Surg Clin North Am [Internet]. 2015;95(3):483–9. Available from: https://doi.org/10.1016/j.suc.2015.02.004
50. Smith CD. Esophageal strictures and diverticula. Surg Clin North Am [Internet]. 2015;95(3):669–81. Available from: https://doi.org/10.1016/j.suc.2015.02.017
51. Affoo RH, Foley N, Garrick R, Siqueira WL, Martin RE. Meta-analysis of salivary flow rates in young and older adults. J Am Geriatr Soc. 2015;63(10):2142–51.
52. Herzberg EG, Lazarus CL, Steele CM, Molfenter SM. Swallow event sequencing: comparing healthy older and younger adults. Dysphagia [Internet]. 2018;33(6):759–67. Available from: http://link.springer.com/10.1007/s00455-018-9898-3

53. Lamster IB, Asadourian L, Del Carmen T, Friedman PK. The aging mouth: differentiating normal aging from disease. Periodontol 2000 [Internet]. 2016;72(1):96–107. Available from: http://doi.wiley.com/10.1111/prd.12131
54. Kendall KA, McKenzie S, Leonard RJ, Gonçalves MI, Walker A. Timing of events in normal swallowing: a videofluoroscopic study. Dysphagia [Internet]. 2000;15(2):74–83. Available from: http://link.springer.com/10.1007/s004550010004
55. Troche MS, Huebner I, Rosenbek JC, Okun MS, Sapienza CM. Respiratory-swallowing coordination and swallowing safety in patients with Parkinson's disease. Dysphagia. 2011;26(3):218–24.
56. Mancopes R, Gandhi P, Smaoui S, Steele CM. Which physiological swallowing parameters change with healthy aging? OBM Geriat [Internet]. 2021;5(1):2101153. Available from: http://www.lidsen.com/journals/geriatrics/geriatrics-05-01-153
57. Namasivayam-MacDonald AM, Barbon CE, Steele CM. A review of swallow timing in the elderly. Physiol Behav [Internet]. 2018;184:12–26. Available from: https://linkinghub.elsevier.com/retrieve/pii/S0031938417303621
58. Robbins J, Hamilton JW, Lof GL, Kempster GB. Oropharyngeal swallowing in normal adults of different ages. Gastroenterology [Internet]. 1992;103(3):823–9. Available from: http://linkinghub.elsevier.com/retrieve/pii/001650859290013O
59. Molfenter SM, Steele CM. Variation in temporal measures of swallowing: sex and volume effects. Dysphagia [Internet]. 2013;28(2):226–33. Available from: http://link.springer.com/10.1007/s00455-012-9437-6
60. Molfenter SM, Steele CM. Temporal variability in the deglutition literature. Dysphagia [Internet]. 2012;27(2):162–77. Available from: http://link.springer.com/10.1007/s00455-012-9397-x
61. Molfenter SM, Lenell C, Lazarus CL. Volumetric changes to the pharynx in healthy aging: consequence for pharyngeal swallow mechanics and function. Dysphagia [Internet]. 2019;34(1):129–37. Available from: http://link.springer.com/10.1007/s00455-018-9924-5
62. Molfenter SM, Leigh C, Steele CM. Event sequence variability in healthy swallowing: building on previous findings. Dysphagia [Internet]. 2014;29(2):234–42. Available from: http://link.springer.com/10.1007/s00455-013-9501-x
63. Nicosia MA, Hind JA, Roecker EB, Carnes M, Doyle J, Dengel GA, et al. Age effects on the temporal evolution of isometric and swallowing pressure. J Gerontol A Biol Sci Med Sci [Internet]. 2000;55(11):M634–40. Available from: https://academic.oup.com/biomedgerontology/article-lookup/doi/10.1093/gerona/55.11.M634
64. Madhavan A, Lagorio LA, Crary MA, Dahl WJ, Carnaby GD. Prevalence of and risk factors for dysphagia in the community dwelling elderly: a systematic review. J Nutr Health Aging [Internet]. 2016;20(8):806–15. Available from: http://link.springer.com/10.1007/s12603-016-0712-3
65. Mateos-Nozal J, Montero-Errasquín B, Sánchez García E, Romero Rodríguez E, Cruz-Jentoft AJ. High prevalence of oropharyngeal dysphagia in acutely hospitalized patients aged 80 years and older. J Am Med Dir Assoc [Internet]. 2020;21(12):2008–11. Available from: https://linkinghub.elsevier.com/retrieve/pii/S1525861020303625
66. Park Y-H, Han H-R, Oh B-M, Lee J, Park J, Yu SJ, et al. Prevalence and associated factors of dysphagia in nursing home residents. Geriatr Nurs (Minneap) [Internet]. 2013;34(3):212–7. Available from: https://linkinghub.elsevier.com/retrieve/pii/S0197457213000633
67. Ghannouchi I, Speyer R, Doma K, Cordier R, Verin E. Swallowing function and chronic respiratory diseases: systematic review. Respir Med [Internet]. 2016;117:54–64. Available from: https://linkinghub.elsevier.com/retrieve/pii/S0954611116301111
68. Roy N, Stemple J, Merrill RM, Thomas L. Dysphagia in the elderly: preliminary evidence of prevalence, risk factors, and socioemotional effects. Ann Otol Rhinol Laryngol [Internet]. 2007;116(11):858–65. Available from: https://doi.org/10.1177/000348940711601112.
69. Brodsky MB, Levy MJ, Jedlanek E, Pandian V, Blackford B, Price C, et al. Laryngeal injury and upper airway symptoms after oral endotracheal intubation with mechanical ventilation

during critical care. Crit Care Med [Internet]. 2018;46(12):2010–7. Available from: http://journals.lww.com/00003246-201812000-00015
70. de Deus Chaves R, de Carvalho CRF, Cukier A, Stelmach R, de Andrade CRF. Sintomas indicativos de disfagia em portadores de DPOC. J Bras Pneumol [Internet]. 2011;37(2):176–83. Available from: http://www.scielo.br/scielo.php?script=sci_arttext&pid=S1806-37132011000200007&lng=pt&tlng=pt
71. Miller AJ. Overview of deglutition and digestion. In: Shaker R, Belafsky PC, Postma GN, Easterling C, editors. Principles of deglutition [Internet]. New York: Springer; 2013. p. 3–17. Available from: http://link.springer.com/10.1007/978-1-4614-3794-9.
72. Winchester J, Winchester CG. Cognitive dysphagia and effectively managing the five systems. Perspect Gerontol [Internet]. 2015;20(3):116–32. Available from: http://pubs.asha.org/doi/10.1044/gero20.3.116
73. Leder SB, Suiter DM, Lisitano WH. Answering orientation questions and following single-step verbal commands: effect on aspiration status. Dysphagia [Internet]. 2009;24(3):290–5. Available from: http://link.springer.com/10.1007/s00455-008-9204-x
74. Jo SY, Hwang J-W, Pyun S-B. Relationship between cognitive function and dysphagia after stroke. Ann Rehabil Med [Internet]. 2017;41(4):564. Available from: http://e-arm.org/journal/view.php?doi=10.5535/arm.2017.41.4.564
75. Yatabe N, Takeuchi K, Izumi M, Furuta M, Takeshita T, Shibata Y, et al. Decreased cognitive function is associated with dysphagia risk in nursing home older residents. Gerodontology [Internet]. 2018;35(4):376–81. Available from: https://onlinelibrary.wiley.com/doi/abs/10.1111/ger.12366
76. Lindgren S, Janzon L. Prevalence of swallowing complaints and clinical findings among 50-79-year-old men and women in an urban population. Dysphagia. 1991;6(4):187–92.
77. Rockwood K, Song X, Mitnitski A. Changes in relative fitness and frailty across the adult lifespan: evidence from the Canadian National Population Health Survey. Can Med Assoc J [Internet]. 2011;183(8):E487–94. Available from: http://www.cmaj.ca/cgi/doi/10.1503/cmaj.101271
78. Clegg A, Young J, Iliffe S, Rikkert MO, Rockwood K. Frailty in elderly people. Lancet [Internet]. 2013;381(9868):752–62. Available from: https://linkinghub.elsevier.com/retrieve/pii/S0140673612621679
79. Fried LP, Tangen CM, Walston J, Newman AB, Hirsch C, Gottdiener J, et al. Frailty in older adults: evidence for a phenotype. J Gerontol A Biol Sci Med Sci [Internet]. 2001;56(3):M146–57. Available from: https://academic.oup.com/biomedgerontology/article-lookup/doi/10.1093/gerona/56.3.M146
80. Mitnitski AB, Mogilner AJ, Rockwood K. Accumulation of deficits as a proxy measure of aging. Sci World J [Internet]. 2001;1:323–36. Available from: http://www.hindawi.com/journals/tswj/2001/321027/abs/
81. González-Fernández M, Humbert I, Winegrad H, Cappola AR, Fried LP. Dysphagia in old-old women: prevalence as determined according to self-report and the 3-ounce water swallowing test. J Am Geriatr Soc [Internet]. 2014;62(4):716–20. Available from: http://doi.wiley.com/10.1111/jgs.12745
82. Nishida T, Yamabe K, Honda S. The influence of dysphagia on nutritional and frailty status among community-dwelling older adults. Nutrients [Internet]. 2021;13(2):512. Available from: https://www.mdpi.com/2072-6643/13/2/512
83. Wang T, Zhao Y, Guo A. Association of swallowing problems with frailty in Chinese hospitalized older patients. Int J Nurs Sci [Internet]. 2020;7(4):408–12. Available from: https://linkinghub.elsevier.com/retrieve/pii/S2352013220301447
84. Shimazaki Y, Nonoyama T, Tsushita K, Arai H, Matsushita K, Uchibori N. Oral hypofunction and its association with frailty in community-dwelling older people. Geriatr Gerontol Int [Internet]. 2020;20(10):917–26. Available from: https://onlinelibrary.wiley.com/doi/10.1111/ggi.14015
85. Cohen SM, Lekan D, Risoli T, Lee H-J, Misono S, Whitson HE, et al. Association between dysphagia and inpatient outcomes across frailty level among patients ≥ 50 years of age.

Dysphagia [Internet]. 2020;35(5):787–97. Available from: http://link.springer.com/10.1007/s00455-019-10084-z
86. Butler SG, Stuart A, Leng X, Wilhelm E, Rees C, Williamson J, et al. The relationship of aspiration status with tongue and handgrip strength in healthy older adults. J Gerontol A Biol Sci Med Sci [Internet]. 2011;66A(4):452–8. Available from: https://academic.oup.com/biomedgerontology/article-lookup/doi/10.1093/gerona/glq234
87. Youmans SR, Stierwalt JAG. Measures of tongue function related to normal swallowing. Dysphagia [Internet]. 2006;21(2):102–11. Available from: http://link.springer.com/10.1007/s00455-006-9013-z
88. Sakai K, Nakayama E, Tohara H, Takahashi O, Ohnishi S, Tsuzuki H, et al. Diagnostic accuracy of lip force and tongue strength for sarcopenic dysphagia in older inpatients: a cross-sectional observational study. Clin Nutr [Internet]. 2019;38(1):303–9. Available from: https://linkinghub.elsevier.com/retrieve/pii/S0261561418300177
89. Namasivayam AM, Steele CM, Keller H. The effect of tongue strength on meal consumption in long term care. Clin Nutr [Internet]. 2016;35(5):1078–83. Available from: https://doi.org/10.1016/j.clnu.2015.08.001
90. Namasivayam-MacDonald AM, Morrison JM, Steele CM, Keller H. How swallow pressures and dysphagia affect malnutrition and mealtime outcomes in long-term care. Dysphagia [Internet]. 2017;32(6):785–96. Available from: http://link.springer.com/10.1007/s00455-017-9825-z
91. Zhao W-T, Yang M, Wu H-M, Yang L, Zhang X, Huang Y. Systematic review and meta-analysis of the association between sarcopenia and dysphagia. J Nutr Health Aging [Internet]. 2018;22(8):1003–9. Available from: http://link.springer.com/10.1007/s12603-018-1055-z
92. Love AL, Cornwell PL, Whitehouse SL. Oropharyngeal dysphagia in an elderly postoperative hip fracture population: a prospective cohort study. Age Ageing [Internet]. 2013;42(6):782–5. Available from: https://academic.oup.com/ageing/article-lookup/doi/10.1093/ageing/aft037
93. Logemann JA, Pauloski BR, Rademaker AW, Lazarus CL, Mittal B, Gaziano J, et al. Xerostomia: 12-month changes in saliva production and its relationship to perception and performance of swallow function, oral intake, and diet after chemoradiation. Head Neck [Internet]. 2003;25(6):432–7. Available from: http://doi.wiley.com/10.1002/hed.10255
94. Rhodus NL, Moller K, Colby S, Bereuter J. Dysphagia in patients with three different etiologies of salivary gland dysfunction. Ear Nose Throat J. 1995;74(1):39–42, 45–8.
95. Rogus-Pulia NM, Logemann JA. Effects of reduced saliva production on swallowing in patients with Sjogren's syndrome. Dysphagia [Internet]. 2011;26(3):295–303. Available from: http://link.springer.com/10.1007/s00455-010-9311-3
96. Furuya J, Suzuki H, Tamada Y, Onodera S, Nomura T, Hidaka R, et al. Food intake and oral health status of inpatients with dysphagia in acute care settings. J Oral Rehabil [Internet]. 2020;47(6):736–42. Available from: https://onlinelibrary.wiley.com/doi/10.1111/joor.12964
97. Takeuchi N, Sawada N, Ekuni D, Morita M. Oral diadochokinesis is related to decline in swallowing function among community-dwelling Japanese elderly: a cross-sectional study. Aging Clin Exp Res [Internet]. 2021;33(2):399–405. Available from: http://link.springer.com/10.1007/s40520-020-01547-7
98. Okamoto N, Morikawa M, Yanagi M, Amano N, Tomioka K, Hazaki K, et al. Association of tooth loss with development of swallowing problems in community-dwelling independent elderly population: the Fujiwara-kyo study. J Gerontol A Biol Sci Med Sci [Internet]. 2015;70(12):1548–54. Available from: https://academic.oup.com/biomedgerontology/article-lookup/doi/10.1093/gerona/glv116
99. Hida Y, Nishida T, Taniguchi C, Sakakibara H. Association between swallowing function and oral bacterial flora in independent community-dwelling elderly. Aging Clin Exp Res [Internet]. 2021;33(1):157–63. Available from: http://link.springer.com/10.1007/s40520-020-01521-3
100. Ikebe K, Matsuda K, Kagawa R, Enoki K, Yoshida M, Maeda Y, et al. Association of masticatory performance with age, gender, number of teeth, occlusal force and salivary flow in Japanese older adults: is ageing a risk factor for masticatory dysfunction? Arch Oral Biol

[Internet]. 2011;56(10):991–6. Available from: https://linkinghub.elsevier.com/retrieve/pii/S0003996911000999
101. Shimazaki Y, Saito M, Nonoyama T, Tadokoro Y. Oral factors associated with swallowing function in independent elders. Oral Health Prev Dent. 2020;18(4):683–91.
102. Koshino H, Hirai T, Ishijima T, Ikeda Y. Tongue motor skills and masticatory performance in adult dentates, elderly dentates, and complete denture wearers. J Prosthet Dent [Internet]. 1997;77(2):147–52. Available from: https://linkinghub.elsevier.com/retrieve/pii/S0022391397702282
103. Ortega O, Parra C, Zarcero S, Nart J, Sakwinska O, Clavé P. Oral health in older patients with oropharyngeal dysphagia. Age Ageing [Internet]. 2014;43(1):132–7. Available from: https://academic.oup.com/ageing/article-lookup/doi/10.1093/ageing/aft164
104. Ortega O, Sakwinska O, Combremont S, Berger B, Sauser J, Parra C, et al. High prevalence of colonization of oral cavity by respiratory pathogens in frail older patients with oropharyngeal dysphagia. Neurogastroenterol Motil [Internet]. 2015;27(12):1804–16. Available from: http://doi.wiley.com/10.1111/nmo.12690
105. Hägglund P, Koistinen S, Olai L, Ståhlnacke K, Wester P, Levring Jäghagen E. Older people with swallowing dysfunction and poor oral health are at greater risk of early death. Community Dent Oral Epidemiol [Internet]. 2019;47(6):494–501. Available from: https://onlinelibrary.wiley.com/doi/abs/10.1111/cdoe.12491
106. Shi T, Denouel A, Tietjen AK, Lee JW, Falsey AR, Demont C, et al. Global and regional burden of hospital admissions for pneumonia in older adults: a systematic review and meta-analysis. J Infect Dis [Internet]. 2020;222(Supplement_7):S570–6. Available from: https://academic.oup.com/jid/article/222/Supplement_7/S570/5372488
107. Welte T, Torres A, Nathwani D. Clinical and economic burden of community-acquired pneumonia among adults in Europe. Thorax [Internet]. 2012;67(1):71–9. Available from: https://thorax.bmj.com/lookup/doi/10.1136/thx.2009.129502
108. Olasupo O, Xiao H, Brown J. Relative clinical and cost burden of community-acquired pneumonia hospitalizations in older adults in the United States—a cross-sectional analysis. Vaccines [Internet]. 2018;6(3):59. Available from: http://www.mdpi.com/2076-393X/6/3/59
109. LaCroix AZ, Lipson S, Miles TP, White L. Prospective study of pneumonia hospitalizations and mortality of U.S. older people: the role of chronic conditions, health behaviors, and nutritional status. Public Health Rep. 1989;104(4):350–60.
110. Corrado RE, Lee D, Lucero DE, Varma JK, Vora NM. Burden of adult community-acquired, health-care-associated, hospital-acquired, and ventilator-associated pneumonia. Chest [Internet]. 2017;152(5):930–42. Available from: https://linkinghub.elsevier.com/retrieve/pii/S0012369217307791
111. Falcone M, Venditti M, Shindo Y, Kollef MH. Healthcare-associated pneumonia: diagnostic criteria and distinction from community-acquired pneumonia. Int J Infect Dis [Internet]. 2011;15(8):e545–50. Available from: https://linkinghub.elsevier.com/retrieve/pii/S1201971211000944
112. Kollef MH, Rello J, Cammarata SK, Croos-Dabrera RV, Wunderink RG. Clinical cure and survival in Gram-positive ventilator-associated pneumonia: retrospective analysis of two double-blind studies comparing linezolid with vancomycin. Intensive Care Med [Internet]. 2004;30(3):388–94. Available from: http://link.springer.com/10.1007/s00134-003-2088-1
113. Kollef MH, Shorr A, Tabak YP, Gupta V, Liu LZ, Johannes RS. Epidemiology and outcomes of health-care-associated pneumonia. Chest [Internet]. 2005;128(6):3854–62. Available from: https://linkinghub.elsevier.com/retrieve/pii/S0012369215496278
114. Wilkinson M, Woodhead MA. Guidelines for community-acquired pneumonia in the ICU. Curr Opin Crit Care [Internet]. 2004;10(1):59–64. Available from: http://journals.lww.com/00075198-200402000-00010
115. Fine MJ, Smith MA, Carson CA, Mutha SS, Sankey SS, Weissfeld LA, et al. Prognosis and outcomes of patients with community-acquired pneumonia. A meta-analysis. JAMA. 1996;275(2):134–41.

116. Chastre J, Fagon J-Y. Ventilator-associated pneumonia. Am J Respir Crit Care Med [Internet]. 2002;165(7):867–903. Available from: http://www.atsjournals.org/doi/abs/10.1164/ajrccm.165.7.2105078
117. Marik PE. Aspiration pneumonitis and aspiration pneumonia. N Engl J Med [Internet]. 2001;344(9):665–71. Available from: http://www.nejm.org/doi/abs/10.1056/NEJM200103013440908
118. van der Maarel-Wierink CD, Vanobbergen JNO, Bronkhorst EM, Schols JMGA, de Baat C. Meta-analysis of dysphagia and aspiration pneumonia in frail elders. J Dent Res [Internet]. 2011;90(12):1398–404. Available from: http://journals.sagepub.com/doi/10.1177/0022034511422909
119. Langmore SE, Terpenning MS, Schork A, Chen Y, Murray JT, Lopatin D, et al. Predictors of aspiration pneumonia: how important is dysphagia? Dysphagia [Internet]. 1998;13(2):69–81. Available from: http://link.springer.com/10.1007/PL00009559
120. Gleeson K, Maxwell SL, Eggli DF. Quantitative aspiration during sleep in normal subjects. Chest [Internet]. 1997;111(5):1266–72. Available from: https://linkinghub.elsevier.com/retrieve/pii/S0012369215469594
121. Huxley EJ, Viroslav J, Gray WR, Pierce AK. Pharyngeal aspiration in normal adults and patients with depressed consciousness. Am J Med [Internet]. 1978;64(4):564–8. Available from: https://linkinghub.elsevier.com/retrieve/pii/0002934378905740
122. Butler SG, Clark H, Baginski SG, Todd JT, Lintzenich C, Leng X. Computed tomography pulmonary findings in healthy older adult aspirators versus nonaspirators. Laryngoscope [Internet]. 2014;124(2):494–7. Available from: http://doi.wiley.com/10.1002/lary.24284
123. Raghavendran K, Mylotte JM, Scannapieco FA. Nursing home-associated pneumonia, hospital-acquired pneumonia and ventilator-associated pneumonia: the contribution of dental biofilms and periodontal inflammation. Periodontol 2000 [Internet]. 2007;44(1):164–77. Available from: http://doi.wiley.com/10.1111/j.1600-0757.2006.00206.x
124. Carrión S, Roca M, Costa A, Arreola V, Ortega O, Palomera E, et al. Nutritional status of older patients with oropharyngeal dysphagia in a chronic versus an acute clinical situation. Clin Nutr [Internet]. 2017;36(4):1110–6. Available from: https://linkinghub.elsevier.com/retrieve/pii/S0261561416301753
125. Fávaro-Moreira NC, Krausch-Hofmann S, Matthys C, Vereecken C, Vanhauwaert E, Declercq A, et al. Risk factors for malnutrition in older adults: a systematic review of the literature based on longitudinal data. Adv Nutr [Internet]. 2016;7(3):507–22. Available from: https://academic.oup.com/advances/article/7/3/507/4653577
126. Serra-Prat M, Palomera M, Gomez C, Sar-Shalom D, Saiz A, Montoya JG, et al. Oropharyngeal dysphagia as a risk factor for malnutrition and lower respiratory tract infection in independently living older persons: a population-based prospective study. Age Ageing [Internet]. 2012;41(3):376–81. Available from: https://academic.oup.com/ageing/article-lookup/doi/10.1093/ageing/afs006
127. Blanař V, Hödl M, Lohrmann C, Amir Y, Egleser D. Dysphagia and factors associated with malnutrition risk: a 5-year multicentre study. J Adv Nurs [Internet]. 2019;75(12):3566–76. Available from: https://onlinelibrary.wiley.com/doi/abs/10.1111/jan.14188
128. Brynes A, Stratton R, Wright L, Frost G. Energy intakes fail to meet requirements on texture modified diets. Proc Nutr Soc. 1998;57:117A.
129. Barone L. An examination of daily dietary intake and swallow function in an older adult population [Internet]. 2017. Available from: https://opencommons.uconn.edu/gs_theses/1112
130. Hudson HM, Daubert CR, Mills RH. The interdependency of protein-energy malnutrition, aging, and dysphagia. Dysphagia [Internet]. 2000;15(1):31–8. Available from: http://link.springer.com/10.1007/s004559910007
131. Azzolino D, Passarelli PC, De Angelis P, Piccirillo GB, D'Addona A, Cesari M. Poor oral health as a determinant of malnutrition and sarcopenia. Nutrients [Internet]. 2019;11(12):2898. Available from: https://www.mdpi.com/2072-6643/11/12/2898

132. Crary MA, Carnaby GD, Shabbir Y, Miller L, Silliman S. Clinical variables associated with hydration status in acute ischemic stroke patients with dysphagia. Dysphagia [Internet]. 2016;31(1):60–5. Available from: http://link.springer.com/10.1007/s00455-015-9658-6
133. Reber E, Gomes F, Dähn IA, Vasiloglou MF, Stanga Z. Management of dehydration in patients suffering swallowing difficulties. J Clin Med [Internet]. 2019;8(11):1923. Available from: https://www.mdpi.com/2077-0383/8/11/1923
134. Whelan K. Inadequate fluid intakes in dysphagic acute stroke. Clin Nutr [Internet]. 2001;20(5):423–8. Available from: https://linkinghub.elsevier.com/retrieve/pii/S0261561401904674
135. Ibrahim JE, Murphy BJ, Bugeja L, Ranson D. Nature and extent of external-cause deaths of nursing home residents in Victoria, Australia. J Am Geriatr Soc [Internet]. 2015;63(5):954–62. Available from: http://doi.wiley.com/10.1111/jgs.13377
136. Kramarow E, Warner M, Chen L-H. Food-related choking deaths among the elderly. Inj Prev [Internet]. 2014;20(3):200–3. Available from: https://injuryprevention.bmj.com/lookup/doi/10.1136/injuryprev-2013-040795
137. Berzlanovich AM, Fazeny-Dörner B, Waldhoer T, Fasching P, Keil W. Foreign body asphyxia. Am J Prev Med [Internet]. 2005;28(1):65–9. Available from: https://linkinghub.elsevier.com/retrieve/pii/S0749379704000777
138. Dolkas L, Stanley C, Smith AM, Vilke GM. Deaths associated with choking in San Diego county. J Forensic Sci [Internet]. 2007;52(1):176–9. Available from: http://doi.wiley.com/10.1111/j.1556-4029.2006.00297.x
139. Wick R, Gilbert JD, Byard RW. Café coronary syndrome-fatal choking on food: an autopsy approach. J Clin Forensic Med [Internet]. 2006;13(3):135–8. Available from: https://linkinghub.elsevier.com/retrieve/pii/S1353113105001811
140. Cichero JAY, Lam P, Steele CM, Hanson B, Chen J, Dantas RO, et al. Development of international terminology and definitions for texture-modified foods and thickened fluids used in dysphagia management: the IDDSI framework. Dysphagia [Internet]. 2017;32(2):293–314. Available from: http://link.springer.com/10.1007/s00455-016-9758-y
141. Brodsky J, Macario A, Mark J. Tracheal diameter predicts double-lumen tube size. Anesth Analg [Internet]. 1996;82(4):861–4. Available from: http://journals.lww.com/00000539-199604000-00032
142. Samuels R, Chadwick DD. Predictors of asphyxiation risk in adults with intellectual disabilities and dysphagia. J Intellect Disabil Res [Internet]. 2006;50(5):362–70. Available from: http://doi.wiley.com/10.1111/j.1365-2788.2005.00784.x
143. Aquila I, Gratteri S, Sacco MA, Nuzzolese E, Fineschi V, Frati P, et al. Could the screening for correct oral health reduce the impact of death due to bolus asphyxia in adult patients? A forensic case report. Med Hypotheses [Internet]. 2018;110:23–6. Available from: https://linkinghub.elsevier.com/retrieve/pii/S0306987717310460
144. Miura H, Yamasaki K, Morizaki N, Moriya S, Sumi Y. Factors influencing oral health-related quality of life (OHRQoL) among the frail elderly residing in the community with their family. Arch Gerontol Geriatr [Internet]. 2010;51(3):e62–5. Available from: https://linkinghub.elsevier.com/retrieve/pii/S0167494309003136
145. Barbe AG, Bock N, Derman SHM, Felsch M, Timmermann L, Noack MJ. Self-assessment of oral health, dental health care and oral health-related quality of life among Parkinson's disease patients. Gerodontology [Internet]. 2017;34(1):135–43. Available from: http://doi.wiley.com/10.1111/ger.12237
146. Lu T-Y, Chen J-H, Du J-K, Lin Y-C, Ho P-S, Lee C-H, et al. Dysphagia and masticatory performance as a mediator of the xerostomia to quality of life relation in the older population. BMC Geriatr [Internet]. 2020;20(1):521. Available from: https://bmcgeriatr.biomedcentral.com/articles/10.1186/s12877-020-01901-4
147. Langmore SE. Evaluation of oropharyngeal dysphagia: which diagnostic tool is superior? Curr Opin Otolaryngol Head Neck Surg. 2003;11(6):485–9.

148. Logemann J, Veis S, Colangelo L. A screening procedure for oropharyngeal dysphagia. Dysphagia. 1999;14:44–51.
149. Carnaby-Mann G, Lenius K. The bedside examination in dysphagia. Phys Med Rehabil Clin N Am [Internet]. 2008;19(4):747–68. Available from: https://doi.org/10.1016/j.pmr.2008.05.008
150. Maccarini AR, Filippini A, Padovani D, Limarzi M, Loffredo M, Casolino D. Clinical non-instrumental evaluation of dysphagia. Acta Otorhinolaryngol Ital. 2007;27(6):299–305.
151. Riquelme L. Frequently asked questions (FAQ) on swallowing screening: special emphasis on patients with acute stroke. ASHA [Internet]. 2006;13(c):1–10. Available from: http://www.asha.org/uploadedfiles/faqs-on-swallowing-screening.pdf
152. Suiter DM, Daniels SK, Barkmeier-Kraemer JM, Silverman AH. Swallowing screening: purposefully different from an assessment sensitivity and specificity related to clinical yield, interprofessional roles, and patient selection. Am J Speech Lang Pathol [Internet]. 2021;29(2S):979–91. Available from: https://doi.org/10.1044/2020_AJSLP-19-00140
153. Belafsky PC, Pryor JC, Allen J, Mouadeb DA, Rees CJ, Postma GN, et al. Validity and reliability of the eating assessment tool (EAT-10). Ann Otol Rhinol Laryngol. 2014;117(12):919–24.
154. Wallace KL, Middleton S, Cook IJ. Development and validation of a self-report symptom inventory to assess the severity of oral-pharyngeal dysphagia. Gastroenterology. 2000;118(4):678–87.
155. Silbergleit AK, Schultz L, Jacobson BH, Beardsley T, Johnson AF. The dysphagia handicap index: development and validation. Dysphagia. 2012;27(1):46–52.
156. Martino R, Maki E, Diamant N. Identification of dysphagia using the Toronto Bedside Swallowing Screening Test (TOR-BSST©): are 10 teaspoons of water necessary? Int J Speech Lang Pathol. 2014;16(3):193–8.
157. Martino R, Silver F, Teasell R, Bayley M, Nicholson G, Streiner DL, et al. The Toronto Bedside Swallowing Screening Test (TOR-BSST) development and validation of a dysphagia screening tool for patients with stroke. Stroke. 2009;40(2):555–61.
158. Depippo KL, Holas MA, Reding MJ. Validation of the 3-oz water swallow test for aspiration following stroke. Arch Neurol. 1992;49(12):1259–61.
159. Suiter DM, Leder SB. Clinical utility of the 3-ounce water swallow test. Dysphagia. 2008;23(3):244–50.
160. Suiter DM, Sloggy J, Leder SB. Validation of the Yale swallow protocol: a prospective double-blinded videofluoroscopic study. Dysphagia. 2014;29(2):199–203.
161. Edmiaston J, Connor LT, Loehr L, Nassief A. Validation of a dysphagia screening tool in acute stroke patients. Am J Crit Care. 2010;19(4):357–64.
162. Edmiaston J, Connor LT, Steger-May K, Ford AL. A simple bedside stroke dysphagia screen, validated against videofluoroscopy, detects dysphagia and aspiration with high sensitivity. J Stroke Cerebrovasc Dis [Internet]. 2014;23(4):712–6. Available from: https://doi.org/10.1016/j.jstrokecerebrovasdis.2013.06.030
163. Liu ZY, Zhang XP, Mo MM, Ye RC, Hu CX, Jiang MQ, et al. Impact of the systematic use of the volume-viscosity swallow test in patients with acute ischaemic stroke: a retrospective study. BMC Neurol. 2020;20(1):1–11.
164. Rofes L, Arreola V, Clavé P. The volume-viscosity swallow test for clinical screening of dysphagia and aspiration. Nestle Nutr Inst Workshop Ser. 2012;72:33–42.
165. Jørgensen LW, Søndergaard K, Melgaard D, Warming S. Interrater reliability of the volume-viscosity swallow test; screening for dysphagia among hospitalized elderly medical patients. Clin Nutr ESPEN [Internet]. 2017;22:85–91. Available from: https://doi.org/10.1016/j.clnesp.2017.08.003
166. Clavé P, Arreola V, Romea M, Medina L, Palomera E, Serra-Prat M. Accuracy of the volume-viscosity swallow test for clinical screening of oropharyngeal dysphagia and aspiration. Clin Nutr. 2008;27(6):806–15.
167. Huckabee ML, McIntosh T, Fuller L, Curry M, Thomas P, Walshe M, et al. The Test of Masticating and Swallowing Solids (TOMASS): reliability, validity and international normative data. Int J Lang Commun Disord. 2018;53(1):144–56.

168. Bonilha HS, Martin-Harris B, O'Rourke AK, Tipnis SV. Radiation exposure in modified barium swallow studies. Curr Opin Otolaryngol Head Neck Surg. 2020;28(6):371–5.
169. Da Silva AP, Lubianca Neto JF, Santoro PP. Comparison between videofluoroscopy and endoscopic evaluation of swallowing for the diagnosis of dysphagia in children. Otolaryngol Head Neck Surg [Internet]. 2010;143(2):204–9. Available from: https://doi.org/10.1016/j.otohns.2010.03.027
170. Bonilha HS, Humphries K, Blair J, Hill EG, McGrattan K, Carnes B, et al. Radiation exposure time during MBSS: influence of swallowing impairment severity, medical diagnosis, clinician experience, and standardized protocol use. Dysphagia. 2013;28(1):77–85.
171. Zammit-Maempel I, Chapple CL, Leslie P. Radiation dose in videofluoroscopic swallow studies. Dysphagia. 2007;22(1):13–5.
172. Langmore SE, Kenneth SMA, Olsen N. Fiberoptic endoscopic examination of swallowing safety: a new procedure. Dysphagia. 1988;2(4):216–9.
173. Miller CK, Schroeder JW, Langmore S. Fiberoptic endoscopic evaluation of swallowing across the age spectrum. Am J Speech Lang Pathol. 2020;29(2S):967–78.
174. Kaynak HK, Çelik Hİ. Ayırma Tipi Mikrofilament İpliklerden Üretilmiş Örme Kumaşların Performans Özelliklerinin İncelenmesi. Tekst ve Mühendis [Internet]. 2016;23(104):238–46. Available from: http://tekstilvemuhendis.org.tr/showpublish.php?pubid=473&type=full
175. Pearson WG, Molfenter SM, Smith ZM, Steele CM. Image-based measurement of post-swallow residue: the normalized residue ratio scale. Dysphagia [Internet]. 2013;28(2):167–77. Available from: http://link.springer.com/10.1007/s00455-012-9426-9
176. Hutcheson KA, Barrow MP, Barringer DA, Knott JK, Lin HY, Weber RS, et al. Dynamic Imaging Grade of Swallowing Toxicity (DIGEST): scale development and validation. Cancer. 2017;123(1):62–70.
177. Goepfert RP, Lewin JS, Barrow MP, Warneke CL, Fuller CD, Lai SY, et al. Grading dysphagia as a toxicity of head and neck cancer: differences in severity classification based on MBS DIGEST and clinical CTCAE grades. Dysphagia. 2018;33(2):185–91.
178. Langmore SE. History of fiberoptic endoscopic evaluation of swallowing for evaluation and management of pharyngeal dysphagia: changes over the years. Dysphagia. 2017;32(1):27–38.
179. Baiju R, et al. Oral health and quality of life: current concepts. J Clin Diagn Res [Internet]. 2017;11(6):ZE21–6. Available from: http://jcdr.net/article_fulltext.asp?issn=0973-709x&year=2017&volume=11&issue=6&page=ZE21&issn=0973-709x&id=10110
180. Furuta M, Yamashita Y. Oral health and swallowing problems. Curr Phys Med Rehabil Rep [Internet]. 2013;1(4):216–22. Available from: http://link.springer.com/10.1007/s40141-013-0026-x
181. Sjögren P, Nilsson E, Forsell M, Johansson O, Hoogstraate J. A systematic review of the preventive effect of oral hygiene on pneumonia and respiratory tract infection in elderly people in hospitals and nursing homes: effect estimates and methodological quality of randomized controlled trials. J Am Geriatr Soc [Internet]. 2008;56(11):2124–30. Available from: http://doi.wiley.com/10.1111/j.1532-5415.2008.01926.x
182. Yoneyama T, Yoshida M, Matsui T, Sasaki H. Oral care and pneumonia. Lancet [Internet]. 1999;354(9177):515. Available from: https://linkinghub.elsevier.com/retrieve/pii/S0140673605755501
183. Son YG, Shin J, Ryu HG. Pneumonitis and pneumonia after aspiration. J Dent Anesth Pain Med [Internet]. 2017;17(1):1. Available from: https://jdapm.org/DOIx.php?id=10.17245/jdapm.2017.17.1.1
184. McNally ME, Martin-Misener R, Wyatt CCL, McNeil KP, Crowell SJ, Matthews DC, et al. Action planning for daily mouth care in long-term care: the brushing up on mouth care project. Nurs Res Pract [Internet]. 2012;2012:1–11. Available from: http://www.hindawi.com/journals/nrp/2012/368356/
185. Pradhan A, Keuskamp D, Brennan D. Pre- and post-training evaluation of dental efficacy and activation measures in carers of adults with disabilities in South Australia – a pilot study. Health Soc Care Community [Internet]. 2016;24(6):739–46. Available from: http://doi.wiley.com/10.1111/hsc.12254

186. Klompas M, Speck K, Howell MD, Greene LR, Berenholtz SM. Reappraisal of routine oral care with chlorhexidine gluconate for patients receiving mechanical ventilation. JAMA Intern Med [Internet]. 2014;174(5):751. Available from: http://archinte.jamanetwork.com/article.aspx?doi=10.1001/jamainternmed.2014.359
187. Price R, MacLennan G, Glen J. Selective digestive or oropharyngeal decontamination and topical oropharyngeal chlorhexidine for prevention of death in general intensive care: systematic review and network meta-analysis. BMJ [Internet]. 2014;348(2):g2197. Available from: https://www.bmj.com/lookup/doi/10.1136/bmj.g2197
188. Klompas M, Li L, Kleinman K, Szumita PM, Massaro AF. Associations between ventilator bundle components and outcomes. JAMA Intern Med [Internet]. 2016;176(9):1277. Available from: http://archinte.jamanetwork.com/article.aspx?doi=10.1001/jamainternmed.2016.2427
189. Chow MCM, Kwok S-M, Luk H-W, Law JWH, Leung BPK. Effect of continuous oral suctioning on the development of ventilator-associated pneumonia: a pilot randomized controlled trial. Int J Nurs Stud [Internet]. 2012;49(11):1333–41. Available from: https://linkinghub.elsevier.com/retrieve/pii/S0020748912001861
190. Sole ML, Penoyer DA, Bennett M, Bertrand J, Talbert S. Oropharyngeal secretion volume in intubated patients: the importance of oral suctioning. Am J Crit Care [Internet]. 2011;20(6):e141–5. Available from: https://aacnjournals.org/ajcconline/article/20/6/e141/3000/Oropharyngeal-Secretion-Volume-in-Intubated
191. Yakiwchuk C, Bertone M, Ghiabi E, Brown S, Liarakos M, Brothwell D. Suction toothbrush use for dependent adults with dysphagia: a pilot examiner blind randomized clinical trial. Can J Dent Hyg [Internet]. 2013;47(1):15–23. Available from: https://ci.nii.ac.jp/naid/10031145553/
192. Unknown. Healthy Populations Institute (HPI). Resources. Retrieved from Brushing Up on Mouth Care: [Internet]. Unknown. 2021 [cited 2021 Jan 4]. Available from: http://brushingup.ca/
193. McNally M. Brushing up on mouth care. 2011. p. 1–70. Available from: https://cdn.dal.ca/content/dam/dalhousie/pdf/dept/ahprc/BrushingUp-OCManual.pdf
194. Yap Ai Ling E. Care for person with swallowing difficulty [Internet]. In: Ministry of Health (Malaysia). 2015 [cited 2021 Mar 30]. Available from: http://www.myhealth.gov.my/en/oral-care-for-person-with-swallowing-difficulty/
195. Cuthbertson BH, Dale CM. Less daily oral hygiene is more in the ICU: yes. Intensive Care Med [Internet]. 2021;47(3):328–30. Available from: http://link.springer.com/10.1007/s00134-020-06261-6
196. Dale CM, Rose L, Carbone S, Smith OM, Burry L, Fan E, et al. Protocol for a multi-centered, stepped wedge, cluster randomized controlled trial of the de-adoption of oral chlorhexidine prophylaxis and implementation of an oral care bundle for mechanically ventilated critically ill patients: the CHORAL study. Trials [Internet]. 2019;20(1):603. Available from: https://trialsjournal.biomedcentral.com/articles/10.1186/s13063-019-3673-0
197. Bolivar-Prados M, Rofes L, Arreola V, Guida S, Nascimento WV, Martin A, et al. Effect of a gum-based thickener on the safety of swallowing in patients with poststroke oropharyngeal dysphagia. Neurogastroenterol Motil [Internet]. 2019;31(11):e13695. Available from: https://onlinelibrary.wiley.com/doi/abs/10.1111/nmo.13695
198. Barbon CEA, Steele CM. Efficacy of thickened liquids for eliminating aspiration in head and neck cancer. Otolaryngol Neck Surg [Internet]. 2015;152(2):211–8. Available from: http://journals.sagepub.com/doi/10.1177/0194599814556239
199. Murray J, Miller M, Doeltgen S, Scholten I. Intake of thickened liquids by hospitalized adults with dysphagia after stroke. Int J Speech Lang Pathol [Internet]. 2014;16(5):486–94. Available from: http://www.tandfonline.com/doi/full/10.3109/17549507.2013.830776
200. Welch MV, Logemann JA, Rademaker AW, Kahrilas PJ. Changes in pharyngeal dimensions effected by chin tuck. Arch Phys Med Rehabil. 1993;74(2):178–81.
201. Mcculloch TM, Hoffman MR, Ciucci MR. High-resolution manometry of pharyngeal swallow pressure events associated with head turn and chin tuck. Ann Otol Rhinol

Laryngol [Internet]. 2010;119(6):369–76. Available from: http://journals.sagepub.com/doi/10.1177/000348941011900602
202. Nagy A, Peladeau-Pigeon M, Valenzano TJ, Namasivayam AM, Steele CM. The effectiveness of the head-turn-plus-chin-down maneuver for eliminating vallecular residue. CoDAS [Internet]. 2016;28(2):113–7. Available from: http://www.scielo.br/scielo.php?script=sci_arttext&pid=S2317-17822016000200113&lng=en&tlng=en
203. Lazarus C, Logemann JA, Gibbons P. Effects of maneuvers on swallowing function in a dysphagic oral cancer patient. Head Neck [Internet]. 1993;15(5):419–24. Available from: http://doi.wiley.com/10.1002/hed.2880150509
204. Bahia MM, Lowell SY. A systematic review of the physiological effects of the effortful swallow maneuver in adults with normal and disordered swallowing. Am J Speech Lang Pathol. 2020;29(3):1655–73.
205. Doeltgen SH, Ong E, Scholten I, Cock C, Omari T. Biomechanical quantification of Mendelsohn maneuver and effortful swallowing on pharyngoesophageal function. Otolaryngol Neck Surg [Internet]. 2017;157(5):816–23. Available from: http://journals.sagepub.com/doi/10.1177/0194599817708173
206. Lazarus C, Logemann JA, Song CW, Rademaker AW, Kahrilas PJ. Effects of voluntary maneuvers on tongue base function for swallowing. Folia Phoniatr Logop [Internet]. 2002;54(4):171–6. Available from: https://www.karger.com/Article/FullText/63192
207. Shaker R, Kern M, Bardan E, Taylor A, Stewart ET, Hoffmann RG, et al. Augmentation of deglutitive upper esophageal sphincter opening in the elderly by exercise. Am J Physiol Liver Physiol [Internet]. 1997;272(6):G1518–22. Available from: https://www.physiology.org/doi/10.1152/ajpgi.1997.272.6.G1518
208. Logemann JA, Rademaker A, Pauloski BR, Kelly A, Stangl-McBreen C, Antinoja J, et al. A randomized study comparing the Shaker exercise with traditional therapy: a preliminary study. Dysphagia [Internet]. 2009;24(4):403–11. Available from: http://link.springer.com/10.1007/s00455-009-9217-0
209. Antunes EB, Lunet N. Effects of the head lift exercise on the swallow function: a systematic review. Gerodontology [Internet]. 2012;29(4):247–57. Available from: http://doi.wiley.com/10.1111/j.1741-2358.2012.00638.x
210. Burkhead LM, Sapienza CM, Rosenbek JC. Strength-training exercise in dysphagia rehabilitation: principles, procedures, and directions for future research. Dysphagia [Internet]. 2007;22(3):251–65. Available from: http://link.springer.com/10.1007/s00455-006-9074-z
211. Robbins JA, Gangnon RE, Theis SM, Kays SA, Hewitt AL, Hind JA. The effects of lingual exercise on swallowing in older adults. J Am Geriatr Soc [Internet]. 2005;53(9):1483–9. Available from: http://doi.wiley.com/10.1111/j.1532-5415.2005.53467.x
212. Robbins JA, Kays SA, Gangnon RE, Hind JA, Hewitt AL, Gentry LR, et al. The effects of lingual exercise in stroke patients with dysphagia. Arch Phys Med Rehabil [Internet]. 2007;88(2):150–8. Available from: https://linkinghub.elsevier.com/retrieve/pii/S0003999306014572
213. Rogus-Pulia N, Rusche N, Hind JA, Zielinski J, Gangnon R, Safdar N, et al. Effects of device-facilitated isometric progressive resistance oropharyngeal therapy on swallowing and health-related outcomes in older adults with dysphagia. J Am Geriatr Soc [Internet]. 2016;64(2):417–24. Available from: http://doi.wiley.com/10.1111/jgs.13933
214. Steele CM, Bayley MT, Peladeau-Pigeon M, Nagy A, Namasivayam AM, Stokely SL, et al. A randomized trial comparing two tongue-pressure resistance training protocols for post-stroke dysphagia. Dysphagia. 2016;31(3):452–61.
215. Wheeler-Hegland KM, Rosenbek JC, Sapienza CM. Submental sEMG and hyoid movement during Mendelsohn maneuver, effortful swallow, and expiratory muscle strength training. J Speech Lang Hear Res. 2008;51(5):1072–87. https://doi.org/10.1044/1092-4388(2008/07-0016). J Speech Lang Hear Res. 2008;51(6):1643.
216. Hegland KW, Davenport PW, Brandimore AE, Singletary FF, Troche MS. Rehabilitation of swallowing and cough functions following stroke: an expiratory muscle strength training

trial. Arch Phys Med Rehabil [Internet]. 2016;97(8):1345–51. Available from: https://doi.org/10.1016/j.apmr.2016.03.027
217. Laciuga H, Rosenbek JC, Davenport PW, Sapienza CM. Functional outcomes associated with expiratory muscle strength training: narrative review. J Rehabil Res Dev. 2014;51(4):535–46.
218. Plowman EK, Watts SA, Tabor L, Robison R, Gaziano J, Domer AS, et al. Impact of expiratory strength training in amyotrophic lateral sclerosis. Muscle Nerve. 2016;54(1):48–53.
219. Rogus-Pulia NM, Plowman EK. Shifting tides toward a proactive patient-centered approach in dysphagia management of neurodegenerative disease. Am J Speech Lang Pathol. 2020;29(2S):1094–109.
220. Arnett SW, Laity JH, Agrawal SK, Cress ME. Aerobic reserve and physical functional performance in older adults. Age Ageing [Internet]. 2008;37(4):384–9. Available from: https://academic.oup.com/ageing/article-lookup/doi/10.1093/ageing/afn022
221. Lewis A, Fricker A. Better oral health in residential care. Professional portfolio: oral health care planning guidelines. Adelaide: South Australian Dental Service; date unknown. Available from: https://www.sahealth.sa.gov.au/wps/wcm/connect/77fd7a004b3323958834ade79043faf0/BOHRC_Professional_Portfolio_Full_Version%5B1%5D.pdf

Xerostomia and Hyposalivation

Rosa María López-Pintor, Lucía Ramírez Martínez-Acitores, Julia Serrano Valle, José González-Serrano, Elisabeth Casañas, Lorenzo de Arriba, and Gonzalo Hernández

Saliva has a critical role in the maintenance of oral health. Although 99% of salivary content is water, saliva also contains immunoglobulins, glycoproteins, electrolytes, digestive enzymes (amylase and lipase), antifungal and antibacterial enzymes, mucins, and leukocytes, among other components. When salivary secretion decreases, the oral cavity becomes dry increasing the risk of oral diseases such as caries, periodontal disease, candidiasis, oral ulcerations, and bacterial sialadenitis. It may also impair individuals' ability to speak, chew, and swallow [1–4]. Salivary secretion is regulated by the autonomic nervous system, especially parasympathetic fibers [3, 5]. It is important to differentiate between xerostomia and hyposalivation. Xerostomia is the subjective feeling of dry mouth, whereas hyposalivation is the objective reduction of salivary flow. In some cases, patients with xerostomia may also suffer from hyposalivation. Similarly, there are patients who present with hyposalivation but may not report dry mouth sensation [6].

Dry mouth is a frequent problem in geriatric patients. There is controversy about whether salivary flow decreases with age [4]. The prevalence of dry mouth increases considerably in older patients, ranging from 17% to 40% in community-dwelling older adults and from 20% to 72% in institutionalized older persons [2, 6]. In this chapter, we will review the etiological factors associated with xerostomia in this age group, as well as its associated oral changes. We will discuss the diagnostic workup for xerostomia and hyposalivation and how to perform individualized treatments for these patients.

R. M. López-Pintor (✉) · L. Ramírez Martínez-Acitores · J. Serrano Valle · J. González-Serrano · E. Casañas · L. de Arriba · G. Hernández
Department of Dental Clinical Specialties, School of Dentistry, Complutense University, Madrid, Spain
e-mail: rmlopezp@odon.ucm.es

© The Author(s), under exclusive license to Springer Nature Switzerland AG 2022
C.-M. Hogue, J. G. Ruiz (eds.), *Oral Health and Aging*,
https://doi.org/10.1007/978-3-030-85993-0_5

1 Causes of Salivary Hypofunction in the Older Patients

There are different causes of xerostomia and hyposalivation. In the following paragraphs, we will review the different causes of dry mouth in geriatric patients.

1.1 Age

It is not clear whether aging itself is associated with salivary gland dysfunction [3]. Studies have shown that acinar cells in salivary glands decrease with aging and are replaced by fatty and connective tissues. Research reveals that acinar cells decrease by 30–40% between 34 and 75 years of age. Despite these age-related changes, epidemiological studies do not show an independent negative effect of aging on salivary flow. Other factors, namely, medication use and certain medical conditions, may be more likely to cause salivary gland dysfunction [2, 3].

The research evidence on the effects of aging on salivary function is mixed. Widely diverse inclusion criteria, different methodologies in the collection of saliva, the way xerostomia was defined, concurrent use of medications, coexisting medical and psychological conditions, and participants from diverse care settings (institutionalized or non-institutionalized) are some of the reasons explaining these divergent results. Longitudinal studies show that the degree of xerostomia increases in a linear pattern in individuals ranging in age between 50 and 65 years. Other studies show that the incidence of xerostomia increases with age. However, there are other studies that do not show significant age-related changes [2].

1.2 Gender

Xerostomia is more common among women. One explanation is that salivary glands in women are usually smaller and, therefore, have a reduced salivary flow reserve. Another factor is that women often take more medications than men. Studies in older individuals show that female sex is a risk factor for hyposalivation after adjustment for age, health status, and use of medications [2].

1.3 Diseases

Different systemic disorders have been associated with salivary gland hypofunction leading to xerostomia or hyposalivation [7]. Table 1 shows a listing of common medical and psychological conditions associated with salivary gland dysfunction.

Table 1 Common medical and psychological conditions associated with salivary gland dysfunction

Rheumatological chronic inflammatory diseases	Sjögren's syndrome Systemic lupus erythematosus Rheumatoid arthritis Scleroderma Primary biliary cirrhosis Mixed connective tissue disease Juvenile idiopathic arthritis
Endocrine disorders	Diabetes mellitus Thyroid disorders Cushing's disease Addison's disease
Neurologic disorders	Parkinson's disease Alzheimer's disease Bell's palsy Stroke
Psychological diseases	Eating disorders (anorexia, bulimia) Depression Anxiety Stress
Salivary gland diseases	Agenesis of salivary glands Ectodermal dysplasia Sialolithiasis Sialadenitis
Genetic disorders	Prader-Willi syndrome Down syndrome Papillon-Lefèvre syndrome Familial amyloidotic polyneuropathy Gaucher disease Hereditary hemochromatosis
Infectious diseases	HIV/AIDS Hepatitis C infection Tuberculosis Human T lymphotropic virus
Metabolic disorders	Dehydrated patients Alcoholism Anemia Patients with chronic renal failure
Others	Fibromyalgia Sarcoidosis Primary biliary cirrhosis Hypertension Fibromyalgia Chronic pancreatitis Graft-versus-host disease Cystic fibrosis Chronic fatigue syndrome Burning mouth syndrome Liver transplant candidates Atrophic gastritis

Rheumatological Diseases
Sjögren's syndrome (SS) is the most common systemic disorder causing hyposalivation [2, 8]. SS is an autoimmune rheumatic disease characterized by a chronic lymphocytic infiltration of salivary and lacrimal glands [3, 9]. It is classified as primary Sjögren's syndrome (pSS) when occurring as an isolated condition or as secondary SS (sSS) when it is associated with a coexisting autoimmune disease [10]. It usually appears in the fourth to fifth decade of life. Although it could manifest at any age, up to 20% of cases appear in older adults [7], and its prevalence is higher in women than men [9]. The most recent criteria were proposed in 2016 by the American College of Rheumatology and the European League Against Rheumatism [11]. The 2016 classification criteria consider, in addition to ocular and oral dryness, the presence of focal lymphocytic sialadenitis of minor salivary glands (focus score of ≥ 1 foci/4 mm^2, weight/score = 3), an anti-SSA/Ro-positive antibody (weight/score = 3), ocular staining score ≥ 5 (or van Bijsterveld score ≥ 4) in at least one eye (weight/score = 1), Schirmer's test ≤ 5 mm/5 min in at least one eye (weight/score = 1), and an unstimulated whole salivary flow rate ≤ 0.1 mL/min (weight/score = 1). A patient with a score ≥ 4 meets criteria for SS. Besides SS, there are other rheumatic diseases that may cause salivary hypofunction. In older patients, the most frequent conditions are rheumatoid arthritis, systemic lupus erythematosus, primary biliary cirrhosis, mixed connective tissue disease, and scleroderma [3, 7].

Endocrine Diseases
Diabetes mellitus (DM) is the most common endocrine disorder associated with xerostomia and low salivary flow rates [3, 12]. This disease is highly prevalent in older patients. DM has become a global epidemic with the overall prevalence among adults increasing considerably over the years [13]. The low levels of saliva could be attributed to alterations in the microcirculation of the salivary glands, damage to the gland parenchyma, degenerative processes of the nerve endings that innervate the glands, dehydration, polyuria, and disturbances in glycemic control [2, 3, 13]. As a consequence of hyposalivation, patients with DM are in a higher risk of developing tooth decay, taste disorders, oral infections (particularly candidiasis), burning mouth syndrome, or periodontal disease [13].

Apart from DM, thyroid dysfunction is one of the most frequent endocrine disorders affecting adults worldwide [14]. It could be classified as either hyperthyroidism or as hypothyroidism. Both diseases have been associated with reduced salivary gland function, more prominent in those patients with hypothyroidism [3, 14]. Alterations in the function of thyroid glands, especially in those patients with hypothyroidism, affect salivary gland function, which in turn could result in dental caries in atypical locations, halitosis, and difficulty in eating, potentially compromising patients' nutritional status and quality of life [14]. Patients with Cushing's or Addison's syndrome may also experience dry mouth and hyposalivation [7].

Neurologic Disorders
Several neurologic disorders are associated with xerostomia and hyposalivation. Parkinson's disease is one of the most common neurologic disorders in older adults.

It is a progressive, chronic, and neurodegenerative condition that affects 1% of adults over the sixth decade of life. Patients with Parkinson's disease may experience xerostomia, either as a side effect of medications or because of the decrease in salivary flow due to disease-related autonomic dysfunction. The resulting hyposalivation coupled with patients' difficulties in performing good oral hygiene increases the risk of developing tooth decay, periodontal disease, and dental loss [6]. Dysphagia is another common symptom of Parkinson's disease, affecting up to 75% of patients. Hyposalivation could contribute to dysphagia, which may further aggravate the feeling of dry mouth [3]. Other neurologic disorders that may cause salivary disorders are Bell's palsy and Alzheimer's disease. Hyposalivation may also appear in patients who have suffered a stroke and demonstrate associated neurological deficits [7].

Psychological Conditions
Depression and anxiety are common disorders in older patients and are frequently associated with xerostomia [7, 15]. These patients usually suffer from dry mouth related to the use of psychoactive drugs prescribed for these conditions, but sometimes, it could have a psychological origin [3, 12]. Other less common disorders that may cause dry mouth are stress and eating disorders such as bulimia and anorexia [7].

Genetic Diseases
Although rare in older adults, several genetic disorders are also associated with salivary gland dysfunction. Among the most common are Prader-Willi syndrome, Gaucher disease, Down syndrome, familial amyloidotic polyneuropathy, hereditary hemochromatosis, and Papillon-Lefèvre syndrome. Other possible genetic malformations associated with hyposalivation include agenesis of the salivary glands and ectodermal dysplasia [3].

Infectious Diseases
Patients with HIV may develop xerostomia and hyposalivation. The introduction of antiretroviral therapies has increased patients' life expectancy and quality of life. In these patients, xerostomia may result from salivary disorders associated with the viral infection or may be drug induced. HIV patients may also develop salivary gland dysfunction due to conditions common in this population including Kaposi sarcoma, intraglandular lymphadenopathy, or non-Hodgkin lymphoma. Hepatitis C is another infection that is associated with salivary disorders due to viral infiltration of the salivary glands. Tuberculosis and human T lymphotropic virus infection are also associated with salivary dysfunction [3, 7].

Other Disorders
Other disorders related to hyposalivation are alcoholism, anemia, dehydration, and chronic renal failure [3]. One of the main oral manifestations of patients undergoing hemodialysis is xerostomia. Moreover, most patients with chronic renal failure suffer from diabetes or hypertension requiring pharmacological therapies, which in turn increase the risk of reductions of salivary flow [16]. Older people are often dehydrated due to different causes. One of the most common is not drinking enough fluids due to physiological and functional decline. Dehydration is a complex

condition and in older adults is associated with a higher risk of morbidity and mortality [17, 18]. Graft-versus-host disease is a condition that may occur after bone marrow transplantation. This syndrome is characterized by a lymphocytic infiltration, mediated by autoreactive T cells, which affect several tissues and organs including the salivary glands. This disease could lead to salivary disorders [3, 7]. Sarcoidosis is a multisystemic disease of unknown etiology, probably due to a dysregulation of the autoimmune system, which leads to the formation of granulomas. In these patients, xerostomia, hyposalivation, and salivary gland swelling could appear [7]. Chronic pancreatitis could also affect the salivary glands. In addition, patients with fibromyalgia, cystic fibrosis, hypertension, chronic fatigue syndrome, burning mouth syndrome, primary biliary cirrhosis, atrophic gastritis and candidates for liver transplant may also experience xerostomia [7].

1.4 Head and Neck Radiotherapy and Chemotherapy

An important cause of xerostomia and hyposalivation in older persons with head and neck cancers is previous or current treatment with radiotherapy. The salivary glands are very radiosensitive to these treatments. Radiation induces a degenerative process leading to a reduction in salivary flow [2, 3]. In many cases, the treatment with radiotherapy induces a total loss of parotid gland salivary flow which may have serious consequences for the oral cavity. Doses greater than 60 grays (Gy) may produce irreversible hyposalivation, while doses of 30–50 Gy produce reversible damage [5]. These alterations in salivary flow may persist for years and in many of these patients may even become irreversible [3]. Chemotherapy can cause xerostomia in up to 50% of patients receiving these treatments. In these patients, normal salivary flow may take between 6 months to 1 year to recover after concluding the treatment [5].

1.5 Drugs

Xerostomia and hyposalivation have been commonly associated with the use of a wide variety of pharmacological agents. More than 400 drugs have been associated with xerostomia. In addition, the risk of xerostomia increases with the number of drugs (polypharmacy), higher doses, drug combinations, and duration of treatment. Some medications produce xerostomia, but do not always cause a reduction in salivary flow [2]. Older patients often take some type of drug on a regular basis to treat a range of chronic conditions. Studies show that 52% of men and 65% of women over 65 years take at least one medication. In addition, between 11% and 24% take more than four medications per day [19]. The concurrent use of multiple medications or polypharmacy has been associated with xerostomia and hyposalivation [1, 3, 7, 19–22]. According to studies, the prevalence of xerostomia in patients older than 65 years increases with the number of prescribed drugs. In fact, 37% of patients taking one drug suffered from xerostomia as compared with 62% and 78% of those taking two or three drugs, respectively [7]. However, there are other studies that showed no association between the degree of xerostomia and the number of drugs received [23]. The duration of treatment may also influence the risk of salivary disorders [1, 19, 22]. According to some studies, patients who take drugs for a longer period of time have lower salivary flow rates [8, 24]. Below we will briefly describe medications often associated with salivary disorders. Table 2 shows all drugs associated with salivary disorders classified according to their mechanism of action following the guidelines of the Anatomical Therapeutic Chemical (ATC) Classification System [25].

Medications Acting on the Central Nervous System

Analgesics such as tramadol, morphine, and paracetamol (acetaminophen) are included in this group. These drugs can reduce salivary flow leading to xerostomia [3, 21, 22]. Among the antiepileptic and psychoactive groups of medications, benzodiazepines are the most often associated with salivary disorders [3]. Benzodiazepine-related drugs and antidepressants have also been associated with salivary disorders [21, 22].

Medications Acting on Muscarinic Receptors

This group includes drugs used for gastrointestinal disorders, urological problems (including urinary frequency, urgency, and incontinence), and chronic obstructive airway diseases. These drugs alter muscarinic receptors, thus increasing xerostomia [20, 22].

Medications Acting on Alpha and Beta Adrenergic Receptors

Alpha-1 drugs used for the treatment of hypertension such as central agents, some beta-blocker agents, and alpha blockers are frequently used in older patients to treat hypertension and benign prostatic hyperplasia. Within this group, there are also nasal preparations including pseudoephedrine. These medications reduce salivary flow increasing xerostomia [20–22]. Alpha-2 adrenergic receptor-blocking drugs such as dexmedetomidine, used to reduce anxiety and delirium in intensive care patients, and brimonidine used for glaucoma have been also associated with xerostomia [20]. Medications acting on beta adrenergic receptors are often used for the treatment of hypertension in older patients. These agents increase the risk of xerostomia [20, 22].

Medications Acting on More than One Receptor Type

There are other drugs acting on several receptors that have been associated with xerostomia: drugs for the treatment of functional gastrointestinal disorders such as prokinetics [22]; drugs to treat neuropathic pain such as antidepressants, sedatives, and hypnotics [22]; opioid drugs such as tapentadol [20–22]; antiepileptics such as carbamazepine [22]; psychoactive medications such as benzodiazepine derivatives and benzodiazepine-related agents [22]; antidepressant drugs such as selective serotonin reuptake inhibitors [21, 22]; and antihistamines for systemic use [22].

Medications that Produce Xerostomia with no Known Mechanism of Action

There are also multiple drugs associated with salivary disorders whose mechanism of action is not yet known such as drugs for acid-related disorders [21],

Table 2 Drugs associated with xerostomia/hyposalivation classified by their mechanism of action according to the Anatomical Therapeutic Chemical (ATC) Classification System

Drugs associated with salivary disorders according to ATC classification			
ATC first, second, and third level	ATC fourth and fifth level	Chemical substance	Site of saliva secretion control
A: Alimentary tract and metabolism			
A02 Drugs for acid-related disorders	A02AA04	Magnesium hydroxide	Not known but clinical effect reported
A03 Drugs for functional gastrointestinal disorders	A03AA07	Dicyclomine/ dicycloverine	Muscarinic receptors
	A03AB05	Propantheline	Muscarinic receptors
A04 Antiemetics and anti-nauseants	A04AD01	Scopolamine	Muscarinic receptors
B: Blood and blood-forming organs			
B01 Antithrombotic agents	B01AC06	Acetylsalicylic acid	Not known but clinical effect reported
C: Cardiovascular system			
C02 Antihypertensives	C02AB01	Methyldopa	Central nervous system
	C02AC01	Clonidine	Central nervous system
	C02AC05	Moxonidine	Central nervous system
	C02AC06	Rilmenidine	Central nervous system
C03 Diuretics	C03AA01	Bendroflumethiazide	Not known but clinical effect reported
	C03AA02	Hydroflumethiazide	Not known but clinical effect reported
	C03AA03	Hydrochlorothiazide	Not known but clinical effect reported
	C03AA04	Chlorothiazide	Not known but clinical effect reported
	C03AA05	Polythiazide	Not known but clinical effect reported
	C03AA06	Trichlormethiazide	Not known but clinical effect reported
	C03AA07	Cyclopenthiazide	Not known but clinical effect reported
	C03AA08	Methyclothiazide	Not known but clinical effect reported
	C03AA09	Cyclothiazide	Not known but clinical effect reported
	C03AA13	Mebutizide	Not known but clinical effect reported

Xerostomia and Hyposalivation

Table 2 (continued)

\multicolumn{4}{l}{Drugs associated with salivary disorders according to ATC classification}
ATC first, second, and third level	ATC fourth and fifth level	Chemical substance	Site of saliva secretion control
C07 Beta-blocking agents	C07AA06	Timolol	Beta-1 adrenergic receptors
	C07AB02	Metoprolol	Beta-1 adrenergic receptors
	C07AB03	Atenolol	Beta-1 adrenergic receptors
	C07AB07	Bisoprolol	Beta-1 adrenergic receptors
C08 Calcium channel blockers	C08DA01	Verapamil	Not known but clinical effect reported
C09 Agents acting on renin-angiotensin system	C09AA01	Captopril	Not known but clinical effect reported
	C09AA02	Enalapril	Not known but clinical effect reported
C10 Lipid-modifying agents	C10A	Lipid-modifying agents plain	Not known but clinical effect reported
G: Genitourinary system and sex hormones			
G04 Urological	G04BD04	Oxybutynin	Muscarinic receptors
	G04BD06	Propiverine	Muscarinic receptors
	G04BD08	Solifenacin	Muscarinic receptors
	G04BD09	Trospium	Muscarinic receptors
H: Systemic hormonal preparations excluded sex hormones and insulins			
H03 Thyroid therapy	H03AA	Thyroid hormones	Not known but clinical effect reported
M: Musculoskeletal system			
M01 Anti-inflammatory and antirheumatic products	M01AX05	Glucosamine	Not known but clinical effect reported
M03 Muscle relaxants	M03BX02	Tizanidine	Alpha-2 adrenergic receptors
M05 Drugs for treatment of bone diseases	M05BA	Bisphosphonates	Not known but clinical effect reported
N: Nervous system			
N01 Anesthetics	N01AH01	Fentanyl	Alpha-2 adrenergic receptors
N02 Analgesics			
N02A Opioids	N02AG02	Morphine	Central nervous system Precise mechanism of action is unknown
	N02AX02	Tramadol	Central nervous system
	N02AX06	Tapentadol	More than one receptor type
N02B Other analgesics and antipyretics	N02BE01	Paracetamol or acetaminophen	Not known but clinical effect reported
N03 Antiepileptics	N03AF01	Carbamazepine	More than one receptor type
N05 Psychoactive			

(continued)

Table 2 (continued)

ATC first, second, and third level	ATC fourth and fifth level	Chemical substance	Site of saliva secretion control
Drugs associated with salivary disorders according to ATC classification			
N05A Antipsychotics	N05AA0	Chlorpromazine	More than one receptor type
	N05AB03	Perphenazine	Muscarinic receptors
	N05AB04	Prochlorperazine	More than one receptor type
	N05AD01	Haloperidol	More than one receptor type
	N05AE03	Sertindole	More than one receptor type
	N05AH02	Clozapine	More than one receptor type
	N05AH03	Olanzapine	More than one receptor type
	N05AL05	Amisulpride	More than one receptor type
	N05AX08	Risperidone	More than one receptor type
	N05AX13	Paliperidone	More than one receptor type
N05B Anxiolytics	N05BA01	Diazepam	Central nervous system
	N05BA06	Lorazepam	Central nervous system
N05C Hypnotics and sedatives	N05CD01	Flurazepam	Central nervous system
	N05CD02	Nitrazepam	Central nervous system
	N05CD03	Flunitrazepam	Central nervous system
	N05CD04	Estazolam	Central nervous system
	N05CD05	Triazolam	Central nervous system
	N05CD06	Lormetazepam	Central nervous system
	N05CD07	Temazepam	Central nervous system
	N05CD08	Midazolam	Central nervous system
	N05CD09	Brotizolam	Central nervous system
	N05CD10	Quazepam	Central nervous system
	N05CD11	Loprazolam	Central nervous system
	N05CD12	Doxefazepam	Central nervous system
	N05CD13	Cinolazepam	Central nervous system
	N05CD14	Remimazolam	Central nervous system
	N05CF01	Zopiclone	Central nervous system
	N05CF04	Eszopiclone	Central nervous system
	N05CF03	Zaleplon	Central nervous system
	N05CF02	Zolpidem	Central nervous system
	N05CM18	Dexmedetomidine	Alpha-2 adrenergic receptors
N06 Antidepressants			

Table 2 (continued)

Drugs associated with salivary disorders according to ATC classification			
ATC first, second, and third level	ATC fourth and fifth level	Chemical substance	Site of saliva secretion control
N06A Antidepressants	N06AA10	Nortriptyline	More than one type of receptor
	N06AB03	Fluoxetine	Central nervous system
	N06AB04	Citalopram	Central nervous system
	N06AB05	Paroxetine	Central nervous system
	N06AB06	Sertraline	Central nervous system
	N06AB10	Escitalopram	Central nervous system
	N06AX12	Bupropion	Central nervous system
	N06AX16	Venlafaxine	Central nervous system
	N06AX21	Duloxetine	Central nervous system
	N06AX23	Desvenlafaxine	More than one type of receptor
	N06AX26	Vortioxetine	More than one type of receptor
N06B Psychostimulant agents used for ADHD and nootropics	N06BA04	Methylphenidate	Central nervous system
P: Antiparasitic products, insecticides, and repellents			
P01 Antiprotozoals	P01BC01	Quinine	Not known but clinical effect reported
R: Respiratory system			
R01 Nasal preparations	R01BA02	Pseudoephedrine	Alpha-1 adrenergic receptors
R03 Drugs for obstructive airway diseases	R03AC03	Terbutaline	Beta-2 adrenergic receptors
	R03AC12	Salmeterol	b2 adrenergic receptors
	R03AC13	Albuterol	b2 adrenergic receptors
	R03BA01	Beclomethasone	Not known but clinical effect reported
	R03BA02	Budesonide	Not known but clinical effect reported
	R03BA03	Flunisolide	Not known but clinical effect reported
	R03BA04	Betamethasone	Not known but clinical effect reported
	R03BA05	Fluticasone	Not known but clinical effect reported
	R03BA06	Triamcinolone	Not known but clinical effect reported
	R03BA07	Mometasone	Not known but clinical effect reported
	R03BA08	Ciclesonide	Not known but clinical effect reported
	R03BA09	Fluticasone furoate	Not known but clinical effect reported
	R03BB01	Glycopyrrolate/ glycopyrronium/ ipratropium	Muscarinic receptors
	R03BB04	Tiotropium	Muscarinic receptors

(continued)

Table 2 (continued)

Drugs associated with salivary disorders according to ATC classification

ATC first, second, and third level	ATC fourth and fifth level	Chemical substance	Site of saliva secretion control
R06 Antihistamines for systemic use	R06AA02	Diphenhydramine	More than one type of receptors
	R06AE07	Cetirizine	More than one type of receptors
	R06AE09	Levocetirizine	More than one type of receptors
	R06AX13	Loratadine	More than one type of receptors
	R06AX19	Azelastine	More than one type of receptors
	R06AX22	Ebastine	More than one type of receptors
	R06AX26	Fexofenadine	More than one type of receptors
S: Sensory organs			
S01 Ophthalmological	S01EA05	Brimonidine	Alpha-2 adrenergic receptors

antithrombotic agents [21], calcium channel blockers [20–22, 26], agents acting on the renin-angiotensin system [21, 26], lipid-modifying agents [21, 26], anti-inflammatory and antirheumatic drugs [21], glucocorticoids used for chronic obstructive airway diseases, antiprotozoals (specifically quinine) [21], and bisphosphonates [21].

1.6 Lifestyle Factors

Modifiable risky behaviors may contribute to the appearance of dry mouth. Among them are excessive consumption of alcohol, tobacco, and caffeinated drinks and use of mouthwashes containing alcohol. Mouth breathing and snoring as seen in obstructive sleep apnea can also increase the risk of xerostomia [27].

2 Impact of Salivary Disorders in the Oral and General Health of Older Patients

Saliva has multiple functions that foster and maintain oral health. Reductions in salivary secretion may lead to alterations in the oral mucosa, caries, and discomfort, reducing patient's quality of life [3, 5, 9, 15, 28, 29]. Next, we will review common consequences of salivary disorders in older adults.

2.1 Changes in Taste

The taste of food stimulates the production of saliva. Saliva in turn dissolves the food to stimulate taste receptors. In addition, components of saliva such as bicarbonate ions can also affect the taste of food. Saliva also protects salivary receptors from atrophy, infection, mechanical damage, and drying out. As a result, when saliva decreases, the taste of food may be altered [28]. The sense of taste often decreases with aging. Several factors may contribute to these changes but among the most well-known are an increasing deterioration of the olfactory senses and side effects of drugs [6]. The research literature is mixed regarding the type, frequency, and severity of age-related losses in taste perception. Some investigators report that bitter taste is the most commonly affected, whereas sweet taste is less impacted by the aging process [30]. According to some authors, older people display a reduction in sensory-specific satiety as compared to younger subjects. This means that the triggers that normally would encourage the intake of different foods are reduced with aging, leading to acceptance of bland and monotonous diets. Others state that older adults compensate for losses in taste perception by increasing their intake of sweet and fatty foods [30]. Taste plays a major role in food perception, and taste disability influences intraoral food processing and perception [31].

2.2 Changes in Mastication, Alterations in the Formation of the Alimentary Bolus, and Swallowing

Saliva lubricates and softens food particles. It also exposes food to salivary enzymes and helps prepare the bolus for subsequent swallowing. Deterioration in the salivary flow rate has been associated with decreased masticatory function in older adults. The masticatory process is influenced by different factors such as the number of teeth, masticatory force, use of dentures, muscular alterations, and salivary flow [6, 28]. When the salivary flow decreases, the number of masticatory cycles increases. Studies show that diets requiring more chewing activity increase salivary flow. Many older patients tend to eat soft diets due to the lack of teeth and the presence of dentures [28, 29].

Saliva also helps in the bolus formation. Salivary enzymes in the mouth begin the digestion of triglycerides and carbohydrates. Saliva moistens the food, and salivary mucins help to bind the food particles and form the alimentary bolus. When there is a reduced salivary flow, the patient needs to drink more fluids to moisten the food which may reduce the cohesiveness of the alimentary bolus [28].

Swallowing is a necessary function for removing excess saliva from the mouth and ingesting solid and liquid food. The salivary flow, viscosity, and composition as well as food textures influence swallowing. When salivary flow decreases, swallowing intervals increase [28]. Oral lesions such as an atrophic, fissured, or dry tongue or the presence of certain infections can impair the patient's ability to swallow food.

Swallowing dysfunction can have an important impact on the nutritional status of older patients [15]. Many older adults who suffer from hyposalivation develop dysphagia [32]. Dysphagia may lead to decreased food and fluid intake leading to negative consequences such as malnutrition, risk of aspiration, and aspiration pneumonia that place the older patient's life at risk [6]. For a more in-depth discussion on the topic of dysphagia, please refer to chapter "Swallowing, Dysphagia, and Aspiration Pneumonia."

A decreased salivation rate is associated with other consequences. Impaired speech among older adults may have a great impact on patients' well-being and quality of life. Reductions in older adults' communication skills may lead to social isolation [6]. The research literature regarding the impact of dry mouth on subjective and objective halitosis is mixed. An utmost reduction in unstimulated saliva has been reported to influence the generation of volatile sulfur compounds that characterize halitosis. Needless to say, this condition in older adults might lead to stigmatization, social isolation, and poor quality of life [6]. As mentioned earlier, reduced salivary flow can alter the taste of food and impair chewing and swallowing processes. As a consequence of reduced salivary flow, patients may not be able to tolerate foods that are more difficult to eat such as raw carrots and meat, potentially decreasing their nutritional intake [29]. In addition, an impaired taste sensation can greatly affect appetite, which can further aggravate older adults' nutritional status [6].

Older patients with reduced salivary flow may also suffer traumatic oral lesions. Saliva plays a fundamental role in the lubrication of the oral mucosa, and certain dry foods such as toast or chips can damage an already dried and friable mucosa. It is also common that patients with dry mouth present with an atrophic, depapillated, fissured, and dry tongue. In addition, these patients may suffer from fissured lips and mucosal ulcers [33]. Patients with hyposalivation often show a poor tolerance to dentures. Saliva forms a protective film that aids in the retention of dentures. When salivary flow decreases, this retention capability is lost. This will considerably influence the nutritional status and quality of life of older patients wearing dentures [33].

2.3 Changes in Biofilm and Their Consequences

When saliva decreases, the oral microbial flora is altered. Concentration of certain microorganisms increases, such as *Lactobacillus acidophilus*, *Streptococcus mutans*, and *Candida albicans*, increasing the risk of caries and candidiasis [15, 28]. However, in certain patients such as patients with SS, it is not clear whether the periodontal flora is altered [34]. In addition, the buffer capacity and clearance effect of saliva decreases, lowering salivary pH which may in turn increase dental demineralization [15, 28]. Cavities appear in the cervical area of the teeth, near the root, and in other atypical locations such as the lingual surfaces, the incisal edges, and the cusps of the teeth [28]. In older adult patients, caries can lead to tooth loss and subsequent edentulism which will further weaken chewing function, worsening nutrition and decreasing quality of life [6]. There is an inverse relationship between salivary flow rates and *Candida albicans* colony-forming units (CFU) among SS patients [35]. The increase of *Candida albicans* may favor the appearance of angular chcilitis, denture stomatitis, and oropharyngeal candidiasis among older adults [6, 35].

3 Diagnosis of Xerostomia and Hyposalivation

To properly diagnose xerostomia and hyposalivation, a complete clinical history, exam, and ancillary tests must be performed [3]. The tests to be performed will depend on the specific pathology and the possible causes of the xerostomia and/or hyposalivation, as we will see below.

3.1 Medical History

When a patient comes to the office complaining of dry mouth, it is critical to perform a complete and detailed medical history. The medical history should include the reason for the consultation, how long the patient has suffered from dry mouth, and associated symptoms. It is important to pay attention to underlying systemic pathologies and drugs associated with dry mouth. In patients with history of head and neck malignancies, it is important to ascertain whether the patient had received radiotherapy or chemotherapy in the past [5, 22, 36, 37]. Asking the patient about dryness in extraoral areas such as the skin and other mucous membranes (ocular, nasopharyngeal, or genital) may uncover underlying systemic pathologies such as SS. Cognitive problems are common in older adults. Therefore, clinicians should always keep in mind the possibility that the patient may have mild cognitive impairment or dementia which in some situations may require adaptations in the history and consideration of secondary sources of information such as caregivers and loved ones [30]. For more details, please refer to "The 3 Ds: Dementia, Delirium, and Depression in Oral Health" chapter in this book.

As mentioned earlier in this chapter, the discomfort associated with dry mouth is often the first and most common symptom reported by patients with xerostomia. It is common that patients reporting dry mouth notice that their saliva has become thicker and viscous or that they need to drink more fluids. They can also suffer functional problems such as difficulties in speaking, eating certain foods, and swallowing. Other frequent symptoms are halitosis and the sensation of burning and/or pain in the tongue. Edentulous patients may also suffer fissures in the corner of the lips or difficulties wearing dentures [30, 31, 38]. Sometimes it can be challenging to differentiate age-related physiological changes in the oral cavity from pathological conditions [30].

3.2 Intraoral and Facial Examination

A careful oral examination is essential to identify clinical signs that may suggest hyposalivation. When the protective function of saliva against different oral insults and infections is lost or diminished, patients may suffer from various xerostomia-associated pathologies such as caries and fungal infections.

Experts have reported several signs during the oral exam that may suggest the presence of dry mouth. The oral mucosa and a gingiva may appear bright, pale, and atrophic on exam [37]. Sometimes, during the oral exploration, the dental mirror will adhere to the oral mucosa or tongue, revealing an absence of saliva accumulation on the floor of the mouth or, when there is some saliva, that it is viscous and with a foamy appearance. In patients with hyposalivation, the tongue appears fissured, lobed, and with an atrophic appearance. The presence of caries is frequent, occurring mainly in the cervical or root areas [37]. Palpation of the salivary glands may detect certain degree of sialomegaly or swelling, which may be uni- or bilateral. The palpation must include extrabuccal and intrabuccal techniques (the bidigital form can be useful). The exit ostium of the glandular ducts should be examined to look for inflammation, and manipulation maneuvers including glandular expression may reveal little or viscous saliva coming out of the glandular orifices [5].

3.3 Sialometry

The degree of salivary glandular dysfunction should also be investigated. It is essential to differentiate whether the patient has xerostomia or hyposalivation. The most commonly used test to determine whether there is a decrease in the amount of saliva is sialometry [6]. There are different types of sialometry depending on whether the saliva from all glands is collected or whether the saliva is collected from individual glands. For clinical diagnosis, whole saliva collection is more useful. Sialometry will not be helpful in determining the cause of dry mouth [3].

The collection of salivary flow must be done first thing in the morning with the patient seated in an upright position. Ninety minutes before the procedure, the patient should not eat, rinse, drink, or smoke. Patients will collect their saliva in a graduated container. There are two types of saliva collection: at rest or unstimulated whole saliva (UWS) and under stimulation or stimulated whole saliva (SWS). When collecting saliva at rest, hyposalivation is defined as a salivary flow of <0.1 mL/min. Saliva should be collected for at least 10 min. The collection of stimulated saliva will require the patient to chew unflavored paraffin wax. Hyposalivation is diagnosed when the saliva flow is <0.5–0.7 mL/min. Stimulated saliva should be collected for at least 5 min [3, 5, 37, 38]. These two techniques are the most widely used. When the cause of dry mouth is medications, the unstimulated saliva is usually reduced, whereas the stimulated saliva values remain normal [5].

3.4 Biopsy of Minor Salivary Glands

Minor salivary gland biopsy may be useful in those older patients who are suspected of having SS (because they also suffer from dry eye) or other non-neoplastic diseases of systemic origin such as sarcoidosis, amyloidosis, or cystic fibrosis. In these conditions, the histological study will show the anatomopathological changes characteristic of each disorder. The biopsy is performed on the inner side of the lower lip [27].

3.5 Questionnaires

There are many available questionnaires for the evaluation of the severity of dry mouth [37]. One of the most widely used is the Xerostomia Inventory which contains 11 items. Each answer is scored using Likert-type options. This questionnaire is very useful to evaluate the degree of dry mouth caused by drugs, which is one of the most frequent causes of xerostomia in the older patient. This questionnaire is also recommended to assess the response to treatment [39]. The question "does your mouth usually feel dry?" has a high sensitivity but low specificity for the diagnosis of hyposalivation [37]. Other questions such as Does your mouth feel dry when eating a meal?; Do you have any difficulty swallowing?; Do you sip liquids to aid in swallowing dry food?; and Does the amount of saliva in your mouth seem to be too little or too much or you do not notice it? are also predictive of hyposalivation [5].

3.6 Other Diagnostic Methods

In some cases, other tests will be necessary to make a correct diagnosis, especially in those patients suffering from enlargement of one or more salivary glands. These tests include imaging techniques such as cone beam CT, magnetic resonance imaging (MRI), sialography, scintigraphy, and ultrasound. Another test used in cases of salivary gland tumors is fine-needle aspiration puncture [3].

In patients who also complain of dry eye, the determination of anti-SSA/SSB (anti-Ro/La) antibodies may be indicated. However, according to the 2016 classification criteria, only anti-SSA/Ro positivity is required. In rheumatic diseases, it is also useful to ask for serum levels of rheumatoid factor and antinuclear antibodies [11].

4 Treatment

The treatment of xerostomia and hyposalivation encompasses a series of interventions, which can range from preventive measures such as good oral hygiene and hydration, through the treatment of some systemic diseases, substitution of certain drugs, and treatment with local measures or systemic drugs. The response to the same treatment can vary in each patient. It is therefore essential that patients receive personalized treatments depending on their needs. In addition, it is advisable to have a dentist follow these patients on a regular basis.

4.1 Preventive Measures

Increasing the daily water intake is probably the first lifestyle measure to implement when trying to reduce symptoms. Preventive measures should include good oral hygiene with fluoride toothpaste and regular visits to the dentist (every 3-4 months) for topical fluoride application and control of dental caries [6, 27]. During these dental appointments, it may be necessary to take radiographs to evaluate the caries risk of each patient, perform professional prophylaxis as needed, counsel the patient on oral hygienic self-care measures, advise patients on the correct use of dentures [6], provide nutritional information, and counsel patients to increase fluid intake in the evenings and avoid spicy, acidic, or hard foods and alcoholic and caffeinated drinks [6, 37].

4.2 Changes or Reduction of Drugs

If the cause of xerostomia is possibly due to drugs, reducing the number of prescribed drugs, reducing the doses, or replacing them with safer pharmacological and non-pharmacological alternatives may be appropriate [6, 27]. In these cases, the patient's primary care clinician should be consulted. Decisions about changing, eliminating, or reducing the dose of the offending drug(s) will always be a shared responsibility between the physician and patient [37].

4.3 Local Measures

Salivary stimulants such as chewing gum or candies and saliva substitutes are commonly used local agents. Chewing gum and candies should be sugar-free to prevent dental caries. These gums often contain xylitol, which reduces cariogenic bacteria. However, individual patient preferences must be considered before recommending specific products for older patients [37, 40]. Studies have shown the efficacy of 1% malic acid spray in the treatment of dry mouth in patients treated with antihypertensives and antidepressants. However, a potential drawback of this treatment is its potential erosive effect on enamel [37]. Saliva substitutes imitate saliva and may provide symptomatic relief. They are commercialized in the form of gel, spray, rinses, or toothpaste and include different tastes and ingredients [37, 41]. They commonly contain xanthan gum, hydroxyethyl cellulose, carboxymethylcellulose, mucins, polyethylene oxide, linseed oil, olive oil, xylitol, and betaine, among others

[27]. They may be the first therapeutic option when there is severe glandular dysfunction, and thus the salivary glands cannot be stimulated. The composition of these substitutes should resemble saliva as much as possible and therefore should have a neutral pH, fluoride, and electrolytes. Patients tend to report greater comfort when using them without significant side effects, although their superiority over placebo is controversial [42–44]. There are other alternative therapies such as electrostimulation [45], acupuncture [46], or hyperbaric oxygen [47], but they are not widely available to all patients.

4.4 Systemic Sialogogues

Pilocarpine and cevimeline are the most well-studied and commonly used drugs to treat xerostomia. These medications are effective only if functioning salivary parenchyma remains [3, 6, 10, 27]. Pilocarpine is a non-selective muscarinic agonist and parasympathetic agent. The recommended dose is 5–30 mg/day, and the usual dose is 5 mg every 8 h for at least 3 months. The use of this drug is associated with a reduction in dry mouth in patients who have received head and neck radiotherapy. The maximum effect occurs after 2–3 months of use [3, 37]. Cevimeline is a selective muscarinic agonist for M1 and M3 receptors. It is longer acting than pilocarpine, and its standard dosing is 30 mg up to three times/day for at least 3 months [37].

These drugs have side effects and interactions and should be used with caution in older patients. Common side effects are sweating, bitter taste, urinary frequency, sialorrhea, gastritis, nausea, vomiting, bradycardia, hypotension, bronchoconstriction, and dyspnea, among others. Before prescribing these drugs, it is appropriate to involve a primary care physician. Moreover, parasympathomimetic drugs may antagonize anticholinergic effects, and as a result, both pilocarpine and cevimeline are contraindicated in patients with cardiovascular disease, asthma, kidney failure, chronic pulmonary disease, and glaucoma, as those patients taking beta adrenergic antagonists [3, 6, 27, 37, 43]. Some of these pathologies are frequent in the older patient, so this type of drugs should be used with caution.

4.5 Treatment of Sjögren's Syndrome

Patients with SS are often treated by rheumatologists. Concurrent lifestyle modifications, local measures, and systemic sialogogues may improve clinical manifestations. Immunomodulatory/immunosuppressive drugs such as glucocorticoids, antimalarials, immunosuppressive agents, intravenous immunoglobulins, and biologics may be helpful in patients with active systemic disease. Treatment should focus on restoring organ function as soon as possible and then establishing a dose capable of maintaining the initial response [10]. Alpha interferon has been used with mixed results [3], while rituximab decreases the glandular lymphocytic infiltrate present in this syndrome. Rituximab is useful in those cases where the patient has residual parenchyma [48]. However, there is no sufficient evidence to recommend one treatment over another nor the duration and dose to be used, so it is necessary to individualize the treatment [10].

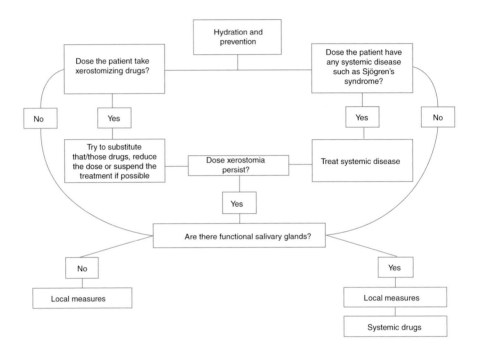

Treatment of xerostomia in the older patient

5 Practical Considerations

We have made a practical guide for dentists (Table 3) including recommendations for the diagnosis and treatment of salivary disorders in the older patient discussed throughout this chapter.

6 Future Research

Salivary alterations in the older patient are frequent. Future studies should further clarify the mechanisms, clinical manifestations, and consequences of chronic systemic diseases and prescription drugs most frequently associated with xerostomia and hyposalivation. The treatment of xerostomia in the older patient is complicated by the concurrent use of drugs indicated for the treatment of a wide variety of chronic medical and psychological conditions. Future research may include

Table 3 Practical considerations for the diagnosis and treatment of the older patient with xerostomia

Diagnosis	
Medical history	Patient's symptoms
	Dryness of other mucous membranes and skin
	Previous and current diseases and whether they are under control
	Record the drugs taken by the patient. Check if these drugs are associated with dry mouth
	Risk factors associated with dry mouth: tobacco, alcohol, caffeinated drinks, toothpastes, and mouthwashes containing irritants
Intraoral examination	Bright and atrophic oral mucosa
	Dental mirror adheres to the oral mucosa or tongue
	Lack of saliva or low saliva viscous and foamy
	Several cavities and oral candidiasis
	Little or viscous saliva coming out of the exist ostium of the glandular ducts
Extraoral examination	Uni- or bilateral swelling of the parotid glands
Diagnostic methods	Sialometry: hyposalivation UWS <0.1 mL/min; SWS <0.5–0.7 mL/min. Advised in all patients
	Biopsy of minor salivary glands: if suspected of SS, sarcoidosis, amyloidosis, and cystic fibrosis
	Imaging techniques: when there is enlargement of the glands
	Blood test: anti-SSA/SSB, rheumatoid factor, antinuclear antibodies, glycemia, thyroid tests
	To assess possible improvement after treatment, use Xerostomia Inventory questionnaire previously to possible treatment
Treatment	
No reduced salivary flow	Preventive measures: drinking more water, no alcohol, no caffeinated drinks, no smoking, good oral hygiene, regular dental visits
	Local measures: topical stimulators and/or substitutes and use of toothpaste and mouthwashes for dry mouth (without lauryl sulfate)
Reduced salivary flow	Take into consideration the previous measures
	Assess with the patient's physician whether the number or dose of drugs associated with salivary disorders can be reduced
	In severe cases, without response to previous measures, with residual glandular function, and in which the patient's health permits, the use of systemic sialogogues should be considered

long-term cohort studies that investigate the use of topical salivary substitutes and stimulators in patients for whom the discontinuation of drugs associated with xerostomia and hyposalivation is not realistic.

7 Conclusions

Salivary dysfunction is common in older adults. These conditions can alter oral function reducing older patients' quality of life. Hyposalivation is associated with caries and fungal infections. The etiology of xerostomia is diverse but in the older patient is usually associated with multiple chronic comorbidities and the prescription of multiple drugs. Dentists and physicians must be aware of the symptoms and signs associated with xerostomia and hyposalivation. The treatment of salivary dysfunction should be individualized according to the identified causes. In the older patient, it is essential to attempt to minimize or eliminate risk factors and to avoid the use of systemic salivary stimulants due to their potential for adverse drug effects. More research is needed to further examine the impact of safe and effective treatment strategies for older patients with salivary disorders.

References

1. Anil S, Vellappally S, Hashem M, Preethanath RS, Patil S, Samaranayake LP. Xerostomia in geriatric patients: a burgeoning global concern. J Investig Clin Dent. 2016;7(1):5–12.
2. Liu B, Dion MR, Jurasic MM, Gibson G, Jones JA. Xerostomia and salivary hypofunction in vulnerable elders: prevalence and etiology. Oral Surg Oral Med Oral Pathol Oral Radiol. 2012;114(1):52–60.
3. Saleh J, Figueiredo MA, Cherubini K, Salum FG. Salivary hypofunction: an update on aetiology, diagnosis and therapeutics. Arch Oral Biol. 2015;60(2):242–55.
4. Smith CH, Boland B, Daureeawoo Y, Donaldson E, Small K, Tuomainen J. Effect of aging on stimulated salivary flow in adults. J Am Geriatr Soc. 2013;61(5):805–8.
5. Pedersen AML, Sorensen CE, Proctor GB, Carpenter GH, Ekstrom J. Salivary secretion in health and disease. J Oral Rehabil. 2018;45(9):730–46.
6. Barbe AG. Medication-induced xerostomia and hyposalivation in the elderly: culprits, complications, and management. Drugs Aging. 2018;35(10):877–85.
7. Han P, Suarez-Durall P, Mulligan R. Dry mouth: a critical topic for older adult patients. J Prosthodont Res. 2015;59(1):6–19.
8. Haldeman SL, Baric JM, Saunders RH, Espeland MA. Hyposalivatory drug use, whole stimulated salivary flow, and mouth dryness in older, long-term care residents. Spec Care Dentist. 1989;9(1):12–8.
9. Moerman RV, Bootsma H, Kroese FG, Vissink A. Sjogren's syndrome in older patients: aetiology, diagnosis and management. Drugs Aging. 2013;30(3):137–53.
10. Ramos-Casals M, Brito-Zeron P, Bombardieri S, Bootsma H, De Vita S, Dorner T, et al. EULAR recommendations for the management of Sjogren's syndrome with topical and systemic therapies. Ann Rheum Dis. 2020;79(1):3–18.
11. Shiboski CH, Shiboski SC, Seror R, Criswell LA, Labetoulle M, Lietman TM, et al. 2016 American College of Rheumatology/European League Against Rheumatism classification criteria for primary Sjogren's syndrome: a consensus and data-driven methodology involving three international patient cohorts. Arthritis Rheumatol. 2017;69(1):35–45.
12. Lopez-Pintor RM, Casanas E, Gonzalez-Serrano J, Serrano J, Ramirez L, de Arriba L, et al. Xerostomia, hyposalivation, and salivary flow in diabetes patients. J Diabetes Res. 2016;2016:4372852.
13. Mauri-Obradors E, Estrugo-Devesa A, Jane-Salas E, Vinas M, Lopez-Lopez J. Oral manifestations of diabetes mellitus. A systematic review. Med Oral Patol Oral Cir Bucal. 2017;22(5):e586–e94.
14. Muralidharan D, Fareed N, Pradeep PV, Margabandhu S, Ramalingam K, Ajith Kumar BV. Qualitative and quantitative changes in saliva among patients with thyroid dysfunction prior to and following the treatment of the dysfunction. Oral Surg Oral Med Oral Pathol Oral Radiol. 2013;115(5):617–23.
15. Ahn-Jarvis JH, Piancino MG. Chapter 14: Impact of oral health on diet/nutrition. Monogr Oral Sci. 2020;28:134–47.

16. Lopez-Pintor RM, Lopez-Pintor L, Casanas E, de Arriba L, Hernandez G. Risk factors associated with xerostomia in haemodialysis patients. Med Oral Patol Oral Cir Bucal. 2017;22(2):e185–e92.
17. Hooper L, Abdelhamid A, Attreed NJ, Campbell WW, Channell AM, Chassagne P, et al. Clinical symptoms, signs and tests for identification of impending and current water-loss dehydration in older people. Cochrane Database Syst Rev. 2015;2015(4):CD009647.
18. Lacey J, Corbett J, Forni L, Hooper L, Hughes F, Minto G, et al. A multidisciplinary consensus on dehydration: definitions, diagnostic methods and clinical implications. Ann Med. 2019;51(3–4):232–51.
19. Sreebny LM, Schwartz SS. A reference guide to drugs and dry mouth-2nd edition. Gerodontology. 1997;14(1):33–47.
20. Smidt D, Torpet LA, Nauntofte B, Heegaard KM, Pedersen AM. Associations between labial and whole salivary flow rates, systemic diseases and medications in a sample of older people. Community Dent Oral Epidemiol. 2010;38(5):422–35.
21. Smidt D, Torpet LA, Nauntofte B, Heegaard KM, Pedersen AM. Associations between oral and ocular dryness, labial and whole salivary flow rates, systemic diseases and medications in a sample of older people. Community Dent Oral Epidemiol. 2011;39(3):276–88.
22. Villa A, Wolff A, Narayana N, Dawes C, Aframian DJ, Lynge Pedersen AM, et al. World Workshop on Oral Medicine VI: a systematic review of medication-induced salivary gland dysfunction. Oral Dis. 2016;22(5):365–82.
23. Wimardhani YS, Annisa W, Rahmayanti F. Medication intake and its influence on salivary profile of geriatric outpatients in Cipto Mangunkusumo Hospital. Dent J. 2012;45(3):138–43.
24. Nederfors T, Dahlöf C, Twetman S. Effects of the beta-adrenoceptor antagonists atenolol and propranolol on human unstimulated whole saliva flow rate and protein composition. Scand J Dent Res. 1994;102(4):235–7.
25. ATC/DDD guidelines of the World Health Organization Collaborating Centre for Drug Statistics Methodology.
26. Nonzee V, Manopatanakul S, Khovidhunkit SP. Xerostomia, hyposalivation and oral microbiota in patients using antihypertensive medications. J Med Assoc Thai. 2012;95(1):96–104.
27. Millsop JW, Wang EA, Fazel N. Etiology, evaluation, and management of xerostomia. Clin Dermatol. 2017;35(5):468–76.
28. Pedersen A, Sorensen CE, Proctor GB, Carpenter GH. Salivary functions in mastication, taste and textural perception, swallowing and initial digestion. Oral Dis. 2018;24(8):1399–416.
29. Peyron MA, Woda A, Bourdiol P, Hennequin M. Age-related changes in mastication. J Oral Rehabil. 2017;44(4):299–312.
30. Cichero JAY. Unlocking opportunities in food design for infants, children, and the elderly: understanding milestones in chewing and swallowing across the lifespan for new innovations. J Texture Stud. 2017;48(4):271–9.
31. Batisse C, Bonnet G, Eschevins C, Hennequin M, Nicolas E. The influence of oral health on patients' food perception: a systematic review. J Oral Rehabil. 2017;44(12):996–1003.
32. Bozorgi C, Holleufer C, Wendin K. Saliva secretion and swallowing-the impact of different types of food and drink on subsequent intake. Nutrients. 2020;12(1):256.
33. Serrano J, López-Pintor RM, Fernández-Castro M, Ramírez L, Sanz M, Casañas E, et al. Oral lesions in patients with primary Sjögren's syndrome. A case-control cross-sectional study. Med Oral Patol Oral Cir Bucal. 2020;25(1):e137–e43.
34. Maarse F, Jager DHJ, Alterch S, Korfage A, Forouzanfar T, Vissink A, et al. Sjögren's syndrome is not a risk factor for periodontal disease: a systematic review. Clin Exp Rheumatol. 2019;37:S225–S33.
35. Serrano J, Lopez-Pintor RM, Ramirez L, Fernandez-Castro M, Sanz M, Melchor S, et al. Risk factors related to oral candidiasis in patients with primary Sjogren's syndrome. Med Oral Patol Oral Cir Bucal. 2020;25(5):e700–e5.
36. Bodineau A, Folliguet M, Séguier S. Tissular senescence and modifications of oral ecosystem in the elderly: risk factors for mucosal pathologies. Curr Aging Sci. 2009;2(2):109–20.

37. Villa A, Connell CL, Abati S. Diagnosis and management of xerostomia and hyposalivation. Ther Clin Risk Manag. 2015;11:45–51.
38. Tanasiewicz M, Hildebrandt T, Obersztyn I. Xerostomia of various etiologies: a review of the literature. Adv Clin Exp Med. 2016;25(1):199–206.
39. Thomson WM, Chalmers JM, Spencer AJ, Williams SM. The Xerostomia Inventory: a multi-item approach to measuring dry mouth. Community Dent Health. 1999;16(1):12–7.
40. Kim HJ, Lee JY, Lee ES, Jung HJ, Ahn HJ, Jung HI, et al. Simple oral exercise with chewing gum for improving oral function in older adults. Aging Clin Exp Res. 2021;33(4):1023–31.
41. Furness S, Worthington HV, Bryan G, Birchenough S, McMillan R. Interventions for the management of dry mouth: topical therapies. Cochrane Database Syst Rev. 2011;(12):CD008934.
42. Barbe AG, Schmidt-Park Y, Hamacher S, Derman SHM, Noack MJ. Efficacy of GUM(R) Hydral versus Biotene(R) Oralbalance mouthwashes plus gels on symptoms of medication-induced xerostomia: a randomized, double-blind, crossover study. Clin Oral Investig. 2018;22(1):169–80.
43. Lopez-Pintor RM, Ramirez L, Serrano J, de Pedro M, Fernandez-Castro M, Casanas E, et al. Effects of Xerostom((R)) products on xerostomia in primary Sjogren's syndrome: a randomized clinical trial. Oral Dis. 2019;25(3):772–80.
44. Sinjari B, Feragalli B, Cornelli U, Belcaro G, Vitacolonna E, Santilli M, et al. Artificial saliva in diabetic xerostomia (ASDIX): double blind trial of aldiamed((R)) versus placebo. J Clin Med. 2020;9(7):2196.
45. Alajbeg I, Falcao DP, Tran SD, Martin-Granizo R, Lafaurie GI, Matranga D, et al. Intraoral electrostimulator for xerostomia relief: a long-term, multicenter, open-label, uncontrolled, clinical trial. Oral Surg Oral Med Oral Pathol Oral Radiol. 2012;113(6):773–81.
46. O'Sullivan EM, Higginson IJ. Clinical effectiveness and safety of acupuncture in the treatment of irradiation-induced xerostomia in patients with head and neck cancer: a systematic review. Acupunct Med. 2010;28(4):191–9.
47. Cankar K, Finderle Z, Jan J. The effect of hyperbaric oxygenation on postradiation xerostomia and saliva in patients with head and neck tumours. Caries Res. 2011;45(2):136–41.
48. Carubbi F, Cipriani P, Marrelli A, Di Benedetto P, Ruscitti P, Berardicurti O, et al. Efficacy and safety of rituximab treatment in early primary Sjögren's syndrome: a prospective, multi-center, follow-up study. Arthritis Res Ther. 2013;15:R172.

Management of Periodontal Disease in Older Adults

Nadia Laniado, Liran Levin, and Ira Lamster

The health and oral health needs of individuals change across the life course. In the oral cavity, the newborn does not have teeth present in the mouth, the first primary teeth begin to erupt between 6 and 9 months of age, and usually the last of the primary teeth exfoliates at 11 or 12 years of age. Beginning with the eruption of the permanent incisors at age 6 or 7, the teeth of the permanent dentition will need to function for 70, 80, or more years and are used multiple times each day, under the harsh conditions of the oral cavity. The maintenance of a functional dentition as a person ages is dependent on many factors, including personal oral hygiene practices and lifelong access to professional dental care. A functional and esthetic dentition, free from infection and pain, allows mastication of a healthy diet and is essential to the physical and emotional well-being of older adults.

This chapter will discuss the management of periodontal disease in the older adult from a holistic perspective. The focus will be on the concerns faced by patients and providers when caring for the oral healthcare needs of older adult patients, with the emphasis on the patient, and less so on specific techniques and procedures. The context will be management of periodontal disease in consideration of overall health, which assumes a larger role as a person ages.

N. Laniado
Department of Dentistry, Albert Einstein College of Medicine, Bronx, NY, USA

L. Levin
Faculty of Medicine and Dentistry, University of Alberta, Edmonton, AB, Canada

I. Lamster (✉)
School of Dental Medicine, Stony Brook University, Stony Brook, NY, USA
e-mail: ibl1@cumc.columbia.edu

1 Introduction

Globally, the prevalence of periodontitis is high. The Global Burden of Disease study identified severe periodontitis as the sixth most prevalent disorder across the globe [1]. Further, both the number of older adults (defined as 65 years of age and older) and the percentage of the population in high income countries that are in this category have increased dramatically in the last decade and are projected to continue to increase in the next few decades [2]. Since the extent and severity of periodontitis are more severe with age, identification and management of older adults with periodontitis is recognized as a significant global public health concern, and the prevalence of oral disease has not improved in the 25-year interval from 1990 to 2015 [3].

The United Nations highlighted this global population shift in its report "World Population Aging 2019" [4]. Highlights from that report include:

1. Almost all countries are seeing an increase in the number and percent of the population who are 65 years of age and older. The current global estimate of the number of older adults is 703 million people.
2. Longevity is also increasing across the globe. A person who reaches 65 years of age can expect to live another 17 years, and that number will increase in the future. Women outlive men by almost 5 years, but that difference will shrink in the future.
3. As populations age, the demands on the public health systems will also increase.
4. Population aging should be managed on the national level by certain policies targeting older adults, including promotion of healthy living, educational programs, universal healthcare, and a gradual rise in the traditional age of retirement.

In the United States, the aging of the population is a public health concern (Fig. 1). The percent of Americans who are 65 years of age and older has increased

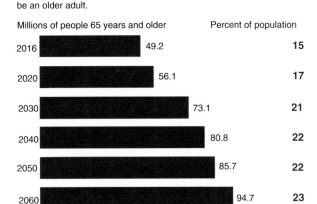

Fig. 1 Projections of the older adult population: 2020 to 2060. (Source: U.S. Census Bureau, 2017 National Population Projections; Vespa et al. [2])

dramatically. In 1960, only 9% of the population was 65 years of age and older. This percentage is projected to increase to 23% by 2060. By 2030, the percent of older adults in the population is projected to equal that of children and teenagers (21%). Further, the number of persons 85 years and older is projected to increase more than three times between 2014 and 2060, from 6 to 20 million [2]. For a more in-depth discussion on the topic, please refer to chapter "Epidemiology of Oral Health Conditions in the Older Population."

Regarding periodontitis, the prevalence in the United States is high and increases with age. The percentage of adults (30 years and older) with periodontitis has been estimated to be 42%, and almost 8% have severe periodontitis [5]. When examined by severity, the percent of individuals with any periodontitis, and the percent with moderate periodontitis, increases with increasing age, while the percentage with severe periodontitis increases until the early 50s and remains between 10 and 15% for older age groups. In addition to increasing age, other risk factors for severe periodontitis include race and ethnicity (Mexican American and non-Hispanic Black) and smoking [5].

Periodontitis is the major cause of tooth loss in older adults [6, 7] and loss of teeth can affect many aspects of a person's life. The ability to masticate normally is essential for consumption of a healthy diet. An intact and disease-free dentition allows for social interaction and avoidance of pain, resulting in better quality of life for older adults. Further, extensive oral disease, specifically periodontitis, has been associated with an increased risk of certain chronic diseases [8].

The importance of "Health in Aging" has been examined in a commentary that overviews the advances in our understanding of healthy aging [9]. Research in the past half century has led to a greater understanding of the biology of aging, how to differentiate aging from disease, as well as biological markers of the aging process. For many of the chronic health conditions that are more prevalent with aging, periodontitis has been documented as a risk factor, including cardiovascular disease [10], diabetes [11], respiratory disease [12], and Alzheimer's disease [13], or as a contributing factor in aging-associated disorders (i.e., frailty) [14]. These association studies have led to experimental studies that are identifying specific mechanisms that provide biologic plausibility for periodontitis as a risk factor for chronic diseases affecting older adults, for example, Alzheimer's disease [15]. For a more in-depth discussion on the topic of dementia, please refer to chapter "The 3 Ds: Dementia, Delirium and Depression in Oral Health."

A major emphasis is the need to reduce the period of disease so that the "health span" becomes as close as possible to the life span. This is an important concept for oral health. Further, Fried and Rowe [6] observed that health disparities will greatly influence this desired outcome. Disparities in access to oral healthcare and financial insecurity are major risk factors for oral diseases across the life course [16]. For a more in-depth discussion on the topic of health disparities, please refer to chapter "Health Disparities in Oral Health."

Periodontal disease, specifically periodontitis, is cumulative, and periodontal support for the dentition is reduced as a person ages, albeit at different rates for different individuals. Similar to many other chronic diseases that are common as a person ages, periodontitis is a chronic disease with periods of exacerbation and remission, but with a trajectory that results in greater extent and severity of disease over time [17]. The result is loss of support for the teeth and ultimately abscess formation and discomfort, with eventual need for tooth extraction with the goal of eliminating infection. Once teeth are lost, replacement is generally required, and many options are available. However, the cost of the most satisfactory solution (dental implants and a prosthetic superstructure) is beyond the financial reach of most of the population even in high income countries and is limited to a very few individuals in low and middle income countries.

The management of periodontal disease/periodontitis in older adults involves consideration of many factors, including:

1. The status of the periodontium, and the dentition, as well as the general condition of the oral cavity including the mucosal surfaces and contiguous structures including the temporomandibular joints and muscles of mastication.
2. Health history/health status, with consideration of chronic diseases. Often consultation with other healthcare providers is necessary. Medication use, both prescription and over the counter, must be evaluated.
3. Dental history/dental status, including the frequency of visits to an oral healthcare provider, and the daily self-care (oral hygiene) regimen.
4. Social, economic, and individual considerations, including health literacy and financial security.

The goal of evaluation and planning is to create a personalized treatment approach that is both appropriate and achievable for each person.

2 Normal Oral Aging Versus True Oral Pathology

Aging is defined as the "process of growing old" but age and pathology are not synonymous. Specifically, it is important to distinguish between the concepts of "chronologic age" and "biologic age." In the former case, we are referring to the passage of time, typically in units of years, and it always increases at a set rate, i.e., an older person has more years lived than a younger person. In contrast, biologic age (also referred to as physiologic or functional age) considers factors besides date of birth such as genetics, lifestyle (exercise, weight, smoking), nutrition, and the presence of other diseases [18]. For a more in-depth discussion on the topic of age-related changes, please refer to chapter "Age-Related Changes in Oral Health."

We now understand that there are "young-old" people whose biological age belies their chronological age. This has spawned a new field of "geroscience" that seeks to understand the mechanisms that make aging a risk factor for chronic disease and that attempts to measure the rate of aging [19, 20]. Because there are often significant variations in the effects and rates of aging, chronologic age and biologic age are often not aligned. This has significant consequences for the management of periodontal disease because treatment decisions should consider the individual variation in general health, host response, and disease expression [21].

Although with increased longevity there is an increased burden of oral disease (dental caries and periodontal disease), chronologic age alone does not have a negative influence on oral health [22]. It is therefore important to distinguish between normal effects of aging and oral disease [23]. In an older adult, normal signs of aging in the mouth would include up to 3 mm of buccal gingival recession, enamel wear and erosion, staining of any fracture lines, and darkening of teeth due to deposition of secondary dentin and enamel thinning [23]. However, in contrast to commonly held notions and beliefs, tooth loss is not a normal consequence of aging [24]. It is not age alone but the cumulative effect of other chronic systemic conditions (i.e., diabetes, osteoporosis), immunologic changes, pharmacologic interventions, functional limitations, and cognitive impairment which may have a negative effect on oral health. Personal situations, including health literacy and self-care, as well as access to professional oral healthcare, also play important roles. For a more in-depth discussion on these topics, please refer to chapters "Health Disparities in Oral Health", "The Role of Oral Health Literacy and Shared Decision Making", and "Barriers to Access Dental Care."

2.1 Salivary Function

Studies have shown that salivary function is well preserved in geriatric populations [25]. Xerostomia (dry mouth) is a condition that is often associated with old age, but it is not a consequence of aging in healthy older adults [26]. The most common cause of xerostomia in older adults are medications such as anticholinergics, tricyclic antidepressants, sedatives and tranquilizers, antihistamines, antihypertensives, and diuretics, which can dry out the oral mucosa and lead to problems with swallowing, mastication, communication, and denture retention [27, 28]. Other causes of xerostomia include several systemic conditions such as Sjogren's disease, HIV/AIDS, diabetes mellitus, and head and neck radiation therapy. A reduction in salivary production impacts the older adult with periodontitis since gingival recession accompanies loss of tooth support, exposing caries-prone root (cementum) surfaces. Overall, quality of life is greatly impacted, and individuals with dry mouth are at increased risk for dental caries, oral candidiasis, and other mucosal disorders. This becomes an even greater concern in older adults, who experience increased severity of periodontitis, accompanied by gingival recession and exposure of vulnerable root surfaces. It is therefore important for clinicians to recognize that dry mouth, although very common among older adults, is not a natural condition of aging and that the appropriate diagnosis must be ascertained to prescribe the appropriate therapy. For a more in-depth discussion on the topic of xerostomia, please refer to chapter "Xerostomia and Hyposalivation."

2.2 Periodontitis and Tooth Retention

Regarding the periodontium, recent surveillance from the National Health and Nutrition Examination Survey (NHANES) has shown that mild and moderate periodontal disease prevalence increases with age due to the cumulative nature of the disease, but interestingly, severe periodontal disease is not associated with increasing age. Periodontitis of moderate severity accounts for the majority of the age-related increase in the prevalence of periodontitis, whereas severe periodontitis prevalence is consistent at 15% or less, even among individuals 65 years and older [5]. This finding is likely attributable to the loss of the teeth at greater risk for periodontitis, and lost teeth are not generally included in periodontal indices.

Healthy aging is associated with good oral health [29]. A study of the oral health of centenarians and their offspring suggests that good oral health is a marker for systemic health and healthy aging [30]. In the Baltimore Longitudinal Study of Aging (BLSA) cohort, researchers found that there was substantial resiliency of the oral cavity during aging and that the oral cavity of healthy older people was comparable to that of healthy younger adults [31]. A study of the association between periodontal disease and mortality from all causes in the VA Dental Longitudinal Study concluded that periodontal status at baseline was a significant and independent predictor of mortality [32]. An interesting dichotomy is at play because aging alone does not contribute to oral pathology, but oral health does affects aging. It appears that it is not just that systemic disease influences oral health but that oral health influences certain chronic diseases [33, 34]. A pro-inflammatory phenotype is believed to be the mechanism underlying associations between periodontal disease and systemic diseases [35]. As noted, the severity of periodontitis is associated with an increased risk for diseases such as cardiovascular disease, diabetes, respiratory diseases, and Alzheimer's disease, as well as certain cancers, specifically lung and colorectal [36, 37].

2.3 Masticatory Function and Cognition

It is not only physical health but also mental health that plays a major role in healthy aging. Cognitive decline is a major concern among older adults, and its impact on oral health has been examined in several studies, although findings are not consistent. The interpretation of these studies is limited due to the bidirectional nature of poor oral health and impaired cognition, i.e., periodontal disease and tooth loss may be both risk factors for cognitive decline and consequences of cognitive decline. A recent systematic review assessing the relationship between oral health and cognitive function in older adults found that there was an association with specific domains of function such as learning and memory, complex attention, and executive function [38]. In the Atherosclerosis Risk in Communities (ARIC) study, a national prospective study of vascular disease among community-dwelling middle-aged adults (45–64 years old), they assessed a 6-year change in cognitive function and multiple oral health measures and behaviors [39]. All measures of cognitive decline were associated with increased odds of tooth loss, but they cautioned that because this was a cross-sectional analysis, the association between cognitive decline and oral health could represent associations in either, or both, directions [39]. A later study of the ARIC cohort, with a final sample of 911 individuals, concluded that although complete tooth loss was significantly associated with lower cognitive performance, the number of teeth and periodontal disease did not predict subsequent cognitive decline over an 8-year period. This contrasts with other studies that have suggested that tooth loss was associated with an increased risk of both dementia and cognitive decline [40]. A mechanism to account for periodontal disease as a direct contributing factor in dementia has been described. Using both murine models and human postmortem tissue samples, the major periodontal pathogen *Porphyromonas gingivalis* and specifically proteases known a gingipains have been identified as etiologic factors in Alzheimer's disease [15].

Increasingly the importance and contribution of masticatory function to oral health and overall health has been examined (Fig. 2). Among older adults, periodontal disease is the greatest cause of masticatory dysfunction [41]. Some recent studies suggest that masticatory dysfunction due to tooth loss and/or muscle weakness may in fact be a risk factor for dementia [41, 42]. Without adequate mastication, there is a lack of stimulation of the central nervous system which leads to atrophy of the hippocampus, the area of the brain which controls learning and memory [43].

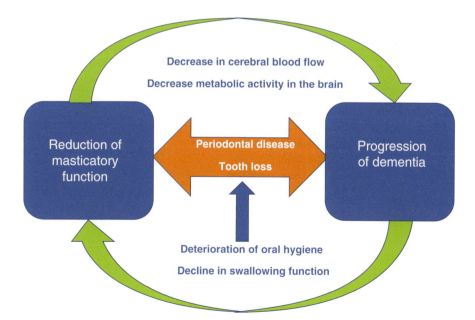

Fig. 2 Relationship between dementia and masticatory function. (Modified from Watanabe et al. (2015). Source: Watanabe et al. [41])

Animal studies support a reciprocal relationship between cognition and mastication such that a decrease in masticatory function due to tooth loss or soft diet may have negative consequences on aspects of cognitive health including spatial memory and learning ability [44]. There are some studies in humans; however, longitudinal studies are necessary to confirm a causal relationship as an explanation for the relationship between masticatory dysfunction and cognitive decline as many factors, including other comorbidities, nutrition, and reverse causation, may be at play.

3 Management of the Older Patient with Periodontal Disease

Periodontal disease is chronic, and the loss of soft and hard tissues is cumulative over the patients' lifetime [45, 46]. Older adults, thus, might present with more advanced cases of attachment and bone loss. The prevalence of periodontitis across the globe is high [1]. Severe periodontitis is most prevalent among adults 65 years or older, Mexican Americans, non-Hispanic Blacks, and smokers [5]. Dental practitioners should be aware of the high prevalence of periodontitis in US older adults and provide preventive care and counseling for this disease. In some cases, general dentists who encounter patients with periodontitis may refer these patients to see a periodontist for specialty care [5]. It is important, as for any patient and at any age, to properly diagnose and treat active periodontal disease as well as to correctly diagnose and maintain periodontal health on a reduced periodontium [47] (Fig. 3). The overarching goal should be to stabilize the periodontal condition by encouraging highly effective home self-care by the patients (or their caregivers when appropriate), eliminating areas of tissue inflammation and more involved periodontal defects, as well as ensuring frequent follow-up and professional maintenance visits. The treatment protocols for reducing inflammation and controlling periodontal disease are very similar in older adults to younger patients and should follow the same rationale [46, 47] (Fig. 4). Special attention should be paid to the manual dexterity of the patients to perform and maintain plaque control at home. Special aids should be provided and practiced individually to make sure proper home self-care is feasible and highly effective [47–50].

In recent years, there has been significant debate over the timing of recall intervals for dental appointments. Maintenance and recall visits should be individually tailored with consideration of the periodontal status, previous attachment loss, home self-care effectiveness, and adherence of the individual [50, 51]. Any deficiencies or concerns in the above parameters should prompt shorter intervals between recall and maintenance visits. The National Institute for Health and Care Excellence (NICE) in the United Kingdom issued guidelines for establishing individualized dental recall intervals [52]. For adults (18 years of age and older), the frequency was suggested to range between 3 and 24 months, dependent upon disease activity and risk factors. For older adults, however, those guidelines may not be appropriate, considering the multitude of factors that must be considered. Rather, consideration should be given to a frequency ranging from 1–2 months, when oral disease is advanced or when proper plaque control is difficult to achieve, to 6–12 months in very

Management of Periodontal Disease in Older Adults

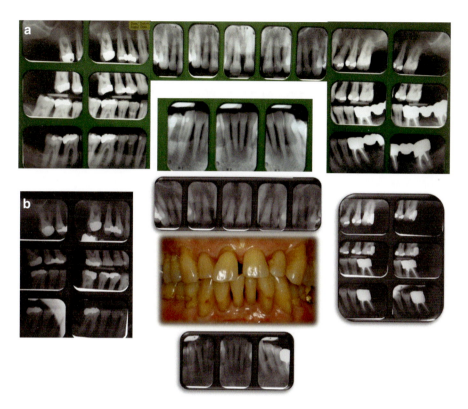

Fig. 3 A 76-year-old patient diagnosed with severe periodontal disease (**a**). Ten years following periodontal treatment (**b**), the dentition is stable, and the patient is well-maintained with no deep pockets or bleeding on probing

well-maintained and periodontally healthy individuals (Fig. 5). Factors that should be accounted for when recommending the frequency of maintenance visits include, among others, (1) oral hygiene and tobacco and alcohol consumption, (2) systemic risk and complicating factors that may influence the patient's periodontal health and their implications, (3) the outcome of previous care episodes and the suitability of previously recommended intervals, (4) the patient's ability to visit the dentist at the recommended interval, and (5) the financial costs to the patient [51]. It is important to realize that older individuals, with increasing complexity of oral and systemic conditions as well as, sometimes, decreasing ability to perform proper home self-care, will require more frequent maintenance visits.

Increasing patient knowledge of risk factors, their ability to modify risk, and providing a way for patients to quantify their risk empower patients to control their periodontal status and might help raise awareness and increase adherence. Some of the risk factors are modifiable, but others are non-modifiable, yet all need to be considered and explained to the patient. For example, plaque control by oral hygiene adherence and effectiveness is a major risk factor for periodontal disease that can be modified with proper education and training. Other risk factors are modifiable but with input from other healthcare providers. Uncontrolled or poorly controlled

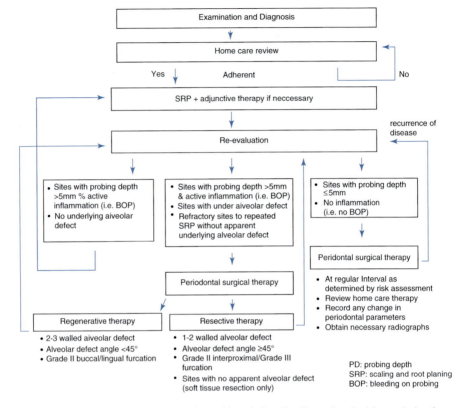

Fig. 4 A decision tree for treating a patient with periodontitis. (Reproduced with permission from Kwon et al. [46])

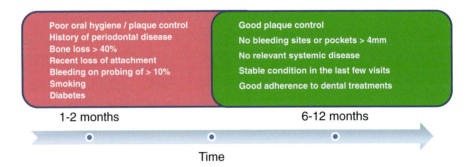

Fig. 5 Factors to be considered when determining frequency of periodontal maintenance visits. The frequency should range from 1–2 months in severe cases or in cases where proper plaque control is difficult to achieve (red box) to 6–12 months in very well-maintained and periodontally healthy individuals (green box)

diabetes is a risk factor for periodontitis, and improved glycemic control will both lessen the risk for systemic complications of diabetes and the risk of further progression of periodontitis [53]. In contrast, there is certainly a genetic component to periodontitis, which is non-modifiable [54]. Consequently, it becomes even more critical to emphasize modifiable risk factors. Goal setting has been recognized as a useful technique for improving oral health, and motivational interviewing is a broader technique that is also valuable in periodontal treatment [55].

4 Social Support and the Periodontium in Older Adults

There is ample evidence in the literature to suggest that social networks and connectedness are important determinants of good health and successful aging [56]. Social support is a modifiable risk factor for disease and thus can and should be addressed in the plan for an older individual's general as well as periodontal health. For older adults who may have limited social networks, this is an area where teledentistry may provide a crucial role and link to healthcare.

Although social support has long been recognized as an important determinant of general health (cardiovascular disease, pulmonary disease, mental health), research has increasingly recognized the impact of social support on clinical measures of oral disease, including periodontitis. Broadly defined, social support systems, also known as social networks, refer to the quality and quantity of social relationships that an individual has in their lives [57].The mechanism by which these networks affect health has been attributed to social norms, the diffusion of health-related knowledge, as well as stress resilience [58].

A few studies, including one of the English Longitudinal Study of Aging (ELSA) cohort, have found an association between structural social support and the number of remaining teeth among older adults [58, 59]. A recent study of individuals of Hispanic/Latino heritage found that US-born individuals with larger social networks had 17% lower odds of moderate-severe periodontal disease than those individuals born outside of the United States [60]. This protective effect of social capital on periodontal disease among the US Hispanic population is supported by other research and suggests that immigrant groups may be at higher risk of periodontal disease due to lack of social connectedness [61, 62].

5 Preserving Teeth or Placing Implant

In the past few decades, dental implants have assumed a fundamental role in periodontal therapy. Dental implants have consistently gained in popularity among providers and patients, sometimes at the expense of treating periodontal disease and retention of teeth. For the older adult population, it is very important to consider several important parameters before deciding to extract a tooth and replace it with a dental implant. There are various considerations when suggesting that older adults proceed with dental implant treatment. These factors include the ability to perform and maintain proper plaque control, the actual need for the implant, some common risk factors for periodontal disease and dental implant failure, as well as the risk for peri-implant diseases. It is also of utmost importance to define and explain the planned maintenance protocol to limit future complications.

5.1 Plaque Control: Current and Future

Plaque control is the most important determinant of long-term success of dental implants [63–65]. Adequate plaque control should be achieved and maintained prior to as well as following dental implant placement. It is important to review and practice home self-care measures prior to placement of dental implants to all patients, but this is even more important when treating an older population that will present with comorbidities and reduced manual dexterity needed to maintain proper plaque control. Proper instruments should be provided and recommended to older individuals who have difficulty using traditional cleaning aids. These might include large-handle toothbrushes, special interdental cleaning aids, and electric toothbrushes. In other cases, the caregivers will play a crucial role in maintaining proper plaque control, and they should be instructed and guided on how to perform proper home self-care. It should be emphasized that the teeth being replaced were lost for a reason, and in most cases, the reason is plaque-related dental diseases. Since plaque control is a crucial component in implant success, proper home self-care practices need to be established prior to implant placement to avoid implant complications that result from the same poor self-care habits that led to the loss of teeth.

When extraction of all teeth is planned, and implant treatment will be provided in the future, the situation allows for observation of the level of self-care. The extractions can be delayed, and the existing detention can be used to educate the patient about plaque control. When there is need for total clearance, the patient probably lost their teeth due to oral disease linked to poor plaque control. If this habit is not corrected, the risk for implant complications or failure increases.

5.2 The Need for Tooth Replacement

The need to provide a dental implant in place of a missing tooth should be carefully assessed and explained to the patient. A single posterior tooth that was missing for years with no apparent consequences might be a good example of a case where an implant is not necessarily indicated. It is well established that, in some cases, bicuspid occlusion or shortened arches can provide proper support for dental and oral functions, and these options should be kept in mind when approaching patients with missing teeth [66]. It was suggested that preserving 20 or more teeth (bicuspid occlusion) enables functions like biting, chewing, and enjoying almost all foods, regardless of the texture. This was established as a goal in some countries to encourage tooth preservation and proper dental care [67]. This concept has been shown to be well-accepted by dental providers and patients, and an analysis of nine systematic reviews concluded that this concept provided satisfactory function [68, 69]. This treatment approach was also determined to be cost-effective [70]. However, support is not universal [71], and there is a need for more long-term studies [68].

Many older patients will present with long-term partial edentulism, and their presenting condition should serve as evidence for the individual need for tooth replacement. The opposing dentition should also be examined carefully when determining the need for a dental implant. It is important to remember that a dental implant is a surgical procedure with possible short- and long-term complications [49, 63, 72], and therefore indications should be carefully weighed in consideration of possible adverse effects.

5.3 The Bone and General Healing Capacity of Older Adults

Overall, studies indicate that implants can be successfully placed in older adults. Since older adults might present with impaired healing capacity due to systemic diseases and altered metabolism, the osseointegration process as well as the soft tissue response around dental implants might be jeopardized. Further, all three stages of gingival/oral mucosal wound healing (inflammation, tissue formation, and remodeling) have been shown to be adversely affected by aging [73]. A variety of factors are involved in the long-term success of the implant, and special consideration should be taken prior to placing implants in older adults to limit the influence of those risk factors [74, 75]. Systemic conditions such as diabetes, osteoporosis, and other diseases that impair bone and soft tissue healing might delay or jeopardize implant success and survival. Specific treatments such as treatment with bisphosphonates might also lead to short- and long-term complications following surgical interventions, and thus, a thorough medical history is of utmost importance.

5.4 Other Diseases and Conditions that Might Influence Success (Diabetes, History of Periodontitis)

Common risk factors for periodontal disease and tooth loss as well as long-term implant survival were discussed previously. While aging itself is not considered a risk factor for implant loss [76], older individuals with a history of periodontal disease are at greater risk for implant failure over time [77–79]. These factors should be all taken into consideration when developing a treatment plan.

5.5 Maintenance Protocol

As discussed above, a maintenance protocol should be tailored to each patient according to an individualized assessment of existing severity of disease, identifiable risk factors, and home self-care and personal characteristics. Patients, especially older adults with dental implants, should be seen more frequently for maintenance visits to maintain adequate health of the dentition as well as to detect and treat early complications as soon as possible [49, 77]. While it is recognized that dental implants and the natural dentition have some important differences in their biologic characteristics, this risk profile should be considered when developing the maintenance protocol for patients with dental implants [80].

5.6 Consideration of Future Implant Complications

While a clinician may observe that an implant is an excellent option when compared to a tooth demonstrating advanced periodontal involvement or extensive caries, the need to consider the possibility of future implant complications is part of the treatment planning process. Peri-implant diseases are becoming more prevalent, and management of these complications, including implant failure, should factor into the treatment approach. A history of periodontal disease is a risk factor for the development of peri-implant disease [81] and should be taken into consideration since many older adult candidates for implant placement have lost their teeth due to periodontitis.

Peri-implant diseases are inflammatory conditions affecting the soft and hard tissues around dental implants. The main clinical characteristic of *peri-implant mucositis* is bleeding on gentle probing where erythema, swelling, and/or suppuration may also be present. *Peri-implantitis* is a plaque-associated pathological condition occurring in tissues around dental implants, characterized by inflammation in the peri-implant mucosa and subsequent progressive loss of supporting bone [82]. Peri-implant complications is a rather new concern, and its prevalence is increasing in recent years [82]. Older adults might be at increased risk for peri-implant diseases [80, 83]. Prevention is the most effective way to mitigate peri-implant disorders, and this begins with proper home self-care and regular professional care. Regular care will also allow for early detection of the disease [65, 84]. Since there is currently no "gold standard" of treatment for peri-implantitis lesions, prevention and early detection are of primary importance.

6 The Dental Office as a Point of Care in the Management and Screening for Systemic Disease

The dental office offers potential as a health location to promote general health and provide screening opportunities for conditions other than oral diseases [85]. Integration of dental professionals into the larger medical care system could advance efforts to identify and control prevalent conditions such as cardiovascular disease, diabetes mellitus, and respiratory disorders, each of which is associated with significant morbidity and healthcare costs [86]. Studies have suggested that a dental office is a suitable setting for the purpose of screening and referrals for these conditions and may result in medical expenditure savings [86–88]. The identified relationship between periodontal diseases and certain chronic systemic conditions should be emphasized and taken into consideration when treating the older adult with periodontitis.

Dental professionals can identify patients who are at risk for chronic systemic diseases and may otherwise not have the opportunity for screening [89, 90]. As an example, assessment of hyperglycemia in clinical dental settings has been widely studied and been found to be effective in identifying patients with previously unidentified hyperglycemia (glycated hemoglobin in the pre-diabetes and diabetes range) [91]. Referral to a medical provider for follow-up evaluation is an essential part of this new professional responsibility.

Promoting oral health might have a significant influence on general health as well, especially regarding cardiovascular diseases and diabetes. In a recent study which assessed the impact of periodontal treatment on diabetes-related healthcare costs in patients with diabetes, it was recommended that periodontitis, a possible complication of diabetes, should receive appropriate attention in diabetes management. The fixed-effect models showed −€12.03 (95% CI − €15.77 to −€8.29) lower diabetes-related healthcare costs per quarter of a year following periodontal treatment compared with no periodontal treatment. The findings of this study provide corroborative evidence for reduced general healthcare costs associated with conservative periodontal treatment in patients [92]. The staff at the dental office can also provide advice and help with other general preventive measures such as dietary consults and lifestyle changes to promote general health. Delivering a global message of overall health promotion may also make it easier to highlight the importance of oral health maintenance [88].

7 Conclusions

In the past, there was a common belief that tooth loss was part of aging, like hair loss, facial wrinkles, and other obvious signs of aging. Furthermore, patients sometimes would easily accept treatment plans that included tooth extraction. That is now changing, as many members of the generation born after the Second World War have enjoyed regular dental care and a complete or near-complete dentition as they age. As a profession, dentists and dental hygienists must constantly emphasize the importance of prevention of dental caries and periodontal diseases and dispel the notion that tooth loss is expected as a person ages.

This is an illogical situation. If a patient is told that a toe needed to be lost, they would demand an explanation and understand how they can prevent similar outcomes in the future. The emphasis on prevention of tooth loss did not exist in the past, but that is changing, and must be consistently reinforced. Patients lose teeth due to caries or periodontal diseases, both of which are plaque-induced and generally preventable. By truly emphasizing prevention, perhaps in the context of a general healthy lifestyle, oral healthcare professionals can change patients' perception and behavior [93]. In that sense, all dental practitioners must be aware of the unique challenges that present when caring for the oral health of older patients. This will require additional emphasis in both pre-doctoral and post-doctoral education.

One critically important consideration is the ability of older adults to afford dental care services. In the United States, dental insurance is often a benefit of employment and is lost when a person retires. The definition of "older adult" has tended to focus on 65 years of age, which is the age when US citizens often consider retirement and become eligible for Medicare insurance. Medicare provides medical benefits but very limited dental benefits and then only for "medically necessary services." Routine preventive dental care is not covered (https://www.medicare.gov/coverage/dental-services). In the United State, less than 30% of older adults have dental insurance [94]. Therefore, retention of teeth, with a focus on teeth at increased risk of being lost due to periodontitis (maxillary and mandibular molars), should begin early in life and be re-assessed as a person enters their adult years. Consequently, older adults are faced with significant out-of-pocket expenses when accessing dental services. This occurs at a time when financial resources are fixed, and the additive effects of dental disease may require more care than earlier in life.

The need for inclusion of oral health benefits for older adults in national health plans must be a part of the solution to the high prevalence of dental disease in older adults [95]. The emphasis on improving the oral health of children in the United States has not been realized by middle-aged and older adults [95, 96]. In the United States, the effort to add basic oral health benefits into the Medicare program is gaining traction [97] with the compelling arguments of improved oral health and quality of life for older adults, as well as the potential for substantial savings in healthcare expenditures [92, 98]. These benefits are primarily associated with the provision of preventive periodontal services. Oral healthcare professionals and dental professional organizations must lead the effort to enact this change.

In conclusion, research and clinical developments over the past 20 years have led to a re-evaluation of the approach to the management of the older patient with periodontitis. The identification of periodontitis as a risk factor for many chronic diseases, as well as the impact of certain chronic diseases and environmental factors (i.e., smoking) on the progression and management of periodontitis, requires a thorough understanding of these conditions, often in close consultation with other healthcare providers. Paradoxically, this situation is complicated by the success realized in reducing tooth loss, resulting in older adults with a greater number of teeth at risk for progression of periodontitis. Further, a reduced or disease-affected detention will negatively impact the quality of life of older adults.

The concern over the available resources to pay for periodontal care further complicates clinical management. The result is the need to develop individualized treatment approaches for each patient. Therefore, these considerations require a comprehensive, multidisciplinary, and interprofessional approach that can redefine the practice of dentistry in a context of health.

Acknowledgments Thanks are expressed to Cynthia Rubiera for assistance with preparation of the manuscript and Olivia Harris for technical support.

References

1. Kassebaum NJ, Bernabe E, Dahiya M, Bhandari B, Murray CJ, Marcenes W. Global burden of severe periodontitis in 1990–2010: a systematic review and meta-regression. J Dent Res. 2014;93(11):1045–53.
2. Vespa J, Medina L, Armstrong DM. Demographic turning points for the United States: population projections for 2020 to 2060. Current population reports. U.S. Census Bureau, Washington, DC, 2020. p. 25–114.
3. Kassebaum NJ, Bertozzi-Villa A, Coggeshall MS, Shackelford KA, Steiner C, Heuton KR, et al. Global, regional, and national levels and causes of maternal mortality during 1990–2013: a systematic analysis for the Global Burden of Disease Study 2013. Lancet. 2014;384(9947):980–1004.
4. United Nations, Department of Economic and Social Affairs, Population Division (2020). World Population Ageing 2019 (ST/ESA/SER.A/444).
5. Eke PI, Thornton-Evans GO, Wei L, Borgnakke WS, Dye BA, Genco RJ. Periodontitis in U.S. adults: National Health and Nutrition Examination Survey 2009–2014. J Am Dent Assoc. 2018;149(7):576–88 e6.
6. Stabholz A, Babayof I, Mersel A, Mann J. The reasons for tooth loss in geriatric patients attending two surgical clinics in Jerusalem. Israel Gerodontol. 1997;14(2):83–8.
7. Hull PS, Worthington HV, Clerehugh V, Tsirba R, Davies RM, Clarkson JE. The reasons for tooth extractions in adults and their validation. J Dent. 1997;25(3–4):233–7.
8. Beck JD, Papapanou PN, Philips KH, Offenbacher S. Periodontal medicine: 100 years of progress. J Dent Res. 2019;98(10):1053–62.
9. Fried LP, Rowe JW. Health in aging – past, present, and future. N Engl J Med. 2020;383(14):1293–6.
10. Liccardo D, Cannavo A, Spagnuolo G, Ferrara N, Cittadini A, Rengo C, et al. Periodontal disease: a risk factor for diabetes and cardiovascular disease. Int J Mol Sci. 2019;20(6):1414.
11. Genco RJ, Graziani F, Hasturk H. Effects of periodontal disease on glycemic control, complications, and incidence of diabetes mellitus. Periodontol 2000. 2020;83(1):59–65.
12. Gomes-Filho IS, Cruz SSD, Trindade SC, Passos-Soares JS, Carvalho-Filho PC, Figueiredo A, et al. Periodontitis and respiratory diseases: a systematic review with meta-analysis. Oral Dis. 2020;26(2):439–46.
13. Dioguardi M, Crincoli V, Laino L, Alovisi M, Sovereto D, Mastrangelo F, et al. The role of periodontitis and periodontal bacteria in the onset and progression of Alzheimer's disease: a systematic review. J Clin Med. 2020;9(2):495. https://doi.org/10.3390/jcm9020495.
14. Castrejon-Perez RC, Borges-Yanez SA. Frailty from an oral health point of view. J Frailty Aging. 2014;3(3):180–6.

15. Dominy SS, Lynch C, Ermini F, Benedyk M, Marczyk A, Konradi A, et al. Porphyromonas gingivalis in Alzheimer's disease brains: evidence for disease causation and treatment with small-molecule inhibitors. Sci Adv. 2019;5(1):eaau3333.
16. Cardoso EOC, Tenenbaum HC. Older adults and the disparity in oral health status; the problem and innovative ways to address it. Isr J Health Policy Res. 2020;9(1):24.
17. Ramseier CA, Anerud A, Dulac M, Lulic M, Cullinan MP, Seymour GJ, et al. Natural history of periodontitis: disease progression and tooth loss over 40 years. J Clin Periodontol. 2017;44(12):1182–91.
18. Jazwinski SM, Kim S. Examination of the dimensions of biological age. Front Genet. 2019;10:263.
19. Kennedy BK, Berger SL, Brunet A, Campisi J, Cuervo AM, Epel ES, et al. Geroscience: linking aging to chronic disease. Cell. 2014;159(4):709–13.
20. Belsky DW, Caspi A, Arseneault L, Baccarelli A, Corcoran DL, Gao X, et al. Quantification of the pace of biological aging in humans through a blood test, the DunedinPoAm DNA methylation algorithm. elife. 2020;9:1–25. https://doi.org/10.7554/eLife.54870.
21. Ebersole JL, Dawson DA 3rd, Emecen Huja P, Pandruvada S, Basu A, Nguyen L, et al. Age and periodontal health - immunological view. Curr Oral Health Rep. 2018;5(4):229–41.
22. De Rossi SS, Slaughter YA. Oral changes in older patients: a clinician's guide. Quintessence Int. 2007;38(9):773–80.
23. Lamster IB, Asadourian L, Del Carmen T, Friedman PK. The aging mouth: differentiating normal aging from disease. Periodontol 2000. 2016;72(1):96–107.
24. Griffin SO, Jones JA, Brunson D, Griffin PM, Bailey WD. Burden of oral disease among older adults and implications for public health priorities. Am J Public Health. 2012;102(3):411–8.
25. Astor FC, Hanft KL, Ciocon JO. Xerostomia: a prevalent condition in the elderly. Ear Nose Throat J. 1999;78(7):476–9.
26. Turner MD, Ship JA. Dry mouth and its effects on the oral health of elderly people. J Am Dent Assoc. 2007;138(Suppl):15S–20S.
27. Sreebny LM, Schwartz SS. A reference guide to drugs and dry mouth–2nd edition. Gerodontology. 1997;14(1):33–47.
28. Barbe AG. Medication-induced xerostomia and hyposalivation in the elderly: culprits, complications, and management. Drugs Aging. 2018;35(10):877–85.
29. Tonetti MS, Bottenberg P, Conrads G, Eickholz P, Heasman P, Huysmans MC, et al. Dental caries and periodontal diseases in the ageing population: call to action to protect and enhance oral health and well-being as an essential component of healthy ageing – consensus report of group 4 of the joint EFP/ORCA workshop on the boundaries between caries and periodontal diseases. J Clin Periodontol. 2017;44(Suppl 18):S135–S44.
30. Kaufman LB, Setiono TK, Doros G, Andersen S, Silliman RA, Friedman PK, et al. An oral health study of centenarians and children of centenarians. J Am Geriatr Soc. 2014;62(6):1168–73.
31. Ship JA, Baum BJ. Old age in health and disease. Lessons from the oral cavity. Oral Surg Oral Med Oral Pathol. 1993;76(1):40–4.
32. Garcia RI, Krall EA, Vokonas PS. Periodontal disease and mortality from all causes in the VA Dental Longitudinal Study. Ann Periodontol. 1998;3(1):339–49.
33. Chapple IL, Bouchard P, Cagetti MG, Campus G, Carra MC, Cocco F, et al. Interaction of lifestyle, behaviour or systemic diseases with dental caries and periodontal diseases: consensus report of Group 2 of the joint EFP/ORCA workshop on the boundaries between caries and periodontal diseases. J Clin Periodontol. 2017;44(Suppl 18):S39–51.
34. Sanz M, Ceriello A, Buysschaert M, Chapple I, Demmer RT, Graziani F, et al. Scientific evidence on the links between periodontal diseases and diabetes: consensus report and guidelines of the joint workshop on periodontal diseases and diabetes by the International Diabetes Federation and the European Federation of Periodontology. J Clin Periodontol. 2018;45(2):138–49.
35. Hajishengallis G. Periodontitis: from microbial immune subversion to systemic inflammation. Nat Rev Immunol. 2015;15(1):30–44.

36. Michaud DS, Lu J, Peacock-Villada AY, Barber JR, Joshu CE, Prizment AE, et al. Periodontal disease assessed using clinical dental measurements and cancer risk in the ARIC study. J Natl Cancer Inst. 2018;110(8):843–54.
37. Lalla E, Papapanou PN. Diabetes mellitus and periodontitis: a tale of two common interrelated diseases. Nat Rev Endocrinol. 2011;7(12):738–48.
38. Nangle MR, Riches J, Grainger SA, Manchery N, Sachdev PS, Henry JD. Oral health and cognitive function in older adults: a systematic review. Gerontology. 2019;65(6):659–72.
39. Naorungroj S, Slade GD, Beck JD, Mosley TH, Gottesman RF, Alonso A, et al. Cognitive decline and oral health in middle-aged adults in the ARIC study. J Dent Res. 2013;92(9):795–801.
40. Batty GD, Li Q, Huxley R, Zoungas S, Taylor BA, Neal B, et al. Oral disease in relation to future risk of dementia and cognitive decline: prospective cohort study based on the Action in Diabetes and Vascular Disease: Preterax and Diamicron Modified-Release Controlled Evaluation (ADVANCE) trial. Eur Psychiatry. 2013;28(1):49–52.
41. Watanabe Y, Hirohiko H, Matsushita K. How masticatory function and periodontal disease relate to senile dementia. Jpn Dent Sci Rev. 2015;51(1):34–40. https://doi.org/10.1016/j.jdsr.2014.09.002.
42. Lin CS. Revisiting the link between cognitive decline and masticatory dysfunction. BMC Geriatr. 2018;18(1):5.
43. Fukushima-Nakayama Y, Ono T, Hayashi M, Inoue M, Wake H, Ono T, et al. Reduced mastication impairs memory function. J Dent Res. 2017;96(9):1058–66.
44. Weijenberg RAF, Delwel S, Ho BV, van der Maarel-Wierink CD, Lobbezoo F. Mind your teeth-the relationship between mastication and cognition. Gerodontology. 2019;36(1):2–7.
45. Chapple ILC, Mealey BL, Van Dyke TE, Bartold PM, Dommisch H, Eickholz P, et al. Periodontal health and gingival diseases and conditions on an intact and a reduced periodontium: consensus report of workgroup 1 of the 2017 world workshop on the classification of periodontal and Peri-implant diseases and conditions. J Clin Periodontol. 2018;45(Suppl 20):S68–77.
46. Kwon T, Lamster IB, Levin L. Current concepts in the management of periodontitis. Int Dent J. 2020:1–15. https://onlinelibrary.wiley.com/doi/epdf/10.1111/idj.12630.
47. Sanz M, Herrera D, Kebschull M, Chapple I, Jepsen S, Beglundh T, et al. Treatment of stage I-III periodontitis-the EFP S3 level clinical practice guideline. J Clin Periodontol. 2020;47(Suppl 22):4–60.
48. Clark-Perry D, Levin L. Systematic review and meta-analysis of randomized controlled studies comparing oscillating-rotating and other powered toothbrushes. J Am Dent Assoc. 2020;151(4):265–75 e6.
49. Kwon T, Salem DM, Levin L. Nonsurgical periodontal therapy based on the principles of cause-related therapy: rationale and case series. Quintessence Int. 2019;50(5):370–6.
50. Kwon T, Levin L. Cause-related therapy: a review and suggested guidelines. Quintessence Int. 2014;45(7):585–91.
51. Dental checks: intervals between oral health reviews. NICE interactive flowchart – Oral and dental health. https://www.nice.org.uk/guidance/cg19.
52. Akram S, D'Cruz L. Implementing NICE guidelines on recall intervals into general practice. Dent Update. 2010;37(7):454–62.
53. Kocher T, Konig J, Borgnakke WS, Pink C, Meisel P. Periodontal complications of hyperglycemia/diabetes mellitus: epidemiologic complexity and clinical challenge. Periodontol 2000. 2018;78(1):59–97.
54. Stabholz A, Soskolne WA, Shapira L. Genetic and environmental risk factors for chronic periodontitis and aggressive periodontitis. Periodontol. 2000;2010(53):138–53.
55. Newton JT, Asimakopoulou K. Managing oral hygiene as a risk factor for periodontal disease: a systematic review of psychological approaches to behaviour change for improved plaque control in periodontal management. J Clin Periodontol. 2015;42(Suppl 16):S36–46.
56. Martire LM, Franks MM. The role of social networks in adult health: introduction to the special issue. Health Psychol. 2014;33(6):501–4.
57. Cattell V. Poor people, poor places, and poor health: the mediating role of social networks and social capital. Soc Sci Med. 2001;52(10):1501–16.

58. Rouxel P, Tsakos G, Demakakos P, Zaninotto P, Watt RG. Social capital and oral health among adults 50 years and older: results from the English longitudinal study of ageing. Psychosom Med. 2015;77(8):927–37.
59. Aida J, Hanibuchi T, Nakade M, Hirai H, Osaka K, Kondo K. The different effects of vertical social capital and horizontal social capital on dental status: a multilevel analysis. Soc Sci Med. 2009;69(4):512–8.
60. Laniado N, Badner VM, Sanders AE, Singer RH, Finlayson TL, Hua S, et al. Social capital and periodontal disease in Hispanic/Latino adults in the United States: results from the Hispanic Community Health Study/Study of Latinos. J Clin Periodontol. 2020;47(5):542–51.
61. Maupome G, McConnell WR, Perry BL. Dental problems and Familismo: social network discussion of oral health issues among adults of Mexican origin living in the Midwest United States. Community Dent Health. 2016;33(4):303–8.
62. Viruell-Fuentes EA, Schulz AJ. Toward a dynamic conceptualization of social ties and context: implications for understanding immigrant and Latino health. Am J Public Health. 2009;99(12):2167–75.
63. Rokaya D, Srimaneepong V, Wisitrasameewon W, Humagain M, Thunyakitpisal P. Peri-implantitis update: risk indicators, diagnosis, and treatment. Eur J Dent. 2020;14(4):672–82.
64. Anner R, Grossmann Y, Anner Y, Levin L. Smoking, diabetes mellitus, periodontitis, and supportive periodontal treatment as factors associated with dental implant survival: a long-term retrospective evaluation of patients followed for up to 10 years. Implant Dent. 2010;19(1):57–64.
65. Clark D, Levin L. Dental implant management and maintenance: how to improve long-term implant success? Quintessence Int. 2016;47(5):417–23.
66. Miyazaki H, Motegi E, Yatabe K, Yamaguchi H, Maki Y. A study of occlusion in elderly Japanese over 80 years with at least 20 teeth. Gerodontology. 2005;22(4):206–10.
67. Morita I. Retained tooth numbers and history of diet and lifestyle in the elderly aged 60, 70 and 80 years. J Dental Health. 1996;46(5):688–706
68. Khan SB, Chikte UM, Omar R. An overview of systematic reviews related to aspects of the shortened dental arch and its variants in adults. Int J Prosthodont. 2017;30(4):357–66.
69. Fueki K, Baba K. Shortened dental arch and prosthetic effect on oral health-related quality of life: a systematic review and meta-analysis. J Oral Rehabil. 2017;44(7):563–72.
70. Levey C, Dunbar C. Shortened dental arch concept shown to be cost effective. Evid Based Dent. 2015;16(1):19–20.
71. Manola M, Hussain F, Millar BJ. Is the shortened dental arch still a satisfactory option? Br Dent J. 2017;223(2):108–12.
72. Cortellini S, Favril C, De Nutte M, Teughels W, Quirynen M. Patient compliance as a risk factor for the outcome of implant treatment. Periodontol 2000. 2019;81(1):209–25.
73. Smith PC, Caceres M, Martinez C, Oyarzun A, Martinez J. Gingival wound healing: an essential response disturbed by aging? J Dent Res. 2015;94(3):395–402.
74. Vignoletti F, Di Domenico GL, Di Martino M, Montero E, de Sanctis M. Prevalence and risk indicators of peri-implantitis in a sample of university-based dental patients in Italy: a cross-sectional study. J Clin Periodontol. 2019;46(5):597–605.
75. Compton SM, Clark D, Chan S, Kuc I, Wubie BA, Levin L. Dental implants in the elderly population: a long-term follow-up. Int J Oral Maxillofac Implants. 2017;32(1):164–70.
76. Becker W, Hujoel P, Becker BE, Wohrle P. Dental implants in an aged population: evaluation of periodontal health, bone loss, implant survival, and quality of life. Clin Implant Dent Relat Res. 2016;18(3):473–9.
77. Monje A, Insua A, Wang HL. Understanding peri-implantitis as a plaque-associated and site-specific entity: on the local predisposing factors. J Clin Med. 2019;8(2):279.
78. Serino G, Hultin K. Peri-implant disease and prosthetic risk indicators: a literature review. Implant Dent. 2019;28(2):125–37.
79. Levin L, Ofec R, Grossmann Y, Anner R. Periodontal disease as a risk for dental implant failure over time: a long-term historical cohort study. J Clin Periodontol. 2011;38(8):732–7.

80. Eggert FM, Levin L. Biology of teeth and implants: the external environment, biology of structures, and clinical aspects. Quintessence Int. 2018;49(4):301–12.
81. Romandini M, Lima C, Pedrinaci I, Araoz A, Soldini MC, Sanz M. Prevalence and risk/protective indicators of peri-implant diseases: a university-representative cross-sectional study. Clin Oral Implants Res. 2021;32(1):112–22.
82. Berglundh T, Armitage G, Araujo MG, Avila-Ortiz G, Blanco J, Camargo PM, et al. Peri-implant diseases and conditions: consensus report of workgroup 4 of the 2017 world workshop on the classification of periodontal and Peri-implant diseases and conditions. J Clin Periodontol. 2018;45(Suppl 20):S286–S91.
83. Schwarz F, Derks J, Monje A, Wang HL. Peri-implantitis. J Periodontol. 2018;89(Suppl 1):S267–S90.
84. Cheung MC, Hopcraft MS, Darby IB. Patient-reported oral hygiene and implant outcomes in general dental practice. Aust Dent J. 2020;66(1):49–60.
85. Levin L. Editorial: medicine and dentistry: different entities? Quintessence Int. 2015;46(5):371.
86. Glick M, Greenberg BL. The role of oral health care professionals in providing medical services. J Dent Educ. 2017;81(8):eS180–eS5.
87. Jontell M, Glick M. Oral health care professionals' identification of cardiovascular disease risk among patients in private dental offices in Sweden. J Am Dent Assoc. 2009;140(11):1385–91.
88. Nasseh K, Greenberg B, Vujicic M, Glick M. The effect of chairside chronic disease screenings by oral health professionals on health care costs. Am J Public Health. 2014;104(4):744–50.
89. Myers-Wright N, Lamster IB, Jasek JP, Chamany S. Evaluation of medical and dental visits in New York City: opportunities to identify persons with and at risk for diabetes mellitus in dental settings. Community Dent Oral Epidemiol. 2018;46(1):102–8.
90. Neidell M, Lamster IB, Shearer B. Cost-effectiveness of diabetes screening initiated through a dental visit. Community Dent Oral Epidemiol. 2017;45(3):275–80.
91. Glurich I, Bartkowiak B, Berg RL, Acharya A. Screening for dysglycaemia in dental primary care practice settings: systematic review of the evidence. Int Dent J. 2018;68(6):369–77.
92. Smits KPJ, Listl S, Plachokova AS, Van der Galien O, Kalmus O. Effect of periodontal treatment on diabetes-related healthcare costs: a retrospective study. BMJ Open Diabetes Res Care. 2020;8(1):e001666
93. Sheiham A, Watt RG. The common risk factor approach: a rational basis for promoting oral health. Community Dent Oral Epidemiol. 2000;28(6):399–406.
94. Raphael C. Oral health and aging. Am J Public Health. 2017;107(S1):S44–S5.
95. Kossioni AE, Hajto-Bryk J, Maggi S, McKenna G, Petrovic M, Roller-Wirnsberger RE, et al. An expert opinion from the European College of Gerodontology and the European Geriatric Medicine Society: European Policy Recommendations on Oral Health in Older Adults. J Am Geriatr Soc. 2018;66(3):609–13.
96. Al-Nasser L, Lamster IB. Prevention and management of periodontal diseases and dental caries in the older adults. Periodontol 2000. 2020;84(1):69–83.
97. Slavkin HC, Santa FG. A national imperative: oral health services in Medicare. J Am Dent Assoc. 2017;148(5):281–3.
98. Jeffcoat MK, Jeffcoat RL, Gladowski PA, Bramson JB, Blum JJ. Impact of periodontal therapy on general health: evidence from insurance data for five systemic conditions. Am J Prev Med. 2014;47(2):166–74.

Management of Caries in Older Adults

Gerry McKenna, Martina Hayes, and Cristiane DaMata

1   Global Epidemiology

Globally we are seeing the effects of an aging population. In many high income countries, as birth rates fall and life expectancy increases, the proportion of older adults within the general population has increased significantly. As fertility rates move towards lower levels, mortality decline, especially at older ages, assumes an increasingly important role in population aging. In low and middle income countries, where low fertility has prevailed for a significant period of time, relative increases in the older population are now primarily determined by improved chances of surviving to old age [1]. Over the next 50 years, life expectancy at birth is projected to increase globally by 10 years, to reach 76 years in 2045–2050. By the end of the next quarter century, life expectancy at birth is expected to reach, on average, 80 years in the more economically developed regions and 71 years in the less economically developed regions. As a result of the generalized shift in the age distribution of mortality towards older groups, more people will survive into their seventh, eighth and ninth decades around the world [2].

G. McKenna (✉)
Centre for Public Health, Queen's University Belfast, Belfast, Northern Ireland, UK
e-mail: G.McKenna@qub.ac.uk

M. Hayes · C. DaMata
Cork University Dental School and Hospital, University College Cork, Cork, Ireland

© The Author(s), under exclusive license to Springer Nature Switzerland AG 2022
C.-M. Hogue, J. G. Ruiz (eds.), *Oral Health and Aging*,
https://doi.org/10.1007/978-3-030-85993-0_7

2 The Oral Health of Older Adults

Epidemiological dental surveys from around the world clearly indicate that tooth retention has increased significantly amongst older adults as they retain their natural teeth into old age [3]. Unfortunately, the cumulative nature of the two main destructive dental diseases: caries and periodontitis, dictate that aging is always likely to be a factor associated with total tooth loss particularly amongst patients in lower socio-economic groups [4]. Clear socio-economic gradients in complete tooth loss have been identified in many countries, including the United Kingdom, Japan, Korea and in Scandinavia [3, 5–7].

Although the overall prevalence of total tooth loss has fallen sharply over recent decades, many patients now become edentate at an older age when they are generally less able to adapt to the limitations of complete dentures. The attitudes of older patients to oral health also appear to have changed as many take advantage of widely available sources of information and demand more from the dental profession. As a result, increasing numbers expect conservative treatment approaches rather than those previously centered around extractions and subsequent replacement of natural teeth [8].

While increasing tooth retention is seen as a leap forward in the oral health of the older population, it also brings with it the challenges of managing chronic dental diseases, including caries and periodontal disease. Due to factors, such as diet, reduced manual dexterity and xerostomia, these chronic diseases can cause considerable pain and suffering amongst older patients and impair oral function [9]. Dental caries remains a problem for this age group with a high prevalence of coronal and root surface caries found amongst old-age populations [10, 11]. In the 1998 UK Adult Dental Health Survey, the proportion of adults with 18 or more sound and unrestored teeth was only 5% amongst those aged 55 years and over [12]. The 2009 UK Adult Dental Health Survey indicated that this figure had improved but still remained at only 13% [12, 13]. The 2009 UK Adult Dental Health Survey reported that 27% of adults aged 65–74 years had evidence of dental caries whilst this figure increased to 40% for those aged 75–84 years [13].

The 1998 UK Dental Health Survey showed that almost 25% of the older adults had 12 or more teeth with a root surface that was either exposed, worn, filled or decayed [12]. The 2009 Survey reported that 73% of all adults had exposed root surfaces, and this increased to 90% for those aged over 55 years. The same survey reported that 11% of 55–64 years old had active root caries compared with 20% of those aged 75–84 years [13].

3 Oral Health in Long-Term Care Facilities (LTCFS)

It is widely reported that the oral health status of older adults within LTCFs is significantly worse than their community living peers [14]. With increasing age, the ability to care for their mouth deteriorates: polypharmacy leads to xerostomia, and diets can become rich in sugars, while good daily oral hygiene is essential for the maintenance of complex dental restorations. All these factors increase the risk of oral disease and directly impact comorbidities.

Unfortunately, a growing proportion of residents in LTCFs are unable to self-care, and with increasing dependency, oral hygiene practices present a significant challenge. Current prevention practices and service provision in LTCFs is often poor. Challenges include inadequate resources and training, and these are compounded by high staff turnover. There is a significant difficulty in obtaining routine dental care due to the very complex needs of institutionalized older people, with a significant proportion suffering from cognitive impairment and dementia. Access to domiciliary dental services is often limited with subsequent admission to hospitals for dental problems which can be distressing for individuals and their families and very costly to the healthcare provider [2].

Within the United Kingdom, the National Institute for Health and Care Excellence (NICE) publishes evidence-based guidelines on all aspects of healthcare. In 2016, NICE published 'Oral health for adults in care homes (NG48)' which included a series of recommendations for LTCFs, including improving access to dental services for LTCF residents, improving the oral health knowledge and skills of care home staff and the implementation of oral health assessments, mouth care plans and daily oral care for all residents [15]. However, adoption of these recommendations has been challenging in many LTCFs as demonstrated by follow-up surveys in the United Kingdom [16]. For a more in-depth discussion on the topic of long-term care, please refer to chapter "Oral Care in Long-Term Care Settings".

4 Dental Caries

Dental caries is a multifactorial, bacterially mediated process that results in the destruction of mineralized tooth tissues. In light of the emergence of the partially dentate older population, there is a need for clinicians to understand the caries disease process in order to establish effective preventive and management regimes. However, older patients can present with some unique etiological considerations which increase their risk of developing dental caries particularly on the root surface [17]. Root caries as 'a cavitation below the cement-enamel junction (CEJ), not usually including the adjacent enamel, usually discoloured, softened, ill-defined and involving both cementum and underlying dentine' [18]. The root surface may be particularly vulnerable to mechanical destruction compared to enamel due to differences in the structure and chemical composition of cementum and dentine. In a population who are frequently exposed to scaling by dental health professionals, the cementum layer is frequently abraded away, exposing the dentine (Fig. 1). Root cementum and dentine are structurally different from enamel and react differently to cariogenic challenges – of note the critical pH of dentine and cementum is approximately 6.4 while that of enamel is 5.5.

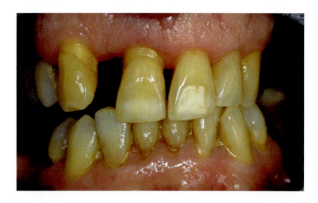

Fig. 1 Exposed root surfaces in a partially dentate older patient

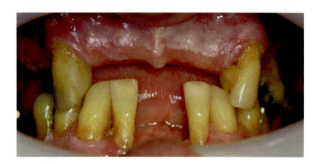

Fig. 2 Root caries in a partially dentate older patient

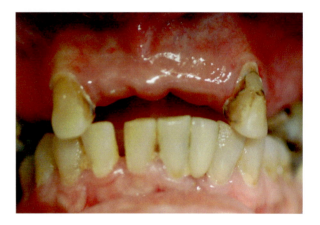

Fig. 3 Root caries in the abutment teeth for a removable partial denture

5 Diagnosing Root Surface Caries

The most common clinical descriptors of root caries are visual-tactile changes in the root surface (Figs. 2 and 3). Colour can range from tan to brown to black, and while color change is indicative of root caries, no correlation has been shown between color and lesion activity. Texture appears to be a better indicator of lesion activity, with active lesions being less resistant to gently probing than quiescent or arrested lesions [19]. Many root caries lesions develop on the proximal surfaces and up to 20% can occur subgingivally [20]. These areas are challenging for the clinician to visualize and to access with a probe. As a result, lesions are often not detected at an early stage. The lesions tend to spread in a wide, circumferential pattern and pain is not a feature until an advanced stage. Frustrating for the dentist and the patient, the first sign of root caries may be a catastrophic fracture of the tooth at the gingival level. The difficulties of detecting this disease in its early stages is a considerable challenge.

6 Risk Assessment

A caries risk assessment should be a part of information gathered in treatment planning for all patients. Given the challenges in detecting root carious lesions early, particular efforts should focus on identifying those older adults at high risk of developing root caries and implement appropriate risk reduction measures. Root caries is a preventable disease; however, access to care, adherence issues, and cost may preclude the use of a preventive intervention on the entire older adult population. This means that one-third of the older adult population bears much of the root caries burden [21]. Therefore, if these individuals could be identified prior to developing the disease, targeted prevention measures could be delivered. A systematic review of root caries risk indicators found that the best predictor of future root caries development was a history of past root caries disease [22]. The clinician should treat any individual with a filled or decayed root surface as a high-risk individual for future disease. Other risk factors which have been identified include older age, number of teeth present, poor plaque control, and wearing removable partial dentures [23].

7 Caries Prevention Strategies for Older Adults

7.1 Oral Hygiene Advice for Older Adults

Beyond the oral cavity, many older people also carry the burden of systemic medical conditions [24]. These can diminish the priority for optimal oral hygiene in the daily routine of some older patients, while others will be dependent on caregivers for mechanical cleaning of the teeth. Many older adults are prescribed a large number of daily medications (polypharmacy), and xerostomia is a side effect of many commonly prescribed drugs [25]. Dry mouth is a major risk factor for dental caries as the protective lubrication of saliva has been removed. For a more in-depth discussion on the topic, please refer to chapter "Xerostomia and Hyposalivation". Loss of manual dexterity, secondary to arthritis or neuromuscular degeneration, presents many older patients with an additional obstacle in maintaining adequate plaque control. Something as simple as holding a toothbrush can be difficult, and manipulation of dental floss or other intricate interdental cleaning aids becomes impossible. Diminishing eyesight can also hinder proper oral hygiene technique. Some patients may be embarrassed to admit to any decline in physical capabilities, and oral health can suffer significantly before appropriate assistance is provided by a caregiver. Dentists and dental hygienists should consider this possibility if they observe a decline in oral hygiene in an older patient and highlight aids such as toothbrush grips, electric toothbrushes and holders for interdental floss and mouthwashes [26].

The simplest home-based measure to reduce caries risk is to incorporate a high-fluoride mouthwash into the daily routine. These are easy to use and do not require a high level of manual dexterity. Alcohol-free mouthwashes are more suitable for patients with dry mouth, and there are a number of mouthwashes specifically formulated to ease the symptoms of xerostomia. Patients should be advised to avoid using carbonated drinks or acidic sweets to alleviate their dry mouth; instead, providers should direct them to an alternative such as sugar-free chewing gum. While many older patients will be aware of the role of sugar in dental disease, the dangers of acid erosion may be less well known amongst this group.

7.2 Fluoride Interventions

High-fluoride mouthwashes can provide an additional source of fluoride, and daily use of 0.2% sodium fluoride mouthwash is frequently recommended for patients judged to be at high risk of developing caries. It may be preferable to ask patients to use the mouthwash at a different time to tooth brushing. This will allow spacing of fluoride exposure throughout the day to maximize its benefit; after lunch or dinner may be suggested as a suitable time to flush out any food debris. High-fluoride toothpaste may also be a useful preventive tool for older patients at high risk of developing caries. A meta-analysis of six randomized controlled trials demonstrated that 2800 ppm fluoride toothpaste resulted in significantly lower caries incidence compared to a 1100 ppm fluoride control [27]. As patients are well used to using toothpaste, a change to a high-fluoride toothpaste should be easily tolerated and 5000 ppm formulations are also available. High-strength-fluoride toothpastes should be kept out of reach of young children, and patients should be encouraged to expectorate after brushing, particularly where assisted toothbrushing is facilitated by a caregiver [28].

7.3 Chlorhexidine Interventions

Older adults often experience more rapid plaque accumulation than younger adults due to the dual effects of gingival recession and reduced salivary function. A number of studies have demonstrated the effectiveness of chlorhexidine 0.12% mouthwash in LTCFs Term Care Facilities to aid oral hygiene and, despite the potential for staining, is a very useful adjunct in older adults who have difficulty in maintaining adequate plaque control through brushing alone. Chlorhexidine works best on a plaque-free surfaces to prevent plaque reforming, but it can also be effective in the presence of plaque [29]. Chlorhexidine mouthwash should be used at a different time to toothbrushing as many brands of toothpaste contain sodium laurel sulphate – a detergent which inactivates chlorhexidine.

7.4 CPP-ACP Intervention

A topical paste containing bioavailable calcium and phosphate has been commercially developed as Recaldent™, which is sold as Tooth Mousse® or as MI Paste Plus® (in combination with 900 ppm fluoride) (GC Corporation, Japan). As it is derived from milk casein, all potential users of Recaldent™ products should be questioned about any possible IgE-mediated casein allergies. These products can be applied at night-time after toothbrushing, and the manufacturers advise application of a pea-sized amount to each arch using a clean dry finger. The paste must be held in the mouth at least 3 minutes, as the longer it is maintained in the mouth with saliva, the more effective it is. After spitting out, patients are advised not to eat or drink for 30 minutes, and rinsing is to be avoided.

7.5 Professionally Administered Interventions

For older patients with a high caries rate or poor adherence with oral hygiene instruction, there are a number of surgery-based interventions available to reduce caries risk. The incorporation of chlorhexidine, fluoride and silver diamine fluoride (SDF) varnishes in the control of dental caries in older patients is a relatively recent development. A protective non-invasive medicament for preventing root caries lesions is of particular interest due to the nature of this destructive dental disease. A recently published systematic review and meta-analysis concluded that SDF provided a protective impact on root caries lesions after 24 months [30]. The application of varnishes is simple, quick and non-invasive and can be used in a domiciliary setting to reduce the development of new caries lesions [31]. Furthermore, it reduces dependence on patient adherence for success, and treatment can be provided by dental care professionals.

8 Challenges in the Operative Management of Root Caries

Root caries lesions may exhibit mixed cavity margins positioned in enamel as well as dentine [32]. Restoration of this cavity type is challenging with respect to the lack of restorative materials, which bond equally well to both dental tissues. The evidence base for the selection of restorative material for the restoration of a root surface lesion is neither plentiful nor convincing. Most of the scientific literature examines lesions restored with amalgam, glass ionomer cement (GIC), resin-modified glass ionomer cement (RMGIC), modified polyacid resins ("compomers") or composite resins. A systematic review published in 2016 concluded that there was insufficient evidence to recommend any specific material [33]. However, failure rates of root caries restorations across all materials were extremely high; 82% of GIC restorations were considered a "failure" after just 24 months. A total of 25% of all composite restorations had developed recurrent caries after 2 years. Despite the poor survival rates of GIC restorations, many authors still conclude that GIC is the material of choice for root caries as conventionally setting glass ionomer cements were associated with protection against secondary caries – even after the filling itself had been lost [34]. Clinical judgement is essential in each individual case, and the choice of restorative material to restore a carious lesion on a root surface is influenced by the location of the lesion, aesthetic requirements of the patient, moisture control and future caries risk.

9 Utilizing Atraumatic Restorative Treatment (ART) for Caries Management in Older Adults

Providing operative dental care to older patients can be challenging, and traditional restorative approaches may not be accessible or even acceptable to some groups. Several authors have pointed out that most economically prosperous countries still prioritize traditional treatment of disease over prevention measures. This is, arguably, excessively costly and does not consider long-term maintenance requirements [35, 36].

In order to avoid further tooth tissue loss and enhance prevention amongst older individuals, minimally invasive dentistry (MID) should always be the first line of treatment for caries. It prioritizes prevention and provides guidance for patients to empower them to be responsible for their own oral health and intervene as conservatively as possible when a surgical approach is judged necessary, thus avoiding unnecessary tooth tissue removal. It was born from the evolvement in the understanding of the caries process and the mechanisms involved in its beginning, progression and control, together with improved dental materials. According to the MID concept, early caries detection and caries risk assessment, remineralization of demineralized enamel and dentine and optimal caries-preventive measures should always be used throughout an individual's life, and operative interventions should only be employed when all of these have failed [37]. In order to decide for a preventive or operative intervention, it is important to differentiate between active and arrested, cavitated and non-cavitated and cleansable and plaque trapping lesions. The type of lesion will influence not only the treatment to be carried out but also the type of material to be used. Cavitated lesions on the root surface that are shallow might become self-cleansable and arrested, and therefore, restoration might not be necessarily recommended. When there is a need for a filling to be placed, cavity preparation should be as minimal as possible to conserve natural tooth tissue.

Atraumatic restorative treatment (ART) is a very effective yet minimally invasive surgical approach for restoration of carious teeth (Fig. 4). It uses hand instruments for

Fig. 4 Root caries restored using ART on 15, occlusal caries on 47 also restored using ART

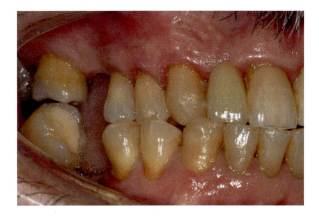

accessing carious lesions and removing decomposed dentine and a high-viscosity glass-ionomer to restore the cavity. Many studies worldwide have demonstrated that ART can achieve high survival rates in single-surface permanent teeth [10, 38, 39]. ART can be used successfully in non-clinical settings, including LTCFs and hospitals, and has been shown to be both cost-effective and acceptable to older adults [40, 41]. Furthermore, ART can be carried out by dental care professionals (DCPs), including therapists and hygienists. The use of DCPs to provide oral care for older people may help to improve access to dental services particularly for patients who are resident in LTCFs [42, 43]. The use of the ART approach could thus result in preventive and restorative care being delivered to a larger number of people compared to traditional restorative approaches. Studies carried out in older adults have demonstrated comparable survival rates for both ART and conventional restorations with glass ionomers [44, 45]. One of the largest studies which compared ART with a conventional restorative technique to treat carious lesions on older patients found that only 8.6% of the ART restorations placed on the root surface failed after 5 years. Overall, failure rates were similar between the ART and the conventional group [10]. Furthermore, the same study found that older adults accept ART well and are happy not to receive anaesthesia or drilling for restoration provision. Dental anxiety is a known barrier for dental attendance, and fearful older adults are less likely to visit a dentist and more likely to avoid or delay dental treatment. The use of ART could change this negative perception of dental treatment and make dental attendance more regular for some patients.

10 Consideration of Caries Development When Replacing Missing Teeth

Previously in this chapter, we have discussed preventive interventions to prevent older adults developing caries including effective mechanical cleaning and the use of fluoride. However, in addition to effective preventative regimes, operative dental treatment can also become an etiological driver for the development of caries. The most common example of this is in the replacement of missing teeth particularly when using a removable partial denture (RPD) [23, 46]. RPDs, which are constructed from acrylic resin, typically cover substantial amounts of the soft tissues and create plaque traps and dead spaces where caries can develop (Fig. 5). Acrylic resin RPDs should be used as transitional prostheses where the remaining teeth are of poor prognosis and additions to the RPD are anticipated in the short to medium term. [47] Where the remaining natural dentition is of a good prognosis and a removable prosthesis is planned, then this should be constructed using a cobalt-chromium framework. This RPD design will provide a prosthesis which is tooth-borne but also minimizes the amount of coverage of the remaining hard and soft

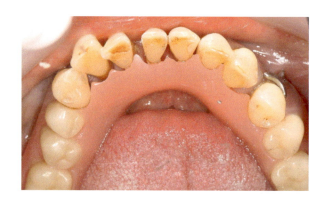

Fig. 5 Lower acrylic resin RPD with extensive coverage of the gingival margins around the remaining natural teeth

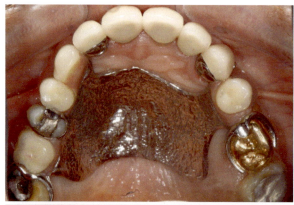

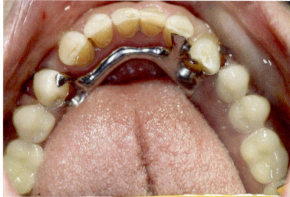

Fig. 6 Upper and lower cobalt-chromium RPDs which have been designed to minimize coverage of the remaining hard and soft tissues

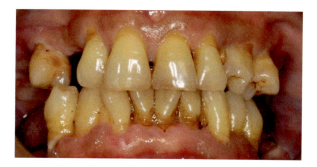

Fig. 7 A shortened dental arch in a partially dentate older patient

tissues (Fig. 6). Whilst a good preventive regime will still be required, the remaining dentition should be less prone to developing caries.

Where replacement of natural teeth is less extensive, then fixed prosthodontics can be considered, either as tooth supported or implant supported restorations. Where systemic medical comorbidities are well controlled, then dental implants can have excellent success rates in older adults [24]. Consideration should also be given to the use of the shortened dental arch concept, where a functional dentition is achieved through retention of natural teeth or using fixed prosthodontics to restore 10 occluding pairs of contacts (Fig. 7). This treatment planning philosophy does not necessitate the use of a RPD and is therefore easier for the patient to maintain and more cost-effective to deliver [48].

11 Conclusions

This chapter has discussed the changing oral health profile of older adults within the population. The emergence of a partially dentate older population is not only a significant advance in terms of oral health but also provides significant challenges for clinicians and patients in managing chronic dental diseases, including caries. Despite root caries being a preventable dental disease, prevalence is very high amongst older adults. Whilst some operative strategies have been discussed, including the application of ART, the most important element is prevention. Interventions using high-fluoride toothpaste and varnish are effective in preventing root caries, and the use of SDF is increasingly promising. Within the context of prevention, clinicians must ensure that they are not adding to the maintenance burden for older patients by providing RPDs, which are plaque retentive and encourage caries development. Alternative approaches should be considered including utilizing the shortened dental arch concept, which provides a functional yet maintainable dentition for older adults.

References

1. UN Department of Economics and Social Affairs. World Population Prospects – Population Division – United Nations. The International Journal of Logistics Management.
2. McKenna G, Tsakos G, Burke FM, Brocklehurst P. Managing an ageing population: challenging oral epidemiology. Primary Dental Care. 2020;9(3):14–7.
3. Steele J, Sullivan IO. Executive summary: adult dental health survey 2009. Health (San Francisco). Published online. 2011.
4. Pearce MS, Thomson WM, Walls AWG, Steele JG. Lifecourse socio-economic mobility and oral health in middle age. J Dental Res. Published online. 2009; https://doi.org/10.1177/0022034509344524.
5. Jung S-H, Tsakos G, Sheiham A, Jae-In R, Watt RG. Socio-economic status and oral health-related behaviours in Korean adolescents. Soc Sci Med. 2010;70(11):1780–8.
6. Aida J, Kondo K, Kondo N, Watt RG, Sheiham A, Tsakos G. Income inequality, social capital and self-rated health and dental status in older Japanese. Soc Sci Med. Published online. 2011; https://doi.org/10.1016/j.socscimed.2011.09.005.
7. Bernabé E, Watt RG, Sheiham A, et al. Childhood socioeconomic position, adult sense of coherence and tooth retention. Community Dent Oral Epidemiol. Published online. 2012; https://doi.org/10.1111/j.1600-0528.2011.00633.x.
8. Cronin M, Meaney S, Jepson NJA, Allen PF. A qualitative study of trends in patient preferences for the management of the partially dentate state. Gerodontology. Published online. 2009; https://doi.org/10.1111/j.1741-2358.2008.00239.x.
9. Hayes M, Da Mata C, Cole M, McKenna G, Burke F, Allen PF. Risk indicators associated with root caries in independently living older adults. J Dent. Published online. 2016; https://doi.org/10.1016/j.jdent.2016.05.006.
10. da Mata C, McKenna G, Anweigi L, et al. An RCT of atraumatic restorative treatment for older adults: 5 year results. J Dent. 2019;83 https://doi.org/10.1016/j.jdent.2019.03.003.
11. Hayes M, Da Mata C, McKenna G, Burke FM, Allen PF. Evaluation of the Cariogram for root caries prediction. J Dent. Published online. 2017; https://doi.org/10.1016/j.jdent.2017.04.010.
12. Kelly M, Steele J, Nuttall N, Bradnock G, Morris J, Nunn J et al. Adult dental health survey: oral health in the United Kingdom 1998. The information centre for health and social care. Published online. 1998.
13. White DA, Tsakos G, Pitts NB, et al. Adult Dental Health Survey 2009: common oral health conditions and their impact on the population. Br Dent J. Published online. 2012; https://doi.org/10.1038/sj.bdj.2012.1088.
14. Karki AJ, Monaghan N, Morgan M. Oral health status of older people living in care homes in Wales. Br Dent J. 2016;51:8–14.
15. Excellence NI of H and C. Improving Oral Health for Adults in Care Homes; 2016.
16. Care Quality Commission. Smiling Matters; 2019.
17. Hayes M, Blum IR, da Mata C. Contemporary challenges and management of dental caries in the older population. Primary Dent J. Published online. 2020; https://doi.org/10.1177/2050168420943075.
18. Jordan H, Sumney D. Root surface caries: review of the literature and significance of the problem. J Periodontol. 1973;44(3):158–63.
19. Lynch E, Beighton D. A comparison of primary root caries lesions classified according to colour. Caries Res. 1994;28(4):233–9.
20. MinQuan D, Han J, BaoJun T, Zhou Y, Wu B, Bian Z. Root caries patterns and risk factors of middle-aged and elderly people in China. Community Dent Oral Epidemiol. 2009;27(3):260–6.
21. Griffin S, Griffin PM, Swann J, Zlobin N. Estimating rates of new root caries in older adults. J Dent Res. 2004;83(8):634–48.
22. Ritter A, Shugars D, Bader JD. Root caries risk indicators: a systematic review of risk models. Community Dent Oral Epidemiol. 2010;38(5):383–97.

23. Hayes M, Da Mata C, Cole M, McKenna G, Burke F, Allen PF. Risk indicators associated with root caries in independently living older adults. J Dent. 2016;51 https://doi.org/10.1016/j.jdent.2016.05.006.
24. Schimmel M, Srinivasan M, McKenna G, Müller F. Effect of advanced age and/or systemic medical conditions on dental implant survival: a systematic review and meta-analysis. Clin Oral Implants Res. 2018;29 https://doi.org/10.1111/clr.13288.
25. de Mata C, McKenna G, Burke FM. Caries and the older patient. Dent Update. 2011;38(6) https://doi.org/10.12968/denu.2011.38.6.376.
26. Hayes M, Allen E, Da Mata C, McKenna G, Burke F. Minimal intervention dentistry and older patients Part 1: risk assessment and caries prevention. Dental Update. Published online. 2014; https://doi.org/10.12968/denu.2014.41.5.406.
27. Bartizek R, Gerlach R, Faller R, Jacobs S, Bollmer B, Biesbrock A. Reduction in dental caries with four concentrations of sodium fluoride in a dentifrice: a meta-analysis evaluation. J Clin Dent. 2001;12(3):57.
28. Kossioni AE, Hajto-Bryk J, Janssens B, et al. Practical guidelines for physicians in promoting oral health in frail older adults. J Am Med Dir Assoc. 2018;19(12) https://doi.org/10.1016/j.jamda.2018.10.007.
29. Slot D, Vaandrager N, Van Loveren C, Van Palenstein Helderman W, Van Der Weijden GA. The effect of chlorhexidine varnish on root caries: a systematic review. Caries Res. 2011;45(2).
30. Grandjean M, Maccarone N, McKenna G, Muller F, Srinivasan M. Silver Diamine Fluoride (SDF) in the management of root caries in elders: systematic review and meta-analysis. Swiss Dent J. 2021;131(5).
31. Jabir E, McGrade C, Quinn G, et al. Evaluating the effectiveness of fluoride varnish in preventing caries amongst long-term care facility residents. Gerodontology. Published online May 24. 2021; https://doi.org/10.1111/ger.12563.
32. Wefel JS, Clarkson BH, Heilman JR. Natural root caries: a histologic and microradiographic evaluation. J Oral Pathol Med. 1985;14(8) https://doi.org/10.1111/j.1600-0714.1985.tb00538.x.
33. Hayes M, Brady P, Burke FM, Allen PF. Failure rates of class V restorations in the management of root caries in adults – a systematic review. Gerodontology. 2016;33(3) https://doi.org/10.1111/ger.12167.
34. de Moor RJG, Stassen IG, van 't Veldt Y, Torbeyns D, Hommez GMG. Two-year clinical performance of glass ionomer and resin composite restorations in xerostomic head- and neck-irradiated cancer patients. Clin Oral Investig. 2011;15(1) https://doi.org/10.1007/s00784-009-0355-4.
35. Meurman JH, McKenna G, Murtomaa H, et al. Managing our older population: the challenges ahead. J Dent Res. 2018;97(10) https://doi.org/10.1177/0022034518784916.
36. Petersen P, Kandelman D, Arpin S, Ogawa H. Global oral health of older people – call for public health action. Community Dent Health. 2010;27:252–62.
37. Frencken JE, Peters MC, Manton DJ, Leal SC, Gordan V, v., Eden E. Minimal intervention dentistry for managing dental caries – a review. Int Dent J. 2012;62(5) https://doi.org/10.1111/idj.12007.
38. da Mata C, Allen PF, McKenna G, Cronin M, O'Mahony D, Woods N. Two-year survival of ART restorations placed in elderly patients: a randomised controlled clinical trial. J Dent. 2015;43(4) https://doi.org/10.1016/j.jdent.2015.01.003.
39. de Amorim RG, Frencken JE, Raggio DP, Chen X, Hu X, Leal SC. Survival percentages of atraumatic restorative treatment (ART) restorations and sealants in posterior teeth: an updated systematic review and meta-analysis. Clin Oral Investig. 2018;22(8) https://doi.org/10.1007/s00784-018-2625-5.
40. da Mata C, Cronin M, O'Mahony D, McKenna G, Woods N, Allen PF. Subjective impact of minimally invasive dentistry in the oral health of older patients. Clin Oral Investig. 2015;19(3) https://doi.org/10.1007/s00784-014-1290-6.

41. da Mata C, Allen PF, Cronin M, O'Mahony D, McKenna G, Woods N. Cost-effectiveness of ART restorations in elderly adults: a randomized clinical trial. Community Dent Oral Epidemiol. 2014;42(1) https://doi.org/10.1111/cdoe.12066.
42. Lundberg A, Hillebrecht A, McKenna G, Srinivasan M. COVID-19: impacts on oral healthcare delivery in dependent older adults. Gerodontology. 2021;38(2) https://doi.org/10.1111/ger.12509.
43. McKenna G, Janssens B, Srinivasan M, Brocklehurst P, Tsakos G. Who is caring for the oral health of dependent institutionalised elderly during the COVID-19 pandemic? Gerodontology. 2020;37(4) https://doi.org/10.1111/ger.12504.
44. Gil-Montoya JA, Mateos-Palacios R, Bravo M, González-Moles MA, Pulgar R. Atraumatic restorative treatment and Carisolv use for root caries in the elderly: 2-year follow-up randomized clinical trial. Clin Oral Investig. 2014;18(4) https://doi.org/10.1007/s00784-013-1087-z.
45. Göstemeyer G, da Mata C, McKenna G, Schwendicke F. Atraumatic vs conventional restorative treatment for root caries lesions in older patients: meta- and trial sequential analysis. Gerodontology. 2019;36(3) https://doi.org/10.1111/ger.12409.
46. Tonetti MS, Bottenberg P, Conrads G, et al. Dental caries and periodontal diseases in the ageing population: call to action to protect and enhance oral health and well-being as an essential component of healthy ageing – consensus report of group 4 of the joint EFP/ORCA workshop on the boundaries be. J Clin Periodontol. 2017;44 https://doi.org/10.1111/jcpe.12681.
47. Allen PF, McKenna G, Creugers N. Prosthodontic care for elderly patients. Dent Update. 2011;38(7) https://doi.org/10.12968/denu.2011.38.7.460.
48. McKenna G, Allen F, Woods N, et al. Cost-effectiveness of tooth replacement strategies for partially dentate elderly: a randomized controlled clinical trial. Community Dent Oral Epidemiol. 2014;42(4) https://doi.org/10.1111/cdoe.12085.

Systemic Disease That Influences Oral Health

Jaisri R. Thoppay and Akhilanand Chaurasia

General health and oral health may interface at many levels [1]. "The oral cavity is the mirror image of systemic health" as highlighted in the US Surgeon General's Report on Oral Health in America 2000 [2]. Many systemic medical conditions may first manifest in the oral cavity [3]. Since the oral cavity is easily accessible, any alterations in systemic health reflected in the mouth can be of diagnostic value. Some interfaces between systemic and oral health are direct [1]. Such clinical oral presentations prompt the clinician to perform a focused evaluation and diagnostic workup [4]. Systemic conditions, for example, may present with symptoms of dry mouth, oral lesions, temporomandibular disorders, or orofacial conditions well before a definitive diagnosis can be made, allowing for an early diagnosis, and management which may in turn improve the patient's prognosis [5, 6]. This chapter offers an overview on the role of systemic diseases in oral health with a focus on common conditions in the geriatric population.

1 Background

Whereas clinical manifestations may be the result of the direct effects of systemic conditions on the oral cavity, indirect effects may be the result of the actions of the non-pharmacological and pharmacological treatments recommended for such conditions [7]. For example, osteoporosis may not have a direct effect on the structures

---

J. R. Thoppay (✉)
Center for Integrative Oral Health, Winter Park, FL, USA
e-mail: jthoppay@inoralhealth.com

A. Chaurasia
Department of Oral Medicine and Radiology, Faculty of Dental Sciences, King George's Medical University, Lucknow, UP, India

of the jaw. However, the antiresorptive medications for the management of osteoporosis may cause osteonecrosis of the jaw in patients with underlying poor oral health. Adverse drug reactions to the administration of certain medications may manifested as erythema multiforme, Steven-Johnson syndrome, anaphylactic stomatitis, intraoral fixed drug eruptions, lichenoid drug reactions, and pemphigoid-like drug reactions [8, 9].

A bidirectional relationship may also occur. There are instances where adverse oral health may lead to complex health conditions and occasionally critical illness. Poor oral health may affect preexisting cardiac conditions, leading to infective endocarditis caused by existing oral microbiota. Both systemic health and quality of life are compromised when edentulism, xerostomia, soft tissue lesions, or poorly fitting dentures influence eating and food choices [10]. Oral and facial pain from dentures, temporomandibular joint disorders, and oral infections may affect social interactions and daily behaviors [11].

Common oral conditions, such as periodontal disease and dental caries, are chronic and associated with multifactorial determinants or risk factors. A causal relationship may be difficult to establish [4, 7]. Furthermore, a cause-and-effect relationship between systemic health and oral disease is not necessarily symmetrical. A well-documented example is the relationship between periodontal disease and diabetes mellitus type II [12, 13]. Patients are more likely to develop periodontal disease as compared to people without diabetes [14]. Poor diabetic control may significantly affect periodontal disease management and prognosis. Treating periodontal disease may reduce oral discomfort, which may assist patients in making better nutritional choices, thereby achieving better glycemic control [15]. A similar bidirectional relationship exists between diabetes, sugar consumption, and dental caries. Another example of an indirect causal relationship in older adults is the combination of periodontal disease and caries causing tooth loss, which subsequently may lead to poor dietary choices resulting in nutritional deficiencies or poor diabetic control.

2 Geriatric Assessment

Geriatric assessment is the multidimensional and multidisciplinary assessment of functional ability, physical health, cognition and mood, and socioeconomic status [16]. In addition to a complete history of presenting oral complaints, geriatric assessment includes a thorough medical and surgical history, medication review, and a geriatric review of systems [11, 17, 18].

A thorough medical history may help:

- Identify patients with undetected systemic diseases that may represent a severe threat to the patient's life or may further complicate dental treatments;
- Identify patients taking drugs that could interact with other prescribed drugs potentially complicating the care plan or provide clues as to whether the patient failed to report an underlying systemic illness;
- Allow the dentist to modify his treatment plan for the patient considering systemic disease or prescribed drugs;

- Provide safe dental care and prevent complications from dental procedures;
- Enable the dentist to communicate with medical consultants regarding the patient's systemic condition; and
- Establish an excellent patient-doctor relationship by showing the patient that we are genuinely interested in their overall well-being.

Oral manifestations of various systemic diseases may look alike, often manifesting as red and white lesions or erythematous oral ulcerations. Such manifestations may be difficult to diagnose solely based on signs and symptoms. Therefore, it is critical to assess the oral as part of the medical history and overall evaluation of systemic health. The figure illustrates a suggested workflow for addressing orofacial complaints. The first visit should start with a detailed history of present illness, past medical, dental, and medication history combined with a comprehensive oral examination complemented with additional diagnostic work-up (Fig. 1).

3 Systemic Health Affecting Oral Health Management

In an outpatient dental setting, managing a medically complex older patient may need modifications to routine dental care. A thorough history is necessary to establish the existence, and nature of any medical problems, assess risk, anticipate any complications, and minimize the chances of any medical emergency while providing appropriate dental treatment. Medical risk assessment requires the following [17]:

- Recognize significant deviations from normal health status that might affect dental management;
- Make an informed judgment on the risk of dental procedures to both outpatients and inpatients; and
- Identify the need for medical consultation.

Several guides have been developed to facilitate the efficient and accurate preoperative assessment of medical risk. The most commonly used are the American Society of Anesthesiologists (ASA) Physical Scoring System (Table 1) and the Goldman's Cardiac Risk Index.

The systemic medical complexity level may correspond to three areas: procedure-related, anesthesia-related, and provider-related. In general, oral health management often requires modifications based on the presence of systemic health conditions. Such modifications depend on the following factors: risk of infection, risk of bleeding, risk of medical complications, and risk of adverse outcomes and any potential drug interactions.

3.1 Risk of Infection

The risk of infection may occur in two clinical situations. First, poorly controlled systemic health can potentially increase the risk of dental infections (e.g., dental decay or periodontal disease). Second, patients with preexisting cardiac conditions

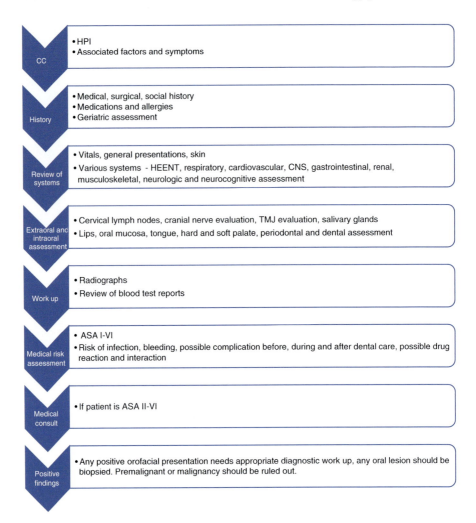

Fig. 1 Geriatric patient evaluation and workup flowchart

may develop infective endocarditis after a dental procedure or from untreated dental conditions that increase the risk of infection. The American Heart Association (AHA) has released guidelines recommending the use of antibiotic prophylaxis for patients with any of the following cardiac conditions or implanted devices [19].

- Prosthetic cardiac valves, including transcatheter-implanted prostheses and homografts
- Prosthetic material used for cardiac valve repairs, such as annuloplasty rings and chords
- History of infective endocarditis
- Cardiac transplant with valve regurgitation due to a structurally abnormal valve

Table 1 American Society of Anesthesiologists' (ASA) physical scoring system for dental treatment and anesthesia

ASA classification	Dental and anesthesia considerations
ASA 1 – Physical status: A patient without systemic disease; a normal patient	Routine dental therapy without modification. Suitable for treatment with anesthetic modality
ASA II – Physical status: A patient with mild systemic disease	Routine dental therapy with possible treatment limitations of special consideration (e.g., duration of therapy, stress of therapy, prophylactic considerations, possible sedation, and medical consultation)
ASA III – Physical status: A patient with severe systemic disease limits activity but is not incapacitating	Dental therapy with possible strict limitations or special consideration Anesthetic modalities generally contraindicated on an outpatient basis
ASA VI – Physical status: A patient with incapacitating systemic disease is a constant threat to life	Emergency dental therapy only with severe limitations or special considerations. Anesthetic modalities in the dental office are contraindicated

- Congenital (present from birth) heart disease (e.g., unrepaired cyanotic congenital heart disease, including palliative shunts and conduits, any repaired congenital heart defect with residual shunts or valvular regurgitation at the site of or adjacent to the site of a prosthetic patch or a prosthetic device)

Patients on immunosuppressant medications or those immunocompromised due to various systemic diseases (e.g., renal failure, transplant recipients, oncology patients receiving chemotherapy) may be at a higher risk of developing postoperative orofacial infections. A complete blood count and differential may also reveal lower absolute neutrophil counts (ANC) of <1500 cells/μL, moderate if 500–1000 cells/mm3, or severe if <500 cells/mm3 [20]. Any neutropenia may indicate the need for proper antibiotic coverage to prevent the risk of acute dental infections or postoperative orofacial infections. Patients with critically low ANC levels may pose a higher risk of infection. Patients with uncontrolled diabetes may also be at a higher risk of infection and poor healing. Hemoglobin A1c and blood glucose levels may provide valuable information to clinicians. Abnormal values should prompt dentists to be careful when performing emergency or essential dental care and only after a thorough discussion with medical consultants. Any elective dental procedures should be deferred until patients are clinically stable. Essential dental care may instead focus on acute pain management and the prevention and management of acute infections.

3.2 Risk of Bleeding

Increased bleeding risk may be due to spontaneous bleeding from periodontal or oral tissues or as a result of peri- and postoperative bleeding associated with certain medications or medical conditions. Spontaneous hemorrhage emanating from the gingival sulcus or bleeding from oral tissues may occur in patients with an underlying systemic disease such as acute leukemia, pancytopenia, thrombocytopenia, hemophilia A and B, liver disease, or hereditary hemorrhagic telangiectasias [21]. Peri- or postoperative bleeding risk may also occur due to prescribed prophylactic aspirin or blood thinners for stroke or cardiovascular prevention. Table 2 shows the suggested dental management for patients receiving anticoagulants [21]. Blood tests related to hemostasis may include prothrombin time, international normalized ratio (INR), partial thromboplastin time, platelet count, clotting time, and bleeding time [22].

3.3 Risk of Medical Complications Before, During, and After a Dental Procedure

Medical complications may occur before, during, or after performing a dental procedure. Potential risks can be prevented by obtaining a thorough history, making appropriate modifications to routine dental procedures, and judiciously requesting consultations. Medical complications should be anticipated, and life-threatening events should be prevented. Although life-threatening emergencies in dental offices are uncommon, many factors may increase the likelihood of emergencies [23]: (1) a larger number of older persons seeking dental care; (2) therapeutic advances in medical and pharmaceutical fields; (3) longer dental appointments; and (4) increasing use of medications in dental practice [24]. Medical events occurring during dental treatments may include syncope, anxiety attacks, postural hypotension, reactions to topical epinephrine, or overdosing with a local anesthetic. In the older adult, syncope may be due to the interaction of coexisting medical problems that may impair cardiovascular and neurogenic compensatory mechanisms. Elevation of the legs and lowering of the head may help reestablish cerebral perfusion and end the syncopal episode. Often, no further treatment is necessary, and the patients rapidly recover. Repeated syncopal episodes in older adults warrant further cardiac evaluation. Other medical events in patients with preexisting conditions are seizures, asthma exacerbations, cardiovascular events [25] (e.g., angina pectoris, myocardial infarction), hyper- or hypoglycemic events, adrenal insufficiency, thyroid storm, or

Table 2 Treatment protocol for patients receiving anticoagulant therapy

Dental treatment risk	Dental treatment protocol
Low	Not necessary to stop anticoagulants
Moderate	Check prothrombin level possible change in anticoagulant medication after the medical consult
High	Defer any dental treatment if possible. For emergency or management to prevent sepsis, the patient may be seen as an inpatient in a hospital set up with a good team

a cerebrovascular event. Falls in older adults are not uncommon and can be prevented in dental settings.

Specific procedures such as nitrous oxide N_2O analgesia are contraindicated in older patients with chronic obstructive pulmonary disease [COPD]. The reason is that these patients may have preexisting alveolar bullae and, as a result, may be at higher risk for bullae rupture. N_2O administration, particularly during prolonged use, may lead to atelectasis and bullae rupture in patients with moderate to severe COPD [26].

3.4 Risk of Adverse Drug Events and Drug Interactions

Anaphylaxis is a severe and potentially life-threatening allergic reaction that may occur in dental practice. Several dental treatment-related medications are associated with anaphylaxis, including mouthwashes, local anesthetics, latex, and antibiotics. Drug-related mucocutaneous eruptions may also manifest in the oral and perioral regions. Table 3 highlights potentially dangerous drug interactions that may be encountered in general dental practices [3, 27, 28].

Furthermore, some drugs used to treat systemic medical conditions may have unintended effects in the oral cavity. A relatively common adverse reaction in the oral cavity is dry mouth or drug-induced xerostomia. Many medications

Table 3 Common prescription drugs in dentistry and their interactions

Drugs	Interacting drugs	Clinical manifestation
Epinephrine in local anesthetics	Beta-blockers	Hypertensive response, palpitations, elevation in blood pressure
	Tricyclic antidepressants	Increased sympathomimetic reaction
	An anesthetic agent such as propofol	Severe hypotension
NSAIDs	Warfarin, aspirin, SSRI	Increased bleeding risk
	ACE inhibitors, beta-blockers, diuretics	NSAIDs decrease the hypotensive effect of drugs
Macrolide antibiotics	Clopidogrel, warfarin,	Increased risk of bleeding
	Calcium channel blockers (CCBs)	Increased and prolonged hypotensive effect
Metronidazole	Warfarin, NSAIDs	Increased risk of bleeding
Azoles	Warfarin	Increased risk of bleeding
	Simvastatin	Muscle toxicity
Penicillin-based antibiotics	Warfarin	Increased risk of bleeding
Opioids	Antihypertensives	Increased and prolonged hypotensive effect

including but not limited to antihistamines, antipsychotics, antiparkinsonian medications, and antihypertensive medications may cause xerostomia by affecting resting salivary flow, while some medications suppress salivary gland acini causing salivary gland hypofunction. For a more in-depth discussion on the topic of xerostomia, please refer to Chapter "Xerostomia and Hyposalivation". Dysgeusia is often reported in patients taking lithium, antidiabetic agents, antibiotics, or chemotherapeutic regimens. Common medications such as nonsteroidal anti-inflammatory drugs [NSAIDS] can interact and cause lichenoid reactions in the oral cavity. Vesiculobullous or ulcerative lesions that mimic other immunologic diseases and reactions may include lichenoid drug reactions (Fig. 2), erythema multiforme (EM), which may present like oral erosive lichen planus, pemphigoid-like, pemphigus-like, and lupus erythematosus (LE)-like reactions [29]. There are case reports of oral adverse drug events caused by drugs such as cyanamide, anticonvulsants, antidiabetics, and antihypertensives [30]. Some medications, such as angiotensin-converting enzyme inhibitors (ACE) inhibitors, may cause oral burning. Antihypertensive medications side effects may include dysgeusia, gingival hyperplasia (nifedipine), lichenoid reactions, salivary hypofunction, and xerostomia [31, 32].

4 Systemic Health Manifesting in Orofacial Areas

Systemic conditions manifesting with oral signs and symptoms are common. Sometimes they may be the first sign or symptom of a specific systemic condition, and hence the dentist may be the first clinician to recognize it. Autoimmune disorders like Sjogren's syndrome may present with salivary gland hypofunction as the single presentation well before other clinical signs and symptoms manifest. Immunological and infectious conditions, hematologic disorders, vitamin deficiencies, endocrinopathies, and psychological disorders can present with oral signs and symptoms [11, 15]. Oral signs such as mucosal inflammation or infection, oral discoloration, decreased salivary flow, dental caries, and bleeding may indicate the presence of a systemic condition. The fact is that many different systemic conditions may present similarly, that is, with oral lesions (red, white), or erosive changes affecting the oral mucosa or periodontal areas, thus increasing the likelihood of a delayed diagnosis or misdiagnosis. Oral lesions commonly present as red, and/or white lesions but with distinguishing clinical characteristics. Coupled with a thorough medical history, oral examination, and judicious use of diagnostic tests that may lead to an early and accurate diagnosis [33]. Clinical competence in detecting abnormalities within the oral cavity, familiarity with typical manifestations of systemic disorders, and knowledge of the pathophysiology of those conditions are essential elements of the comprehensive orofacial exam [17]. A thorough history, review of systems, and a meticulous extraoral and intraoral exam will play a critical role in ensuring an early diagnosis. In the following sections, we will review oral manifestations in different organ systems.

Fig. 2 Lichenoid drug reaction secondary to NSAIDS

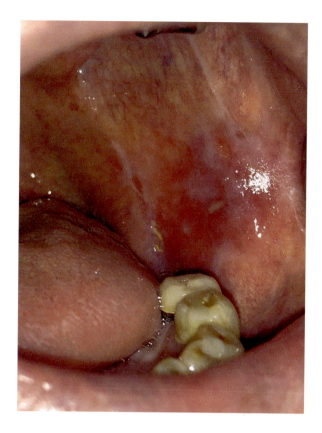

4.1 Gastrointestinal Disorders

Oral presentations such as granulomas or ulcerations in orofacial areas are easily visualized and aid in the recognition of inflammatory conditions such as Crohn's disease. The oral microbiome is a unique feature of the gastrointestinal tract. The oral cavity is a suitable environment for microbial agents due to its stable medium with optimal temperature, neutral pH, and salivary flow. The interaction between oral diseases and systemic conditions, such as in cardiovascular disease, head and neck cancers, and diabetes mellitus, may alter the oral microbiome either due to the disease process itself or due to disease management. Systemic medical conditions themselves may contribute to an altered oral microbiome. Table 4 lists oral manifestations of common gastrointestinal conditions [3, 33–36].

4.2 Renal Disorders

Renal failure can be due to end-organ damage secondary to many systemic disorders. Patients with renal failure often present with oral complications that may significantly impact older individuals receiving dental care. Orofacial manifestations

Table 4 Oral manifestations of gastrointestinal diseases

Gastrointestinal disease	Oral structure	Presenting signs and symptoms
Inflammatory bowel disease – Crohn's disease, ulcerative colitis	Vestibule and buccal mucosa	Oral ulcers, linear ulcerations, cobblestoning of buccal mucosa, mucosal tags, pyostomatitis vegetans
	Gingiva	Orofacial granulomas, granulomatous gingivitis
	Lips	perioral edema, cheilitis granulomatosis, angular cheilitis
	Tongue	Fissuring of the dorsum, mucosal tags
Celiac disease [spruce]	Oral mucosa	Aphthous ulcers
	Tongue	Atrophic, painful tongue with glossodynia – often related to secondary effect due to malabsorption of hematinics
Hepatitis, jaundice	Oral mucosa	Icterus of oral mucosa, which is readily seen on the palate and the sublingual mucosa, mucosal discoloration (yellow) caused by jaundice, petechiae, and ecchymoses caused by liver dysfunction, lichen planus associated with hepatitis C (in certain geographical regions), enlarged major salivary glands
Cirrhosis	Oral mucosa, tongue	Glossitis, angular cheilitis, mucosal discoloration, increased provenance of oral cancer, sialadenosis, increased periodontal disease
GERD (gastroesophageal reflux disease)	Oral mucosa, teeth	Oral burning, dysgeusia, halitosis, eroded teeth on the lingual surfaces

of renal disease and its treatments (e.g., dialysis and renal transplantation) include enlarged salivary glands, which are often asymptomatic, salivary gland hypofunction, parotitis, xerostomia, halitosis, dysgeusia, macroglossia, periodontal disease, pale mucosa (related to malabsorption of hematinics and low erythropoietin production), petechiae and ecchymosis, opportunistic candidiasis, glossitis, dysesthesia, glossodynia, and drug-induced gingival hyperplasia (Fig. 3). Patients on corticosteroids or immunosuppressive agents used to treat rejection in renal transplants or autoimmune renal conditions, may develop opportunistic dental infections or changes in jaw bone trabeculations. Steroid-related melanosis of the oral mucosa may be seen in patients on chronic steroid use [37–39].

4.3 Cardiovascular Disorders

Pain during angina and/or myocardial infarction may refer to the left mandible and occasionally presents as jaw or dental pain. A thorough temporomandibular evaluation along with an oral exam may serve to clarify the etiology of jaw-related pain or odontogenic pain and facilitate a prompt referral to medical care when a cardiovascular event is suspected. Cerebrovascular disease may also present with oral

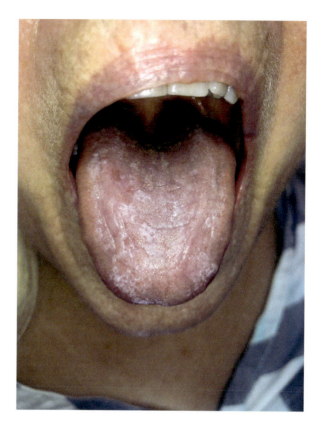

Fig. 3 Oral candidiasis and glossitis

manifestations, including weak palate, flaccid tongue, paralysis of orofacial muscles, slurred speech, dysphagia, and poor oral hygiene on the affected side.

4.4 Endocrine Disorders

Oral manifestations of diabetes include a higher incidence of dental caries, glossodynia, oral burning, xerostomia with salivary gland hypofunction, poor wound healing, higher prevalence of periodontal disease, opportunistic oral candidiasis, and acute exacerbation of oral infections [14, 15, 40, 41]. Extraoral and intraoral findings of hypothyroidism may include a puffy face, enlarged lips, gingival edema and macroglossia [42]; in hyperthyroidism, tardive dyskinesia and oral tremor may also occur [42].

4.5 Hematologic Diseases

Anemia is the most common hematological condition in older people and often presents with angular cheilitis, atrophic glossitis, oral burning, and pale mucosal pallor [43]. Patients with neutropenia or leucopenia may display oral ulcerations, exacerbation of dental infections, severe periodontal disease, and periodontal infections. These patients may also show a higher incidence of oral candidiasis and herpetic infections [20]. Individuals suffering from leukemia may present with an oral mucosa with ulcerations, opportunistic infections, mucosal bleeding, tongue bleeding, ecchymoses, petechiae, gingival and periodontal disease, gingival enlargements due to leukemic infiltrates, and gingival bleeding [44]. Dentists treating older patients with multiple myeloma, a condition that is more common with aging, may observe single or multiple "punched-out" or mottled radiolucent lesions on dental/facial radiographs, soft tissue plasma cell tumors, non-odontogenic pain mimicking dental pain, or trigeminal neuralgia. Patients with myeloma receiving antiresorptive medications may also develop medication-induced osteonecrosis of the jaw [45].

4.6 Neurocognitive Disorders

Patients with severe cognitive impairment are at increased risk for caries, periodontal disease, and oral infection because of decreased ability to engage in home oral care. In addition to poor oral hygiene, patients with Alzheimer's disease and related dementias have an increased prevalence of dental caries, periodontal disease, oral candidiasis, and salivary gland hypofunction [46, 47]. Those with Parkinson's disease may suffer from alterations of oral motor functions leading to drooling secondary to difficulties in swallowing. These patients often drool due to impaired swallowing secondary to muscle weakness and pooling of saliva, which may further increase the prevalence of dental caries and periodontal disease [48, 49]. Patients with Parkinson's may also suffer from oral burning; dysphagia; slow speech; tardive dyskinesia (involuntary oral-facial movements including lip-smacking, grimacing, tongue flittering), caused by long-term therapy with levodopa; tremors of the head, lips, and tongue; angular cheilitis; xerostomia; and salivary gland hypofunction secondary to the use of anticholinergic medications.

4.7 Respiratory Disorders

Patients with COPD on inhalation corticosteroids may develop candidiasis, periodontitis, and smoking-related intraoral findings (i.e., xerostomia, lesions including nicotine stomatitis, halitosis, tooth stain) [7]. Patients with tuberculosis may develop oral lesions (i.e., solitary ulcerations), enlarged cervical or submandibular lymph nodes, or scrofula [7]. Patients with asthma may develop fungal infections secondary to extended antibiotic use and hyperpigmentation of the mucosa from chronic steroid inhaler use (Fig. 4) [50].

Fig. 4 Hyperpigmentation of hard and soft palate after chronic inhaler use

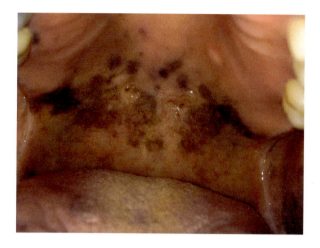

4.8 Autoimmune Disease

Lupus erythematosus may show a characteristic butterfly, malar rash on the cheeks and bridge of the nose, oral lichenoid lesions, xerostomia with salivary gland hypofunction, periodontal disease, caries, and oral candidiasis [5, 51, 52]. Individuals with Sjogren's syndrome may suffer from xerostomia with salivary gland hypofunction, dysphagia, dysphasia, lobulated tongue oral lesions, oral candidiasis, oral burning due to dry lips and mucosa, minor salivary glands with lymphocytic foci, and acinar destruction (Fig. 5), [5, 53]. Patients with fibromyalgia may present with orofacial pain and temporomandibular disorders with trigger zones [54].

5 Conclusions

In this chapter, we have reviewed how many systemic medical conditions may first manifest in the oral cavity. Since the oral cavity is easily accessible, any alterations in systemic health reflected in the mouth can be of diagnostic value. According to the US Census, by 2060 the number of US adults aged 65 years or older is expected to reach 98 million, or 24% of the population. This older population have a high prevalence of chronic medical conditions with systemic manifestations including the oral cavity. The design and implementation of comprehensive community oral healthcare programs for this growing number of older adults will certainly present numerous challenges. It will be critical to develop and implement feasible and comprehensive oral health status assessments and treatments for older patients with oral manifestations of systemic disease. Eliciting pertinent and relevant information about a patient's current medical and physical status and taking an accurate,

Fig. 5 Lobulated tongue

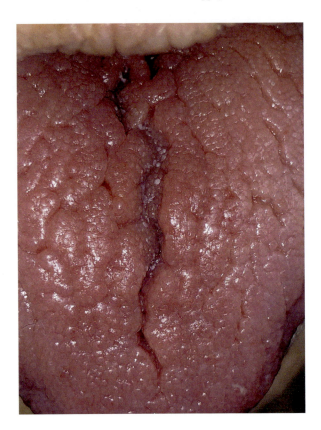

relevant, and concise medical history will ensure the prompt and accurate diagnosis of older patients with systemic conditions compromising the oral cavity. This process may require a close working relationships with medical providers and other healthcare professionals as part of an interprofessional approach for managing older adults with oral manifestations of systemic disease.

References

1. Fiorillo L. Oral health: the first step to well-being. Medicina (Kaunas). 2019;55(10):676.
2. Oral health in America: a report of the Surgeon General. J Calif Dent Assoc. 2000;28(9):685–95.
3. Tavares M, Lindefjeld Calabi KA, San Martin L. Systemic diseases and oral health. Dent Clin N Am. 2014;58(4):797–814.
4. Kane SF. The effects of oral health on systemic health. Gen Dent. 2017;65(6):30–4.
5. Saccucci M, et al. Autoimmune diseases and their manifestations on oral cavity: diagnosis and clinical management. J Immunol Res. 2018;2018:6061825.
6. Villa A, Connell CL, Abati S. Diagnosis and management of xerostomia and hyposalivation. Ther Clin Risk Manag. 2015;11:45–51.

7. Johnson NW, Glick M, Mbuguye TN. (A2) Oral health and general health. Adv Dent Res. 2006;19(1):118–21.
8. Femiano F, et al. Oral manifestations of adverse drug reactions: guidelines. J Eur Acad Dermatol Venereol. 2008;22(6):681–91.
9. Hernández-Salazar A, et al. Epidemiology of adverse cutaneous drug reactions. A prospective study in hospitalized patients. Arch Med Res. 2006;37(7):899–902.
10. Shtereva N. Aging and oral health related to quality of life in geriatric patients. Rejuvenation Res. 2006;9(2):355–7.
11. Ástvaldsdóttir Á, et al. Oral health and dental care of older persons-A systematic map of systematic reviews. Gerodontology. 2018;35(4):290–304.
12. Kudiyirickal MG, Pappachan JM. Diabetes mellitus and oral health. Endocrine. 2015;49(1):27–34.
13. Ship JA. Diabetes and oral health: an overview. J Am Dent Assoc. 2003;134 Spec No:4s–10s.
14. Lalla E, Papapanou PN. Diabetes mellitus and periodontitis: a tale of two common interrelated diseases. Nat Rev Endocrinol. 2011;7(12):738–48.
15. Cervino G, et al. Diabetes: Oral health related quality of life and oral alterations. Biomed Res Int. 2019;2019:5907195.
16. Tatum Iii PE, Talebreza S, Ross JS. Geriatric assessment: an office-based approach. Am Fam Physician. 2018;97(12):776–84.
17. Greenberg BL, Glick M. Assessing systemic disease risk in a dental setting: a public health perspective. Dent Clin N Am. 2012;56(4):863–74.
18. Ortíz-Barrios LB, et al. The impact of poor oral health on the oral health-related quality of life (OHRQoL) in older adults: the oral health status through a latent class analysis. BMC Oral Health. 2019;19(1):141.
19. Wilson W, et al. Prevention of infective endocarditis: guidelines from the American Heart Association: a guideline from the American Heart Association Rheumatic Fever, Endocarditis and Kawasaki Disease Committee, Council on Cardiovascular Disease in the Young, and the Council on Clinical Cardiology, Council on Cardiovascular Surgery and Anesthesia, and the Quality of Care and Outcomes Research Interdisciplinary Working Group. J Am Dent Assoc. 2008;139 Suppl:3s–24s.
20. Fillmore WJ, Leavitt BD, Arce K. Dental extraction in the neutropenic patient. J Oral Maxillofac Surg. 2014;72(12):2386–93.
21. Lu SY, Lin LH, Hsue SS. Management of dental extractions in patients on warfarin and antiplatelet therapy. J Formos Med Assoc. 2018;117(11):979–86.
22. Cocero N, et al. Direct oral anticoagulants and medical comorbidities in patients needing dental extractions: management of the risk of bleeding. J Oral Maxillofac Surg. 2019;77(3):463–70.
23. Frichembruder K, Santos CMD, Hugo FN. Dental emergency: scoping review. PLoS One. 2020;15(2):e0222248.
24. Malamed SF. Medical emergencies in the dental surgery. Part 1: preparation of the office and basic management. J Ir Dent Assoc. 2015;61(6):302–8.
25. Kufta K, Saraghi M, Giannakopoulos H. Cardiovascular considerations for the dental practitioner. 2. Management of cardiac emergencies. Gen Dent. 2018;66(1):49–53.
26. Chi SI. Complications caused by nitrous oxide in dental sedation. J Dent Anesth Pain Med. 2018;18(2):71–8.
27. Hersh EV, Moore PA. Three serious drug interactions that every dentist should know about. Compend Contin Educ Dent. 2015;36(6):408–13; quiz 414, 416.
28. Hersh EV. Adverse drug interactions in dental practice: interactions involving antibiotics. Part II of a series. J Am Dent Assoc. 1999;130(2):236–51.
29. Yuan A, Woo SB. Adverse drug events in the oral cavity. Oral Surg Oral Med Oral Pathol Oral Radiol. 2015;119(1):35–47.
30. Al-Hashimi I, et al. Oral lichen planus and oral lichenoid lesions: diagnostic and therapeutic considerations. Oral Surg Oral Med Oral Pathol Oral Radiol Endod. 2007;103 Suppl:S25.e1–12.

31. Cockburn N, et al. Oral health impacts of medications used to treat mental illness. J Affect Disord. 2017;223:184–93.
32. Wolff A, et al. A guide to medications inducing salivary gland dysfunction, xerostomia, and subjective Sialorrhea: a systematic review sponsored by the world workshop on oral medicine VI. Drugs R D. 2017;17(1):1–28.
33. Bhalla N, et al. Oral manifestation of systemic diseases. Dent Clin N Am. 2020;64(1):191–207.
34. Taylor VE, Smith CJ. Oral manifestations of Crohn's disease without demonstrable gastrointestinal lesions. Oral Surg Oral Med Oral Pathol. 1975;39(1):58–66.
35. Carrozzo M, Scally K. Oral manifestations of hepatitis C virus infection. World J Gastroenterol. 2014;20(24):7534–43.
36. Watanabe M, et al. Oral soft tissue disorders are associated with gastroesophageal reflux disease: retrospective study. BMC Gastroenterol. 2017;17(1):92.
37. Sowell SB. Dental care for patients with renal failure and renal transplants. J Am Dent Assoc. 1982;104(2):171–7.
38. Proctor R, et al. Oral and dental aspects of chronic renal failure. J Dent Res. 2005;84(3):199–208.
39. Jover Cerveró A, et al. Dental management in renal failure: patients on dialysis. Med Oral Patol Oral Cir Bucal. 2008;13(7):E419–26.
40. Borgnakke WS, et al. Is there a relationship between oral health and diabetic neuropathy? Curr Diab Rep. 2015;15(11):93.
41. Carrington J, Getter L, Brown RS. Diabetic neuropathy masquerading as glossodynia. J Am Dent Assoc. 2001;132(11):1549–51.
42. Chandna S, Bathla M. Oral manifestations of thyroid disorders and its management. Indian J Endocrinol Metab. 2011;15(Suppl 2):S113–6.
43. Vucicevic-Boras V, et al. Lack of association between burning mouth syndrome and hematinic deficiencies. Eur J Med Res. 2001;6(9):409–12.
44. Lynch MA, Ship II. Oral manifestations of leukemia: a postdiagnostic study. J Am Dent Assoc. 1967;75(5):1139–44.
45. Feitosa ÉF, et al. Oral health status of patients with multiple myeloma. Hematol Transfus Cell Ther. 2020;42(2):166–72.
46. Gao SS, Chu CH, Young FYF. Oral health and care for elderly people with Alzheimer's disease. Int J Environ Res Public Health. 2020;17(16):5713.
47. Aguayo S, et al. Association between Alzheimer's disease and oral and gut microbiota: are pore forming proteins the missing link? J Alzheimers Dis. 2018;65(1):29–46.
48. Koszewicz M, et al. The characteristics of autonomic nervous system disorders in burning mouth syndrome and Parkinson disease. J Orofac Pain. 2012;26(4):315–20.
49. Jeter CB, et al. Parkinson's disease oral health module: interprofessional coordination of care. MedEdPORTAL. 2018;14:10699.
50. Steinbacher DM, Glick M. The dental patient with asthma. An update and oral health considerations. J Am Dent Assoc. 2001;132(9):1229–39.
51. De Rossi SS, Glick M. Lupus erythematosus: considerations for dentistry. J Am Dent Assoc. 1998;129(3):330–9.
52. Brennan MT, et al. Oral manifestations of patients with lupus erythematosus. Dent Clin N Am. 2005;49(1):127–41. ix
53. Napenas JJ, Rouleau TS. Oral complications of Sjogren's syndrome. Oral Maxillofac Surg Clin North Am. 2014;26(1):55–62.
54. Rhodus NL, et al. Oral symptoms associated with fibromyalgia syndrome. J Rheumatol. 2003;30(8):1841–5.

The 3 Ds: Dementia, Delirium and Depression in Oral Health

Natasha Resendes, Iriana Hammel, and Christie-Michele Hogue

1 Epidemiology, Assessment, and Management

1.1 Dementia

Dementia is a disorder characterized by a decline in cognition involving one or more cognitive domains (learning and memory, language, executive function, complex attention, perceptual-motor, social cognition) [3]. Mild cognitive impairment (MCI) is a precursor condition, as shown in Table 1.

The person with dementia may show a gradual decline in cognitive function. Individuals may become forgetful especially for recent events. They must be reminded to perform healthy oral self-management behaviors. They may misplace their toothbrush or flossing aids. Individuals may have problems understanding oral health professionals' instructions or having difficulties expressing themselves or finding the right word. They may at times appear confused. Even if they remember to perform their daily activities, they may have trouble conducting self-care

---

N. Resendes
Department of Medical Education, University of Miami Miller School of Medicine, Miami VA Healthcare System, Geriatric Research, Education and Clinical Center (GRECC), Miami, FL, USA

I. Hammel (✉)
Miami VA Healthcare System, Geriatric Research, Education and Clinical Center, Miami, FL, USA

Division of Geriatrics and Palliative Medicine, University of Miami Miller School of Medicine, Miami, FL, USA
e-mail: ish29@miami.edu

C.-M. Hogue
Department of Dental Services - VA Healthcare System, Division of Geriatrics and Gerontology, Emory University School of Medicine, Atlanta, GA, USA

© The Author(s), under exclusive license to Springer Nature Switzerland AG 2022
C.-M. Hogue, J. G. Ruiz (eds.), *Oral Health and Aging*,
https://doi.org/10.1007/978-3-030-85993-0_9

Table 1 Comparing mild cognitive impairment and dementia

Mild cognitive impairment	Mild dementia
Objective evidence of low performance in *one or more* cognitive domains that is greater than expected for the patient's age and educational background	Objective evidence of low performance in *more than one* cognitive domain that is greater than expected for the patient's age and educational background
Does not substantially interfere with daily activities, although complex functional previously tasks, such as paying bills, preparing a meal, or shopping, may take more time or be performed less efficiently. Independence in daily life is preserved, with minimal aids or assistance	Significant interference with the ability to function at work or at usual activities but still able to carry out basic activities of daily living (bathing, dressing, personal hygiene) and participate in some pastimes, chores, and social functions

Not explained by delirium or major psychiatric disorder

activities requiring assistance or at least caregiver supervision. These cognitive symptoms may be accompanied by changes in behavior, which may further impair oral self-care and disrupt patient and caregiver routines. Depression and apathy are among the most common behaviors which may lead to disinterest or inconsistency in performing oral hygiene. Particularly challenging is the issue of shared decision-making. Although patients with mild to moderate dementia may be able to retain the ability to make decisions, as the disease progresses, the caregiver or surrogate may have to be increasingly involved in the decision-making progresses regarding oral healthcare interventions. For a more in-depth discussion on these topics, please refer to chapters "Ethical Considerations", and "The Role of Oral Health Literacy and Shared Decision Making".

The available evidence suggests that the etiology of dementia in older adults is complex and likely multifactorial, probably encompassing genetic, environmental, and lifestyle factors [4]. As the population ages, the overall burden of dementia is increasing worldwide. More than 5.2 million Americans are living with Alzheimer's disease or 1 in 8 Americans over the age of 65 have AD [4]. Prospective studies employing mild cognitive impairment (MCI) criteria at the outset have tended to report results of the incidence of MCI in the 10%–20% range [5]. It is estimated that by 2050, the number of people with Alzheimer's disease may nearly triple, from 5 million to as many as 16 million [6]. Therefore, we could extrapolate that at least 1 in 8 patients over the age of 65 seen in dental offices has cognitive impairment. The numbers may be lower since these patients tend to seek oral care less often than the general population. The most common types of dementia [7–9] and their clinical and pathological features are described in Table 2.

Other neurodegenerative disorders can also cause dementia, including Parkinson's disease, progressive supranuclear palsy, corticobasal degeneration, multisystem atrophy, and Huntington disease. Mixed dementia refers to the coexistence of more than one dementia-producing pathology, most commonly Alzheimer's disease and vascular dementia. Less common etiologies include alcohol-related dementia, chronic traumatic encephalopathy, normal pressure hydrocephalus (NPH), chronic subdural hematoma, and other central nervous system (CNS) illnesses (e.g., prion diseases, HIV infection) [7–9]. The assessment and diagnosis of dementia is multi-faceted, and its component are listed elsewhere in Table 3.

Table 2 Types of distinct dementia

Dementia type	Early characteristics	Pathology	Distribution
Alzheimer's disease	Slow, progressive decline in cognition (especially memory) and behaviors (apathy, depression)	Cortical amyloid plaque and neurofibrillary tangles	50–75%
Vascular dementia	Stepwise or gradual progression of cognition	Cerebrovascular disease, single infarcts in critical areas or more diffuse multi-infarct disease	20–30%
Dementia with Lewy bodies	Marked fluctuations in cognition, visual hallucinations, Parkinsonism	Cortical Lewy bodies	<5%
Frontotemporal dementia	Personality changes, mood changes, disinhibition, language difficulties	Damage limited to frontal and temporal lobes. No single pathological changes	5–10%

Table 3 Components of assessment for dementia

Assessment	Notes
History and physical	History and physical including functional status, social and family history, and a complete neurological examination
Cognitive screening tools	Mini-Cog©, Folstein Mini-Mental State Examination (MMSE), Montreal Cognitive Assessment (MoCA), Test Your Memory (pooled sensitivity of 75 to 92 percent and a specificity of 81 to 91 percent)
Neuropsychological testing	Determine etiology and severity
Depression screening	Depression can also worsen cognitive impairment in patients
Laboratory tests and imaging	TSH, vitamin B12, folate, RPR, HIV, brain imaging (CT or MRI) or amyloid PET scan of the brain

Management: The cornerstone of dementia management is non-pharmacological therapy and supportive care, including control of vascular risk factors [10], cognitive rehabilitation, nutrition counseling, and exercise and physical activity programs and caregiver support [11, 12]. The pharmacological treatment of AD consists of acetylcholinesterase inhibitors (donepezil, galantamine, rivastigmine) and memantine [11].

1.2 Delirium

Delirium is an acute disorder of attention and cognition in older adults that is common, serious, costly, under-recognized, and often fatal. A formal cognitive assessment and history of acute onset of symptoms are necessary for diagnosis [13]. Early recognition and treatment of the underlying cause of delirium is of great importance due to poor outcomes. Patients with delirium who present to the emergency department have an approximately 70% increased risk of death during the first 6 months after the visit [14]. Delirium at admission to post-acute care is associated with a five-time increased risk of mortality at 6 months [15]. In older patients with dementia, delirium is associated with increased rates of cognitive decline [16–18], institutionalization, and mortality [19]. Delirium is mostly found in hospitalized patients, with the highest incidence rates noted in intensive care units and in postoperative and palliative care settings. The prevalence of delirium in the community is low (1–2%) [13], but since many studies involving delirium excluded patients with baseline dementia, the incidence and prevalence of delirium are likely underestimated. Since it is possible, albeit rare, for a delirious patient to be seen in a dental office for oral care, it becomes important to recognize delirium and refer the patient immediately to the emergency department for evaluation. Delirium should be suspected when the patient's confusion and/or agitation has had an acute onset according to the caregiver and the patient manifests inattention (core features of delirium), as well as either disorganized thinking or an altered level of consciousness [20].

Although a single factor can lead to delirium, the etiology of delirium in older adults is usually multifactorial [21]. In vulnerable patients, such as those with underlying dementia and multimorbidity, a seemingly benign insult (e.g., a dose of an opioid narcotic) might be enough to precipitate delirium. Conversely, in a young, healthy patient, delirium will develop only after exposure to a series of noxious insults, such as general anesthesia, major surgery, several psychoactive drugs, a stay in intensive care, or sleep deprivation. Screening for delirium in hospitalized patients should be done routinely on medical and surgical wards, but especially in ICU and postoperative patients, who have the highest incidence of delirium.

Management of delirium is focused on treating the underlying etiology and using non-pharmacological strategies, cognitive rehabilitation, drug reduction, drug-sparing approaches (i.e., substitution for less toxic alternatives), treatments targeted toward neuroprotection, improvement of sleep hygiene, and reduction of pain and stress (including complementary and alternative medicine) [21].

1.3 Depression

Depression is the most common psychiatric disorder in the general population [22] and the most common mental health condition in patients seen in primary care [23–26]. A systematic review and meta-analysis published in 2010, which included 24 studies based on the community-based older adults population aged 75 years and older, found that the prevalence of major depression ranged from 4.6% to 9.3% and that of depressive disorders from 4.5% to 37.4% [27]. The current view of the etiology of depression focuses on the alteration of three major monoamine neurotransmitters: serotonin (5-hydroxytryptamine, 5HT), norepinephrine (NE), and dopamine (DA). Other genetic and environmental factors, such as adverse life events including childhood trauma, impact the risk for developing major depression [28].

In the older adult population, depression mainly affects those with chronic medical illnesses and cognitive impairment. Depression causes suffering, family disruption and disability, worsens the outcomes of many medical illnesses, and increases mortality [29]. For a diagnosis of major depression to be made, the Diagnostic and Statistical Manual of Mental Disorders (DSM-V) state that either depressed mood or loss of interest or pleasure must be present. Although not part of the diagnostic criteria, late-life major depression is often associated with bodily changes and cognitive impairment. Non-demented older people with major depression often have difficulties with concentration, speed of mental processing, and executive function [30, 31]. These deficits improve, but may not completely resolve, after remission of late-life depression [32–34].

In the absence of screening, it is estimated that only 50 percent of patients with major depression are identified [34]. This makes screening for depression very important. Short screening instruments include the Patient Health Questionnaire-9 (PHQ-9), the Patient Health Questionnaire-2 (PHQ-2), the Beck Depression Inventory for Primary Care (BDI-PC), and the 5-Item World Health Organization Well-Being Index (WHO-5). These can be self-administered by patients preceding their appointment or while in the waiting area.

The first-line treatment of depression consists of the combination of psychotherapy and antidepressant medication. Successful management of depression in late life is dependent upon several factors: addressing comorbid conditions, tailoring non-pharmacological and pharmacologic interventions to the individual patient, monitoring therapy for side effects and effectiveness, and close follow-up. Consultation with a psychiatrist should be considered for patients who have failed multiple trials of antidepressants or who prefer non-pharmacologic treatment [28].

2 The Importance of Cognition and Mood on Oral Health

2.1 Dementia

Oral health and cognitive health seem to have a bidirectional relationship. Some evidence suggests that patients with periodontal disease and normal cognition at baseline may be at higher risk for developing cognitive impairment. A single prospective cohort study showed that cognitively intact subjects at baseline who had elevated antibodies to periodontopathic microorganisms compared to cognitively intact patients without elevated antibodies were more likely to develop MCI and dementia on follow-up [35] (Level of Evidence 4). On the other hand, an expert review [36] suggests that cognitive decline frequently causes behavioral changes that may directly affect oral health. For example, patients with cognitive impairment may exhibit loss of interest and ability to complete oral self-care behaviors such as brushing and flossing. Failing to perform routine oral self-care may lead to a rapid development of hard and soft tissue diseases that result in further deterioration of function and increased dental pain and suffering. While there is no evidence in the literature that oral pain leads to increased levels of depression or delirium in older adults, it is reasonable to assume from other evidence in chronic pain in other areas that it does. As the functional status of patients with dementia declines, a person's self-esteem and confidence may also decline [37], which may further impair oral health.

Two systematic reviews reveal the association between dementia and gum disease. A systematic review encompassing 10 cohort studies, 2 controlled trials, 14 cross-sectional, and 10 case control including 5687 participants in 38 settings [37] showed that older people with dementia had high scores for gingival bleeding, periodontitis, and plaque formation and needed assistance with oral care. This was corroborated by another systematic review of 56 cohort studies, including 8301 participants in 58 settings [38], that showed that individuals with dementia were more likely to present with gingival bleeding or inflammation and suffer from periodontal disease than people without dementia. This evidence confirms that adults with dementia are more vulnerable to gingivitis and periodontal diseases probably as a result of a decline in the patients' ability to perform oral self-care behaviors and other preventive measures (Level of Evidence 1).

The level of evidence linking dementia to dental caries and tooth loss compared to healthy controls is not as robust. A systematic review of 16 cohort studies including 803 participants in 10 settings found mixed results. Some studies showed that the number of teeth and periodontal disease were associated with risk of cognitive decline or incident dementia, whereas others did not find an association [39]. Another systematic review of 28 cohort studies including 4620 participants in 74 settings showed that those with dementia had a significantly fewer number of teeth, more carious teeth, significantly worse oral hygiene, and significantly poorer periodontal health [40] (Level of Evidence 2). The latest evidence from these systematic reviews suggests that patients with cognitive impairment may have fewer and more carious teeth.

The impact of poor oral health in patients with dementia may also have wider impacts on healthcare utilization and mortality. In a systematic review of 11 cross-sectional studies, the most common reasons for preventable dental hospital admissions in patients with dementia were dental caries, followed by embedded or impacted teeth [41]. A control trial in German nursing homes randomized 219 residents to either an intervention group that consisted of dental health education and ultrasonic baths for denture cleaning ($n = 144$) or a usual care, control group ($n = 75$). The study showed that those with higher plaque record had higher mortality, suggesting the benefits of the intervention [42] (Level of Evidence 4).

In summary, dementia and cognitive decline are risk factors for poor oral healthcare outcomes. Those in later stages of the disease tend to have more plaque accumulation, gingivitis, attachment loss, dental caries, and poor denture hygiene. Evidence-based interventions to address these deficits are addressed later in the chapter.

2.2 Delirium

There have not been studies on whether delirium is associated with an increased risk of poor oral healthcare outcomes. Based on evidence observed in patients with dementia, these patients will likely be uncooperative during their delirium, and we can speculate that they will have similar outcomes to those with dementia. However, there is no research literature that characterizes the oral health status of patients with delirium. As patients with delirium may be unable to perform oral self-care activities by themselves, it would be reasonable to assume that appropriate oral healthcare interventions may be effective.

2.3 Depression

Late-life depression has been consistently associated with disinterest in performing oral hygiene behaviors, leading to poor health outcomes. According to a systematic review of 26 studies, including 42,357 patients from diverse, mainly community-dwelling clinical settings [43], severity of depression, medication, and medical comorbidity were the most important medical barriers influencing the oral health of people diagnosed with depression. A systematic review [44] of 57 studies of oral health that included samples from 38–4769 mental health consumers found that the prevalence of suboptimal oral health was 61% among individuals with serious mental illnesses. The following outcomes were seen in most patients: xerostomia, gross caries, decayed teeth, and periodontal disease. In a systematic review of 26 cohort studies, including 334,503 adult patients from 32 settings [45], psychiatric diagnoses were associated with increased dental decay in dental surfaces and missing teeth. In a separate meta-analysis of 25 studies of 5076 psychiatric patients and 39,545 controls from hospitalized and community surveys, people with serious mental illness had greater odds of having lost all their teeth compared with those without mental illness [46]. This was corroborated by a systematic review of 16 studies [47], showing that depression in adults and older adults increased the odds of tooth loss and edentulism. However, the generalizability to older adults with depression is limited, because these systematic reviews only featured a small number of studies including older adults. More cohort studies of older adults with depression are needed to determine whether these associations persist.

3 Oral Health Assessment

Older adults with cognitive impairment (especially those in long-term care institutions) are not often evaluated and managed by dental health professionals. As an alternative, experts proposed that oral examinations should be supplemented with oral health assessments and screenings conducted by trained nurses and other formal caregivers. These professionals can monitor institutionalized residents' oral health, evaluate oral hygiene care interventions, trigger calls for dentists when required, assist with individualized oral care plans, and assist with triaging and prioritizing residents' for a higher level of dental care [48]. A systematic review of 4 studies including 440 patients from 3 countries and 4 settings [49] looked at the use of instruments that nurses and other formal caregivers can use when evaluating residents' oral health. The results revealed that successful oral assessments by nursing staff required appropriate staff training and education by dental professionals.

The Brief Oral Health Status Examination (BOHSE) is a comprehensive, validated, and reliable screening tool that nurses and caregivers can use with cognitively impaired, institutionalized residents [50]. The BOHSE covers ten oral hygiene categories—lymph nodes, lips, tongue, cheek/roof of mouth, gums, saliva, natural teeth, artificial teeth, chewing position, and oral cleanliness. Using a penlight, tongue depressor, and gauze, trained staff can examine and grade the status of the oral cavity, surrounding tissues and natural or artificial teeth.

Other useful oral assessment tools that nurses and caregivers of institutionalized persons with dementia can use include the Index of Activities of Daily Oral Hygiene and the Mucosal Plaque Score [50]. Experts have proposed several strategies that staff can implement to facilitate patients and caregivers' cooperation with periodontal care in older adults with dementia (Table 4). These approaches centered on dispelling misconceptions, scheduled appointments at convenient times, strategic length of appointments, continuity of care among dental staff, and proper communication techniques such as the VERA framework outlined in Table 5 [51].

Table 4 Expert opinion strategies to engender cooperation for periodontal care

Dispel patients' and caregivers' attitudes and misconceptions regarding the ability of the dental team to cope with the symptoms of dementia by providing an environment where patients and caregivers feel comfortable
Appointments should be scheduled at the time of day that best suits the patient and caregiver
Long appointments are best avoided and, for patients with moderate dementia, are best kept to under one hour
Continuity of care is important for those with individuals with dementia, so try to have the same hygienist and dentist attend the patient
Use measures that ease the patient, interpret communication, and respond appropriately to patient's needs

Table 5 VERA framework

V = Validate, accepting that the behavior exhibited has a value to the person and isn't just another symptom of dementia
E = Emotion, paying attention to the emotional content of what the person's saying
R = Reassurance, can be as simple as saying "it'll be okay" and smiling, holding their hand
A = Activity, people with dementia need to feel occupied, active, see if you can engage them in some related activity

4 Interventions to Improve Oral Health in Persons with Cognitive Impairment

Most randomized controlled trials of oral health interventions for patients with dementia took place in long-term care settings. Dental expert opinion suggests that the management techniques that have worked in institutionalized patients may also work for persons with cognitive impairment living in the community.

In a systematic review of 8 cohort studies and 1 randomized control trial including 531 patients in LTC settings [52], the use of battery-powered devices improved the oral health status of nursing home residents with dementia. However, only one study was a randomized control trial, whereas all the others lacked appropriate controls. Of note, the randomized control trial did show an improvement in residents' oral health status. Multicomponent interventions may be especially effective for patients with cognitive impairment. The Managing Oral Hygiene Using Threat Reduction (MOUTh) intervention consists of 3 components: (1) an evidence-based mouth-care protocol for older adults with natural dentition and dentures, (2) recognition of care-resistant behaviors, and (3) strategies to reduce threat perception during the provision of mouth care. The MOUTh intervention employs strategies to prevent and reduce care-resistant behaviors including the following: establishing rapport by approaching the resident at or below eye level with a pleasant and calm demeanor; providing mouth care in front of a sink and in front of a mirror (to access procedural or implicit memories); avoiding elderspeak (a type of sing-song "baby talk"); chaining, which involves starting the mouth care and having the older adult finish the task; cueing by using gestures, pantomimes, and short, one-step commands; distraction; bridging, where the older adult is asked to hold a toothbrush during mouth care; rescue, where a second experimental staff provider may replace the first experimental mouth care provider if care-resistant behaviors escalate; and hand-over-hand, which involves either the older adult placing his or hand over that of the experimental mouth care provider or the experimental mouth care provider gently guiding the older adult's hands. In a randomized trial of 101 older nursing home residents with dementia and care-resistant behaviors, those patients receiving the MOUTh intervention had twice the odds of allowing mouth care and completing oral hygiene activities as compared with usual care controls with an established mouth care protocol [53]. The intervention also allowed staff to provide longer duration of mouth care to these residents. The investigators reported only small reductions in the intensity of care resistant behaviors and a small improvement in oral health.

In summary, this evidence suggests that the use of battery powered devices and multicomponent strategies aimed at reducing care-resistant behaviors will improve the oral health status of older adults with dementia in long-term care settings.

5 Interventions to Improve Oral Health in Persons with Depression

There is a paucity of evidence from randomized controlled trials on dental interventions in patients with depression. A study of a brief educational 10-minute video and educational brochure compared to the brochure alone significantly decreased the plaque record in patients with mental illness, both community-dwelling and institutionalized patients [54]. However, this trial in Korea did not include patients over 65 years old, so its generalizability to the population of older adults is limited. Expert opinion from dentists suggest that the appropriate dental management of geriatric patients with depression necessitates the use of anticaries agents containing fluoride, saliva substitutes, and special precautions when prescribing analgesics and local anesthetics [55].

6 Practical Considerations and Recommendations for Management of Patients with Cognitive Impairment and Mood Disorders

6.1 Simple Advice on Key Issues Based on Expert Opinion [56]

Prior to dental appointments, caregivers should be contacted 1 week to 2 weeks in advance of the appointment to update the patients' health, dental, and pharmacologic history.

6.2 During Dental Appointments

Due to the impact of dementia, delirium, and depression on oral health status, oral health professionals should consider assessing older adult patients for cognitive impairment and depression on the first visit and at least yearly thereafter with one of the screening tools listed in Table 6.

6.3 Communication

When communicating with older adults, use simple, short sentences and a soft tone of voice. Patients with dementia should be encouraged to express their ideas and feelings regarding their oral health. Asking a patient about her hobbies, favorite sports teams, or family may facilitate care and adherence, which helps foster rapport

The 3 Ds: Dementia, Delirium and Depression in Oral Health

Table 6 Practical screening for dementia, delirium, and depression disorders

Condition	Screening tool	Rationale	Validity
Dementia	Test Your Memory (TYM), Self-Administered Gerocognitive Exam (SAGE)	Self-administered	Better correlation than MMSE with neuropsychological testing [57]
Depression	PHQ-2	Short, quick to administer	Sensitivity comparable with the PHQ-9 in most populations [58]
Delirium	3D-CAM	Easy to administer	The sensitivity [95% CI] of 3D-CAM was 95% [84%, 99%] and the specificity was 94% [90%, 97%] [59]

and engagement with the shared decision-making process. Nonverbal communication, such as direct eye contact, empathetic facial expressions, and supportive body postures, may assist in communicating with patients with dementia. Patting the patient's shoulder and smiling can help decrease anxiety and increase cooperation. Demonstrating the procedures to be performed can alleviate fear and encourage cooperation. Even though caregivers should be involved in the decision-making process, the dentists should always address the patients during the interview.

6.4 Involvement of Caregivers

Based on expert opinion [56], the most beneficial advice for treating an older adult with dementia, delirium, and depression is the involvement of the older adults' caregivers. The older patient's caregiver is an essential asset to the dental office, because they are a source of familiarity in an unfamiliar environment, enable an accurate dental and medical history, assist in consolidating information that the older adult may not be able to articulate, provide continuity from appointment to appointment when the patient forgets details regarding their treatment plan, remind the patient about their future dental appointments, and provide support and reminders of oral daily, self-care behaviors such as when to brush or floss.

6.5 Managing Care-Resistant Behaviors at the Dental Office

With the aid of a caregiver, first use evidence-based behavioral approaches such as those described in the MOUTH intervention described earlier. If the behavior is not controlled with these interventions, based on expert opinion, sedation or general anesthesia may be necessary. Informed consent should be obtained if restraints are used [56]. Sedation may enable dental professionals to treat patients effectively and perform all required dental treatments during a single appointment, thereby saving time, cost, and inconvenience for patients and caregivers.

6.6 Oral Self-Care-Resistant Behaviors

Explain oral self-care in simple language: (1) Brush and floss your teeth every day; brushing and flossing help remove dental plaque, a sticky film of bacteria (germs). If plaque builds up on your teeth, it can cause tooth decay or gum disease. (2) Brush your teeth with fluoride toothpaste twice a day. Brush after breakfast and before bed. (3) Floss between your teeth every day. If you have trouble flossing, ask your dentist about using a special floss-aids instead. Techniques such as the teach-back and the use of written handouts may complement these interventions. Teach-back is a way to make sure the healthcare provider explained information clearly by asking a patient (or family member) to explain—in their own words—what they need to know or do and to check for understanding and, if needed, re-explain and check again. Research has shown that this technique may promote adherence, quality of care, and patient safety. For a more in-depth discussion on the teach-back technique, please refer to chapter "The Role of Oral Health Literacy and Shared Decision Making".

7 Future Research Agenda

There is a paucity of cohort studies characterizing the clinical presentation of patients with dementia in community-based dental clinics. Studies are needed on the validity of the Brief Oral Health Status Examination in community-dwelling older adults with dementia. Research into the efficacy of caregiver education programs, use of electronic toothbrushes, and replications of the MOUTH intervention in diverse community settings may provide valuable information to clinicians. Also given the paucity of data in older adults with depressive disorder, trials on the effect of educational programs on the plaque record of older adults specifically with depression are needed, and whether treatment of depression is associated with better oral healthcare outcomes. We need more studies in healthcare institutions on the effects of delirium on oral health status.

8 Conclusions

In this chapter, we presented a brief overview of cognitive and mood disorders in older adults including dementia, depression, and delirium, explored the relationship of oral health and these conditions, and offered advice on clinical interventions. One in 8 patients over the age of 65 seen in dental offices has cognitive impairment and over 35% have depressive disorders. Cognitive disorders such as dementia and depression lead to higher rates of caries, gum disease, tooth loss and edentulism. We discussed how the assessment and management of oral conditions may be adapted to patients with cognitive and mood disorders (i.e., by involving caregivers) and gave oral health clinicians practical advice on how they should screen with validated screening tools (i.e., PHQ-2, 3DCAM, SAGE questionnaires) and manage these disorders in their dental practice by employing strategies to Engender Cooperation for Periodontal Care (i.e., such as the VERA Framework). We presented evidence that suggests that the use of battery powered devices and multicomponent strategies aimed at reducing care-resistant behaviors will improve the oral health status of older adults with dementia in long-term care settings. Finally, we formulated an agenda for future research to obtain a better understanding of how dementia, delirium, and depression impact oral health and the interventions that may be needed to address these conditions in the older population. We need more studies on the impact of delirium, depression, and dementia and their respective treatments on patients' oral health across the healthcare spectrum.

References

1. Organization, W.H. Mental Health of older adults 2017 [cited 2020]; Available from: https://www.who.int/news-room/fact-sheets/detail/mental-health-of-older-adults. Accessed 30 Nov 2020.
2. Brennan LJ, Strauss J. Cognitive impairment in older adults and oral health considerations: treatment and management. Dent Clin N Am. 2014;58(4):815–28.
3. Knopman DS, et al. Practice parameter: diagnosis of dementia (an evidence-based review). Report of the quality standards Subcommittee of the American Academy of Neurology. Neurology. 2001;56(9):1143–53.
4. Dubois B, et al. Preclinical Alzheimer's disease: definition, natural history, and diagnostic criteria. Alzheimers Dement. 2016;12(3):292–323.
5. Manly JJ, et al. Frequency and course of mild cognitive impairment in a multiethnic community. Ann Neurol. 2008;63(4):494–506.
6. Tanner P. Dementia: prevalence, risk factors and management strategies. Nova Science Publishers, Inc; 2014.
7. Petersen RC, et al. Practice parameter: early detection of dementia: mild cognitive impairment (an evidence-based review). Report of the quality standards Subcommittee of the American Academy of Neurology. Neurology. 2001;56(9):1133–42.
8. Caselli RJ. Current issues in the diagnosis and management of dementia. Semin Neurol. 2003;23(3):231–40.
9. Knopman DS, Boeve BF, Petersen RC. Essentials of the proper diagnoses of mild cognitive impairment, dementia, and major subtypes of dementia. Mayo Clin Proc. 2003;78(10):1290–308.
10. Small SA, et al. Selective decline in memory function among healthy elderly. Neurology. 1999;52(7):1392–6.
11. Reisberg B, et al. Memantine in moderate-to-severe Alzheimer's disease. N Engl J Med. 2003;348(14):1333–41.
12. Qaseem A, et al. Current pharmacologic treatment of dementia: a clinical practice guideline from the American College of Physicians and the American Academy of Family Physicians. Ann Intern Med. 2008;148(5):370–8.
13. Inouye SK, Westendorp RG, Saczynski JS. Delirium in elderly people. Lancet. 2014;383(9920):911–22.

14. Han JH, et al. Delirium in the emergency department: an independent predictor of death within 6 months. Ann Emerg Med. 2010;56(3):244–252.e1.
15. Marcantonio ER, et al. Outcomes of older people admitted to postacute facilities with delirium. J Am Geriatr Soc. 2005;53(6):963–9.
16. Fong TG, et al. Delirium accelerates cognitive decline in Alzheimer disease. Neurology. 2009;72(18):1570–5.
17. Fong TG, et al. Adverse outcomes after hospitalization and delirium in persons with Alzheimer disease. Ann Intern Med. 2012;156(12):848–56. w296
18. Gross AL, et al. Delirium and long-term cognitive trajectory among persons with dementia. Arch Intern Med. 2012;172(17):1324–31.
19. United States Department of Health and Human Services Agency for Health Care Policy and Research. Recognition and initial assessment of Alzheimer's disease and related dementias. In: Clinical practice guidelines, number 19; 1996.
20. Oh ES, et al. Delirium in older persons: advances in diagnosis and treatment. JAMA. 2017;318(12):1161–74.
21. Kessler RC, et al. Development of lifetime comorbidity in the World Health Organization world mental health surveys. Arch Gen Psychiatry. 2011;68(1):90–100.
22. Spitzer RL, Kroenke K, Williams JB. Validation and utility of a self-report version of PRIME-MD: the PHQ primary care study. Primary care evaluation of mental disorders. Patient health questionnaire. JAMA. 1999;282(18):1737–44.
23. Ansseau M, et al. High prevalence of mental disorders in primary care. J Affect Disord. 2004;78(1):49–55.
24. Linzer M, et al. Gender, quality of life, and mental disorders in primary care: results from the PRIME-MD 1000 study. Am J Med. 1996;101(5):526–33.
25. Roca M, et al. Prevalence and comorbidity of common mental disorders in primary care. J Affect Disord. 2009;119(1–3):52–8.
26. Luppa M, et al. Age- and gender-specific prevalence of depression in latest-life--systematic review and meta-analysis. J Affect Disord. 2012;136(3):212–21.
27. Saveanu RV, Nemeroff CB. Etiology of depression: genetic and environmental factors. Psychiatr Clin North Am. 2012;35(1):51–71.
28. Alexopoulos GS. Depression in the elderly. Lancet. 2005;365(9475):1961–70.
29. Lockwood KA, Alexopoulos GS, van Gorp WG. Executive dysfunction in geriatric depression. Am J Psychiatry. 2002;159(7):1119–26.
30. Elderkin-Thompson V, et al. Neuropsychological deficits among patients with late-onset minor and major depression. Arch Clin Neuropsychol. 2003;18(5):529–49.
31. Butters MA, et al. Changes in cognitive functioning following treatment of late-life depression. Am J Psychiatry. 2000;157(12):1949–54.
32. Murphy CF, Alexopoulos GS. Longitudinal association of initiation/perseveration and severity of geriatric depression. Am J Geriatr Psychiatry. 2004;12(1):50–6.
33. Nebes RD, et al. Persistence of cognitive impairment in geriatric patients following antidepressant treatment: a randomized, double-blind clinical trial with nortriptyline and paroxetine. J Psychiatr Res. 2003;37(2):99–108.
34. Mitchell AJ, Vaze A, Rao S. Clinical diagnosis of depression in primary care: a meta-analysis. Lancet. 2009;374(9690):609–19.
35. Sparks Stein P, et al. Serum antibodies to periodontal pathogens are a risk factor for Alzheimer's disease. Alzheimers Dement. 2012;8(3):196–203.
36. Venete A, et al. Relationship between the psychosocial impact of dental aesthetics and perfectionism and self-esteem. J Clin Exp Dent. 2017;9(12):e1453–8.
37. Delwel S, et al. Oral hygiene and oral health in older people with dementia: a comprehensive review with focus on oral soft tissues. Clin Oral Investig. 2018;22(1):93–108.
38. Lauritano D, et al. Oral health status and need for oral care in an aging population: a systematic review. Int J Environ Res Public Health. 2019;16(22):4558.

39. Wu B, et al. Association between oral health and cognitive status: a systematic review. J Am Geriatr Soc. 2016;64(4):739–51.
40. Foley NC, et al. A systematic review examining the oral health status of persons with dementia. JDR Clin Trans Res. 2017;2(4):330–42.
41. Acharya A, et al. Dental conditions associated with preventable hospital admissions in Australia: a systematic literature review. BMC Health Serv Res. 2018;18(1):921.
42. Klotz AL, et al. Is compromised oral health associated with a greater risk of mortality among nursing home residents? A controlled clinical study. Aging Clin Exp Res. 2018;30(6):581–8.
43. Stepović M, et al. Barriers affecting the oral health of people diagnosed with depression: a systematic review. Zdr Varst. 2020;59(4):273–80.
44. Matevosyan NR. Oral health of adults with serious mental illnesses: a review. Community Ment Health J. 2010;46(6):553–62.
45. Kisely S, et al. The oral health of people with anxiety and depressive disorders - a systematic review and meta-analysis. J Affect Disord. 2016;200:119–32.
46. Kisely S, et al. A systematic review and meta-analysis of the association between poor oral health and severe mental illness. Psychosom Med. 2015;77(1):83–92.
47. Cademartori MG, et al. Is depression associated with oral health outcomes in adults and elders? A systematic review and meta-analysis. Clin Oral Investig. 2018;22(8):2685–702.
48. Pearson A, Chalmers J. Oral hygiene care for adults with dementia in residential aged care facilities. JBI Libr Syst Rev. 2004;2(3):1–89.
49. Manchery N, et al. Are oral health education for carers effective in the oral hygiene management of elderly with dementia? A systematic review. Dent Res J (Isfahan). 2020;17(1):1–9.
50. Chalmers JM, Pearson A. A systematic review of oral health assessment by nurses and carers for residents with dementia in residential care facilities. Spec Care Dentist. 2005;25(5):227–33.
51. Cerajewska TL, West NX. Dementia friendly dentistry for the periodontal patient. Part 1: recognising and assessing patients with dementia. Br Dent J. 2019;227(7):563–9.
52. Rozas NS, Sadowsky JM, Jeter CB. Strategies to improve dental health in elderly patients with cognitive impairment: a systematic review. J Am Dent Assoc. 2017;148(4):236–245.e3.
53. Jablonski RA, et al. Randomised clinical trial: efficacy of strategies to provide oral hygiene activities to nursing home residents with dementia who resist mouth care. Gerodontology. 2018;35(4):365–75.
54. Mun SJ, et al. Reduction in dental plaque in patients with mental disorders through the dental hygiene care programme. Int J Dent Hyg. 2014;12(2):133–40.
55. Friedlander AH, et al. Dental management of the geriatric patient with major depression. Spec Care Dentist. 1993;13(6):249–53.
56. Alabdullah J, Almuntashiri A. Strategies for safe and effective treatment of patients with Alzheimer disease. Dimen Dental Hygiene. 2020;18(7):32–5.
57. Brown J, et al. Self administered cognitive screening test (TYM) for detection of Alzheimer's disease: cross sectional study. BMJ. 2009;338:b2030.
58. Bruce ML, et al. Reducing suicidal ideation and depressive symptoms in depressed older primary care patients: a randomized controlled trial. JAMA. 2004;291(9):1081–91.
59. Marcantonio ER, et al. 3D-CAM: derivation and validation of a 3-minute diagnostic interview for CAM-defined delirium: a cross-sectional diagnostic test study. Ann Intern Med. 2014;161(8):554–61.

Oral Care in Long-Term Care Settings

Ronald Ettinger and Leonardo Marchini

1 Introduction

The US population is aging, and the most recent data available suggest that in 2018 persons over 65 made up 16% of the total population [1, 2]. The older population has been projected to grow in number and percentage reaching 22% in 2050 [3]. As these people age, 34% of them will become frail and functionally dependent, that is, they will not be able to maintain their independence, and will require either home health services or long-term care services and other supports (LTSS) sometime during their life span [4]. In 2010, it was estimated that 10.9 million persons who lived in the community needed LTSS; half of them were over the age of 65. In addition, there were 1.8 million persons living in long-term care facilities (LTCF), the majority of which were older adults [5]. In 2019, it was noted that approximately 1.5 million persons were now living in nursing homes, and 65.6% were women, while 7.8% were over the age of 95 years, 33.8% were between 85 and 94 years, 26.4% were between 75 and 84 years, 16.5% were between 65 and 74 years, and 15.5% were under the age of 65 [6]. In general, nursing home residents need help with instrumental activities of daily living (IADLs) and at least one activity of daily living (ADLs). Consequently, many need help with daily oral hygiene and are more likely to have poorer oral health than persons of a similar age living independently [7–9].

The current cohort of older Americans is keeping their teeth for longer, as edentulism rates have declined to 17.6% for persons 65 years and older [10, 11].

R. Ettinger (✉)
Department of Prosthodontics, College of Dentistry, University of Iowa, Iowa City, IA, USA
e-mail: ronald-ettinger@uiowa.edu

L. Marchini
Department of Preventive and Community Dentistry, College of Dentistry, University of Iowa, Iowa City, IA, USA

© The Author(s), under exclusive license to Springer Nature Switzerland AG 2022
C.-M. Hogue, J. G. Ruiz (eds.), *Oral Health and Aging*,
https://doi.org/10.1007/978-3-030-85993-0_10

However, this rate varies by state, by income, and by education [11]. Currently, the majority of residents in long-term care facilities (LTCFs) are dentate [12], and it has been shown that poor oral health impacts a person's quality of life [13], by putting them at risk for pain and infection [14]. Also, it has been reported that lack of oral hygiene can precipitate aspiration pneumonia [15, 16]. Although this information has been known for some time, the provision of daily oral care and oral services for persons living in LTCFs is still poor [17], as communication between healthcare providers and dentists in LTCF is inadequate [18].

Most investigators who have attempted to introduce an adequate oral hygiene care program within LTCFs have failed once the supporting funding ceases. The main reasons for this failure are lack of an organizational culture within LTCFs to prioritize oral healthcare, which translates to the absence of enforcement of existing regulations/guidelines (OBRA 1987) [19]. Many LTCFs are understaffed and in addition the direct care workers (nurses' aides) are underpaid, overworked, and undereducated [17, 20]. Unfortunately, many of them have poor oral health themselves, so they are not motivated to care for the oral health of the residents. Therefore, the quality of any oral healthcare program in a LTCF will depend upon the importance the director of nursing and the administrator place on the oral health of the residents [19].

There have been many modes of delivery of dental care services in LTCFs. The method most acceptable for dentists has been transporting residents to a local dental practice, which will accept these patients. This method is inconvenient and costly for nursing homes, because they must designate a staff member to accompany the resident to the appointment. Therefore, nursing homes would prefer it if the residents' family members were willing to transport them [21]. To provide services in the nursing home, the simplest method has been emergency care only using a tackle box, which contains enough instruments and supplies for the extraction of teeth and the adjustment of dentures. The next level, which includes more comprehensive care, uses portable equipment that can perform preventive procedures and simple restorations. At the next level, the dental provider would use mobile equipment, which is set up in the nursing home for a period of time, and allows the dentist to do comprehensive care, including more complex procedures. Mobile vans have been equipped to visit nursing homes, but their use is limited by geography and the weather, because it requires taking the residents from the home to the van for care.

This chapter will expand on the details of the LTCFs population and their oral health problems. It will discuss dental care delivery systems, which have evolved, and define possible advantages and disadvantages of each of these systems and how these have been impacted by the COVID-19 pandemic.

2 Description of Long-Term Care Facilities and Their Population

Traditionally, nursing homes were used to provide services for frail and functionally dependent older adults, as well as younger adults with disabilities, who were unable to support themselves independently in their daily lives. With the advent of the Affordable Care Act (ACA), a new term for nursing homes was defined as long-term care services and supports (LTSSs). This new term includes both institutionally and noninstitutionally based care, which includes adult day services, home health agencies, hospice, nursing homes, and assisted living facilities (ALF) and similar residential care communities [22].

Within the long-term care population, there are two major groups of residents. The first group are those who live in the facilities and receive long-term care, the second group are those who are admitted for post-acute care, usually following a stay in the hospital. The two groups have different clinical characteristics, as well as different sources of funding for their stay in the LTCFs [23]. The first group need permanent help with their activities of daily living, while the second group need help for a limited period of time to recover from their illnesses and should be able to return to their communities. The funding for the first group is either by out-of-pocket or by private nursing home insurance, or, if they become very poor, they may qualify for Medicaid, the US government healthcare insurance for the poor. The second group of older adults are usually funded by Medicare, the government healthcare insurance for Americans over 65 years of age, for up to 100 days, after a medically necessary hospital stay of at least 3 consecutive days. If the recovery time needs to be longer, then the cost will need to be financed either by out-of-pocket, by private insurance, or by Medicaid [24].

The traditional pool of family caregivers has changed due to decreasing family size and increasing employment rates among women, which has resulted in an increasing need for paid long-term care services for frail and functionally dependent family members. In the past, family members with early to middle stage dementia who were at risk, and living by themselves, were cared for by their families. However, this situation has changed as there is nobody at home during the day to care for these persons [22]. Consequently, these older adults with frailty would have three options. If the family can afford it, then they can employ a caretaker to come to the home or, if it is available, the older adults can go to an adult day care center. The third option is a long-term care facility, which can vary from residential care communities to a traditional nursing home [22].

Data from the National Longitudinal Caregiver Study [25] reported that the caregivers' reasons for placing dependents in LTCFs were related to the need for more skilled care (65%), the deterioration of caregiver's health (49%), the dependents' dementia-related behaviors (46%), and the need for more assistance (23%). For persons living at home, cognitive impairment and incontinence are common reasons for families to place their relatives in LTCFs, because dealing with these conditions severely impacts the life satisfaction of the family and caregivers. The majority of these frail and functionally dependent older adults have maintained some natural teeth. These natural dentitions need continuing daily oral hygiene care, which they may or may not get adequately when residing in a LTCF [17].

3 Oral Health Problems Among Residents of LTCFS

There is very little current data on the dental status of LTCFs residents, as there has not been a national study since 1997 [26, 27]. However, there are some regional studies in which the dentate status among LTCFs residents has been reported and varies from 53% in Kentucky [9] to nearly 80% in Florida [12] (see Table 1). The increased retention of teeth has resulted in a need for maintenance of these heavily restored dentitions (Figs. 1 and 2), which sometimes results in a need for complex restorations [10].

Many of the LTCFs residents are taking multiple medications to treat their numerous medical problems. It has been reported that over 400 medications have some potential for causing hyposalivation and xerostomia [30, 31]. The effects of these conditions on the heavily restored dentitions are increased plaque levels, resulting in new coronal caries, recurrent caries, root caries, and an exacerbation of periodontal disease (Fig. 3). These oral diseases can cause a decrease in oral health-related quality of life [31]. Poor eyesight, decreased hand-eye coordination, reduced

Table 1 Dentate status of residents in long-term care facilities in the USA

Author	Year	State	Percentage dentate
Murray et al. [12]	2006	Florida	79.6
Bush et al. [9]	2010	Kentucky	53.3
Chen et al. [28]	2013	Minnesota	69.9
Caplan et al. [29]	2017	Iowa	67.0
Marchini et al. [17]	2018	Iowa	77.8

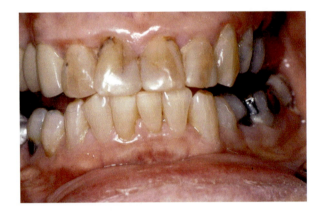

Fig. 1 Intraoral view of an 82-year-old female resident with a heavily restored dentition, who is still able to maintain oral hygiene at an acceptable level, although there is evidence of plaque accumulation and localized marginal gingivitis

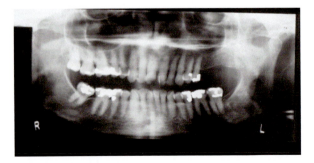

Fig. 2 Orthopantomograph of the same 82-year-old resident pictured in Fig. 1, showing her heavily restored dentition

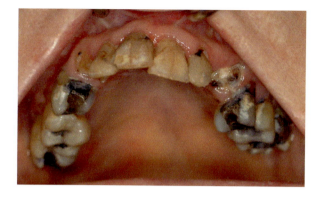

Fig. 3 Intraoral view of 68-year-old female resident, showing plaque accumulation resulting in coronal and root caries and periodontal disease, in an already heavily restored dentition with a history of taking multiple medications with xerostomic potential

manual dexterity, and cognitive impairment can cause increased plaque levels, which can lead to higher levels of oral disease unless appropriate daily oral hygiene routines are provided by LTCFs staff [32, 33]. For a more in-depth discussion on the topics of xerostomia, periodontal disease, and cognitive impairment, please refer to chapters "Xerostomia and Hyposalivation", "Management of Periodontal Disease in Older Adults", and "The 3 Ds: Dementia, Delirium and Depression in Oral Health".

However, there is data to show that the daily oral hygiene support by staff in LTCFs is often poor or inadequate [17, 34]. The reasons for this dilemma are that the primary caregivers are nurses' aides, who often have poor oral health themselves and are inadequately trained to carry out oral hygiene procedures for residents, especially those who resist care. In addition, the nurses' aides are underpaid and overworked, and many LTCFs are understaffed, which results in inadequate oral healthcare for the residents. There have been several attempts to improve oral hygiene routines in LTCFs [17, 20]. The most successful has been the hiring of a dental hygienist either part-time or full-time to help with daily oral healthcare [35]; however, most LTCFs are not prepared to pay for these services, as dental care is not reimbursable through the health insurance of Medicare, unlike physical therapy, speech therapy, or occupational therapy [36, 37]. Another successful approach has been to designate one of the nurses' aides as the "oral health specialist" and, after some training, to have them spend at least 50% of their time caring for the oral health of the residents [38]. Unfortunately, when the grant money runs out for such a program, so does the support of the LTCF. Another problem is the high rate of turnover of LTCFs staff. If a training program exists within the LTCF, unless it is repeated on a continuous basis, the resignation of the current staff will dilute the commitment of the nurses' aides to an oral hygiene program; and when the new staff are hired, they have not benefited from the training program nor from the cooperative environment previously achieved [39].

Consequently, many reports have found poor oral health among LTCFs residents [17, 40, 41]. The consequences of an inadequate dentition can be inability to chew food adequately that can result in poor nutrition [42], as well as difficulties with communication [43], and declining systemic health, such as poor glycemic control

[44], increased risk for cardiovascular disease [45], and aspiration pneumonia [46]. The microbial colonization of hard surfaces, such as teeth and/or dentures, allows for formation of biofilms. These biofilms if left undisturbed due to a lack of oral hygiene change from gram-positive and mostly aerobic to gram-negative and anaerobic, which if inhaled can cause aspiration pneumonia, which is the leading cause of death in LTCFs [47]. There are several studies that have shown that daily oral hygiene for residents decreases the incidence of aspiration pneumonia in LTCFs [46]. For a more in-depth discussion on this topic, please refer to chapter "Swallowing, Dysphagia, and Aspiration Pneumonia".

The COVID-19 pandemic has negatively influenced access to care for LTCFs residents, because currently many facilities will not allow healthcare practitioners into their premises, unless they are salaried staff. LTCFs are reluctant to send their residents to other healthcare facilities, unless the resident requires emergency care or hospitalization, which rarely includes oral healthcare. The consequences for the residents' oral health are an exacerbation of their caries and periodontal disease, especially because oral hygiene routines have been disrupted due to COVID-19 social distancing protocols [48, 49]. The emergency approval of COVID-19 vaccines and its currently availability for healthcare providers and LTCFs residents will change the negative impact of isolation on the residents and should allow them to regain access to regular oral healthcare.

4 Types of Oral Health Services for LTC Patients

Historically, there have always been a few dedicated dentists who have been prepared to care for residents in LTCFs, by either having them transported to their dental offices or by visiting them at their residences [50]. The reluctance of the majority of dentists to care for these persons has been studied over time, and a series of barriers have been identified [50, 51]. The barriers include lack of training in geriatric dental medicine, the cost in terms of time and efficiency caring for these patients, the complexity of the residents medical and pharmacological regimens, as well as the complexity of dealing with deteriorating, heavily restored dentitions [51, 52]. Additionally, some dentists may also be negatively influenced by the prevalent ageist culture in modern societies, predisposing them against caring for this age group who requires more time and also challenges the culture of efficient practice management [53].

Some families of residents in LTCFs are also reluctant for their relatives to receive dental care because it is expensive, and unless they have private dental insurance or are covered by Medicaid, all costs are out-of-pocket. Medicare does not cover routine dental care, only some oral surgical procedures [37]. Another reason for families' reluctance for providing dental care for their relatives is because they believe that such care will disrupt the life of their relatives [50]. Some older adults with frailty may have had bad childhood experiences with dental care and consequently may fear or distrust dentists [10]. Many residents may have low dental health literacy [54], which impacts their understanding of the importance of dental care and daily oral hygiene routines, such as tooth brushing and the use of fluoridated toothpaste, which means they may not brush their own teeth regularly or they may resist help with oral hygiene.

Finding a nearby dentist who is prepared to treat LTCF residents may also be a barrier, as the accessibility of dentists' office may be a problem, even if he/she is willing to care for the residents. Some such office barriers include not having ramps, wheelchair accessible elevators, doors wide enough to accommodate wheelchairs, and operatories that are wheelchair accessible [55]. The staff of such an office needs to be sensitive to patients with vision and hearing disabilities, as well as knowing how to safely transfer patients.

The time of day to appropriately schedule residents may depend on their medical problems. For instance, patients with chronic heart failure are best seen in the morning, because they are strongest after a night's rest. Residents with arthritis need time to have their joints unstiffen; therefore, late morning to early afternoon are more appropriate appointment times for these patients. Mid- to late morning is appropriate for residents with dementia, as they may become more confused and sundown as the day progresses. Several residents may be underweight and may need appropriate support, such as pillows, egg crate foam, etc., to sit comfortably in the dental chair. These patients cannot tolerate long procedures, and their appointments should not exceed 2 hours, which must include travel time, as well as the time in the dental office [21].

Many practitioners may not want to treat LTCF residents, because they may become frustrated as these patients are unable to maintain their daily oral hygiene, and consequently their oral health may decline no matter what treatment is provided by the dentist. Their oral health may be further impacted by xerostomia caused by the medications they are using, their visual impairment, as well as their lack of manual dexterity [56].

Many residents do not have relatives living nearby and require the LTCF to transport them to the dentist's office, which incurs expenses for the facility. These expenses include providing an appropriate vehicle or a driver and/or a nurses' aide to accompany the resident, which means the aide is not available for duties within the facility. An alternative to transporting the resident is to provide care within the LTCF. One advantage is that many residents with frailty do not cope well with being transported out of their environment. Also, residents who are incontinent or catheterized are more easily treated within the LTCF [21].

The simplest mode of dental care for LTCFs residents is the use of a "tackle box" (Fig. 4). The tackle box contains equipment and supplies that allow the dentist to adjust dentures and do simple extractions [21]. A simple but necessary procedure would be to show the nurses' aides how to put the residents' name on their dentures. The simplest method is to abrade the surface of the denture and write the resident's name on the denture with a marking pencil and then to cover the area with two layers of clear nail varnish. This technique will allow the name to remain for 12–18 months. The "tackle box" can be used to treat caries using atraumatic restorative treatment (ART) technique, which includes silver diamine fluoride (SDF)

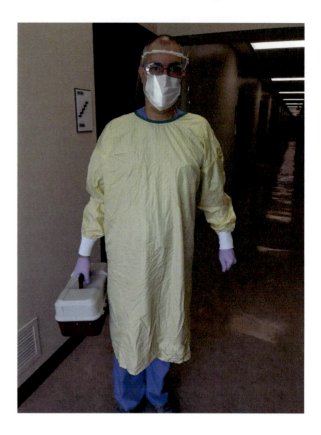

Fig. 4 Dentist visiting a long-term care facility, with the appropriate PPE, carrying a tackle box to provide a denture adjustment for a resident

applications and glass ionomer restorations [57]. These procedures require only hand instruments and do not generate aerosols, reducing the risk of COVID-19 infection [36]. For a more in-depth discussion on the topic of caries management, please refer to chapter "Management of Caries in Older Adults".

At the next level is commercial portable dental equipment, which allows the dentist to do the procedures described previously as well as direct restorations using rotary instruments, surgical extractions, and rest preparations for removable partial dentures (RPD). This equipment is not usually capable of sustained use but is efficient for intermittent procedures (Fig. 5). Some dental associations have bought this kind of equipment, which can be utilized at no cost by their members.

However, mobile equipment is now available, which is as effective as traditional dental office equipment (Fig. 6). This equipment allows the dentist to see multiple patients with comparable efficiency to a traditional dental office and provide comprehensive treatment. The advantage of this equipment is that it can be easily transported and timely installed in a facility, which allows providers to waste a minimum of their time prior to caring for residents, making it more cost-efficient for the dentist [57].

Especially equipped vans (Fig. 7) have been designed with dental chairs and other equipment. However, for a frail, functionally dependent or cognitively

Fig. 5 An Example of a portable dental unit (Aseptic Transport II, Aseptico, Inc Woodinville, WA 98072)

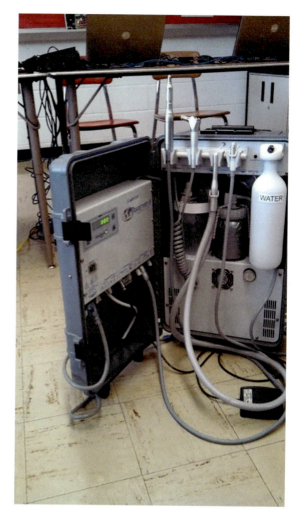

impaired persons, moving them from the LTCF to the mobile van can create serious risks or precipitate inappropriate behaviors. In hot weather, there is a risk of hyperthermia. In cold weather, there is a risk of falls, as well as hypothermia. Also, the van needs to be wheelchair accessible either with a ramp or a lift. Another disadvantage of the mobile van is related to their power source, which usually requires a 220-volt connection, and water lines that may freeze in the winter [57] If the van and the vehicle are directly connected, when the engine needs to be serviced, the equipment becomes unavailable, which further increases the cost of service.

Some large LTCFs that have a high proportion of private pay residents are able to provide in-house dental facilities for their residents, which allow the oral healthcare practitioners to have similar surroundings to a dental office and that is designed to care for at-risk and wheelchair-bound patients. To make such an on-site dental

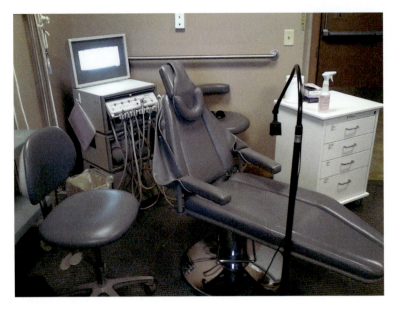

Fig. 6 An example of mobile equipment from DNTL (ProCart II) set up in a room in a nursing home with a portable chair and light, which is used by the University of Iowa's Geriatric Mobile Unit Program

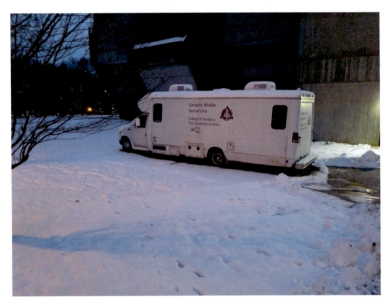

Fig. 7 The van used by the Geriatric Mobile Unit Program parked outside of nursing home, in the Iowa winter, showing the problems that weather can pose to such a program

facility economically feasible, the LTCF should have at least 150 to 200 residents. To be flexible, these programs should also have some portable equipment to be able to treat residents in their rooms if they are bedridden [21]. In some cases, these operatories may be shared with podiatry and occasionally with hair dressing shops. These LTCFs may be able to employ a hygienist either full- or part-time to care for the residents, providing the state regulations allow indirect supervision by a dentist [57]. In Table 2, the advantages and disadvantages of different types of dental care delivery systems for LTCFs are summarized.

The most important service a consultant dentist needs to instigate in a LTCF is to develop a continuing and functioning oral hygiene program within the facility. Educating the director of nursing (DON) and the administrator to support such a program is not easy as previously discussed. This program should also include the help of the LTCF dietician to reduce the residents' intake of refined sugars and other carbohydrates, as well as discouraging the residents from snacking between meals or consuming sugary treats and carbonated beverages.

In-service programs for nurses' aides should begin by asking them what barriers they face when providing daily oral hygiene care for the residents. It helps to provide hands-on training with residents, especially showing the aides how to manage care-resistant behaviors, such as refusing oral care, kicking, hitting, biting, spitting, or inability to understand what is happening and/or to follow directions. The program should then describe basic communication techniques, as can be seen in Table 3.

Table 2 Advantages and disadvantages of different types of dental care delivery systems for LTCFs

Type of program	Advantages	Disadvantages
Transport to practice	Dentist has all equipment Cost-effective for dentists Cost-effective for LTCF if family transports the resident	Office needs architectural changes to accommodate wheelchairs Not cost-effective for LTCF if responsible for transportation Maybe stressful for residents
"Tackle box"	No additional equipment costs Ease of portability Cost-effective for LTCFs Less stressful for residents	Time-consuming for dentist Limited range of treatment options
Portable equipment	Ease of portability Ease of set-up Cost-effective for home Less stressful for residents	Time-consuming for dentist Limited range of treatment options Cost of equipment
Mobile equipment	Cost-effective for home Still portable Less stressful for residents	Time-consuming for dentist High cost of equipment Transportation and set up time
In-house facility	Cost-effective for dentist Less time consuming for dentist Less stressful for residents	High cost of equipment for LTCF

Table 3 Basic communication techniques to be used with care-resistant residents

Basic communication techniques
Be patient, respectful, and gentle when approaching the resident
Avoid removing the resident from his/her favorite activity
Address the resident by his/her name
Always smile
Keep eye contact, preferably at the resident's eye level
Approach the resident from the front; move slowly
Introduce yourself to the resident
Use plain language and short sentences
Provide only one instruction at a time
Briefly explain what you are doing and why you are doing it, and repeat it as necessary
Be sure to provide constant encouragement and abundant and immediate positive reinforcement for good behavior

If the resident does not voluntarily cooperate in toothbrushing, it may be helpful to simply touch the lips and teeth with a toothbrush, which may trigger a reflex related to toothbrushing. If there is further resistance, Jane Chalmers [58] has summarized in detail techniques that have been used to manage oral hygiene care for residents with dementia. One such technique for helping to clean a person's teeth who will not open his/her mouth is to take a toothbrush; bend it back at a 45° angle; slide the bent toothbrush into the angle of the mouth, holding it against the cheek, to break the perioral muscles spasm; and allow for the removal of plaque and debris. Some other techniques, which have been described to communicate with residents with challenging behaviors, are shown in Table 4.

When discussing with nurses' aides, the reasons why they were reluctant to brush residents' teeth was a fear of being bitten and punched. To protect themselves, nurses' aides can be shown how to approach the resident from the side, gain his/her attention, and then move behind him/her, cup the chin with one hand, and slowly bring the brush to the mouth with the other hand. This allows the nurses' aide to protect themselves from being kicked or punched as they can control the residents' hands. If the resident has a rocking chair in his/her room, it is very useful to place a foot on the rocker, tip it back, and bring the resident back toward the caregiver's abdomen, which gives easier access to the mouth, from a more protected position (Fig. 8).

If the resident is agitated, it is important for the caregiver to determine if the resident is at risk of self-injury or of hurting others, prior carrying out oral healthcare at this time. The caregiver may try distraction and/or rescuing techniques, but if the resident does not respond, then the procedure should be aborted for another more convenient time when the patient is less agitated.

If the resident has a permanent nasogastric tube and is bedridden, many caregivers do not believe that the resident needs oral hygiene care. However, even though the resident is not eating, he/she is still generating biofilm, which if undisturbed increases the risk of aspiration pneumonia. Many of these residents cannot follow instructions and will not open their mouths to allow their teeth to be brushed. To overcome this problem, it is possible to insert a tongue depressor between the teeth

Oral Care in Long-Term Care Settings

Table 4 Techniques to communicate with residents with challenging behaviors

Name of the technique	Description of the technique	Example
Rescuing	A second caregiver comes to deliver care, as the first caregiver leaves or steps back	The resident resists having the teeth brushed by one caregiver. A second caregiver takes over the resident's care.
Distraction	The resident can be distracted by singing a favorite song, by holding an item (such as a blanket or a doll), by watching a TV show or other video on YouTube	A resident is agitated during dental care. The resident is offered a doll or soft blanket as a distraction and this usually calms him/her down.
Bridging	The resident's sensory connection to the activity can be improved by having he/she hold the same object that is being used by the caregiver	Have the resident hold a toothbrush while the caregiver brushes his/her teeth with another toothbrush
Hand over hand	The resident is guided in an activity by the caregiver placing his/her hand over the resident's hand, in order to complete the task	Have the resident hold a toothbrush and then the caregiver places his/her hand over resident's hand and guides the toothbrushing
Chaining	A caregiver starts an oral healthcare activity and then lets the patient finish it	The caregiver places the resident's denture in his/her hand and encourages him/her to return the denture into his/her mouth

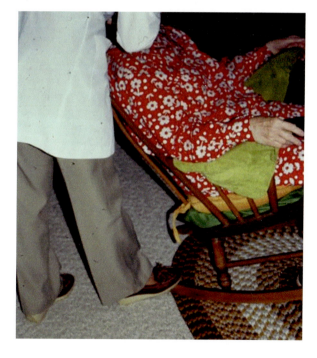

Fig. 8 A resident sitting in a rocking chair; the caregiver is tipping the chair backward to improve access to the mouth while brushing the residents' teeth

and then slide another one underneath it and keep adding them until the mouth is opened wide enough to insert a toothbrush. If that toothbrush is attached to suction, the mouth can be cleaned, the tongue brushed, and chlorhexidine sprayed to prevent dental diseases.

The development of a preventive program may help to reduce the effects of xerostomia and plaque accumulation in the residents' dentitions. The use of prescription high concentration fluoride toothpastes, such as toothpastes with 5000 ppm fluoride content, and no alcohol, or 0.12% chlorhexidine rinses have been shown to help reduce caries and periodontal disease [3]. Residents who are in a semicomatose state need to have their teeth, tongue, and gums wiped 2–3 times/day with moist gauze or glycerin and/or 10% solution of bicarbonate of soda to remove the coating which forms on these tissues [21]. The residents' lips should also be lubricated with lanolin to prevent drying and cracking. For care-resistant residents, the use of chlorhexidine in atomizers, which can be squirted into the buccal mucosa, has been shown to be efficacious [59].

5 Influence of the COVID-19 Pandemic on Oral Health Services for LTCFS Residents

In addition to the abovementioned barriers, residents of LTCFs are now facing new barriers related to the COVID-19 pandemic, which is caused by the severe acute respiratory syndrome coronavirus 2 (SARS-Cov-2). The major risk factors for poorer COVID-19 outcomes have been identified as older age and comorbidities [60], for instance, the case fatality rate for individuals aged 80+ has been reported to be about 22% [61].

LTCFs have become high-risk sites for COVID-19 infection and transmission. Many LTCFs have had outbreaks of COVID-19 around the USA, which may be caused by asymptomatic shedding of the virus, a lack of adequate personal protective equipment (PPE) for the staff, limited tracing of COVID-19 positive staff, and the limited testing of residents and staff [6, 62]. Unfortunately, many direct care workers in LTCFs have received inadequate training on how to protect themselves and others from COVID-19 infection. Also, many live in homes with multiple generations of family members, which reduces social distancing, and many must rely on public transportation to reach the LTCFs. These social issues heighten the staffs' risk of being infected by SARS-Cov-2, which has resulted in widespread virus outbreaks in LTCFs [49, 63]. As cognitively impaired residents now constitute a large proportion of residents in American LTCFs, many will not observe precautions related to COVID-19, such as wearing masks and maintaining social distancing, and so are at higher risk of getting infected and infecting others [6].

Another unintended consequence of the pandemic is that nurses' aides are avoiding providing daily oral hygiene help for residents, because they are afraid of getting infected by the residents' saliva, which increases plaque levels in residents and results in more untreated dental disease [36].

LTCFs have improvised new infection control protocols as a result of COVID-19, such as forbidding group activities and reducing or barring visitors, which includes dentists and other non-salaried providers [6]. During these months of LTCFs lockdowns, elective dental treatment has been postponed, and the consequences will be increased severity of dental disease among residents [3].

The use of tele-dentistry has emerged as a method to triage residents either to monitor their dental problems, to prescribe analgesics or antibiotics, and, if necessary, to refer residents to a hospital with a dental department for extractions. There have been reports that neglected dental infections may result in a hospital admission requiring the administration of IV antibiotics for facial swelling due to a dental abscess [3]. However, some cognitively impaired residents are not easily transferred to a hospital. The policy of some LTCFs is that if a resident leaves the facility, the LTCF will require that the resident quarantines outside the facility for 14 days before he/she can return. Many families have become very stressed because they are unable to visit their family members who are residing in a LTCF and to safely provide healthcare for the resident outside of the facility.

6 The Integration of Oral Healthcare in LTC Services

In the 1980s, as a result of a federal class action lawsuit, due to decades of scandals caused by inappropriate care and lack of regulations, the Congress mandated a study of nursing home regulations, which was led by the Institute of Medicine. This resulted in the Omnibus Budget Reconciliation Act of 1987 (OBRA-87) [64]. These regulations required LTCFs to have a dentist affiliated with the facility and that each resident has a dentist of record and an annual dental in service [1]. Unfortunately, nursing home assessors did not routinely inspect each resident to determine their oral health problems; consequently, the nursing homes ignored these regulations. In 1990, Medicare and Medicaid introduced new regulations, including new standards of care, which were resident-focused and outcome-oriented. This process resulted in a range of new federal enforcement measures, which required Medicare and Medicaid to certify nursing facilities to use a standardized, reproducible, comprehensive functional assessment tool for all residents and to develop individualized care plans. As a consequence, the Resident Assessment Instrument (RAI) was developed under the supervision of the Health Care Financing Administration (HCFA), which included the Minimum Data Set (MDS) [64]. However, several studies have indicated that the MDS dental assessments identified very few oral health problems and that even when problems were identified, it did not result in dental care, as the nurse assessors still do not inspect the resident's oral health [6, 65].

It is clear that dentistry has been missing in geriatric interprofessional teams [66], in part because dental education has been separated from medical and allied healthcare training programs. The impact of oral health on the older patient's well-being is not fully understood by non-dental healthcare professionals. A possible solution would be to develop geriatric interprofessional education (IPE) courses [67]. The World Health Organization (WHO) defines IPE as "when two or more professions learn with, about and from each other to enable effective collaboration and improve health outcomes." The WHO then defines interprofessional collaborative practice as "when multiple health workers from different professional backgrounds provide comprehensive services by working with patients, their families, caregivers, and communities to deliver the highest quality of care across settings" [68]. Interprofessional care for frail and functionally dependent older adults is critical due to the complexity of their healthcare needs and the small number of specialists available to consult and treat them [69, 70].

An example of a government sponsored program to improve the oral health of residents in LTCFs is Australia's "Better Oral Health in Residential Care Model." The basis of this program was to change the perception of healthcare workers that oral health was the responsibility of dental professionals and to make healthcare workers understand that it was the responsibility of the healthcare team. This model advocates for sharing roles among nurses, primary care providers, nurses' aides, and dental professionals to implement four key oral health-related processes, which "include oral health assessment, oral healthcare planning, daily oral hygiene support, and dental assessment and treatment" [71].

However, due to the existing limitations in geriatric clinical education in dental schools, many dentists are not familiar or comfortable using portable and mobile equipment to treat residents in LTCFs [72]. Many studies [50, 51] have shown that some dentists are prepared to care for these patients in their private practices but that can create problems for the patients and the LTCFs with regard to added stresses for the patients and transportation problems for the facilities. Another barrier for the dentist is that they are inadequately reimbursed for the additional time required to travel to and from the LTCFs and the extra time it takes to care for these older adults with frailty due to their limited ability to cooperate during treatment.

Possible strategies to mitigate these problems to train and allow allied oral healthcare professionals, such as expanded function dental hygienist and dental therapists, to provide care for the residents under indirect supervision of a consulting dentist [3]. The use of tele-dentistry to diagnose some oral lesions would reduce traveling time for the residents and dentists, allowing for more efficient and cost-effective care for this population [73].

7 Some Solutions to Problems Caused by COVID-19

Tele-dentistry (Fig. 9) has become an important tool to remotely assess frail and functionally dependent older adults who might not be able to come to the office due to COVID-19 and related isolation or quarantine [74]. This technology can be used to remotely assess a LTCF resident who has acute dental needs and is isolated. Such a resident may need a prescription for analgesics, or for antibiotics if there is any

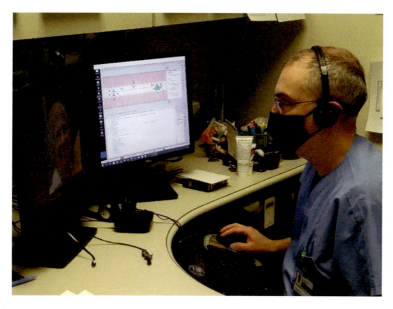

Fig. 9 A tele-dentistry consultation with a resident of a long-term care facility to determine her chief complaint, in order to decide if it is necessary for the dentist to visit the facility or if the resident needs to be referred to the dental practice. Please, note that she is a patient of record and that the dentist has access to her electronic dental records

sign of infection, such as facial swelling. If necessary, a referral may be required to transport the resident to a hospital emergency department that has a dental service.

Using this technology legally requires the dentist to appropriately identify the patient, e.g., by confirming their name and date of birth, which requires the dentist to have the patient's clinical records available. It may also require a staff member or the patient's legal advocate to be present in order to inform the patient/legal advocate about the limitations associated with tele-dentistry. At the end of the remote appointment using tele-dentistry, the dentist must keep detailed notes of the appointment. Dentists should avoid using tele-dentistry to consult with patients who are not patients of record, unless the patient has been referred to them.

Frail and functionally dependent older adult patients residing in LTCFs and their care providers should also be educated about the mitigation strategies that are being used in dental practices to improve infection control and aimed at minimizing COVID-19 transmission. These strategies include initial contact by telephone or tele-dentistry apps to identify the patient and their chief complaint, including asking about the existence of any COVID-19 symptoms. If the dentist refers the resident to his/her dental practice, the resident's temperature will be taken, and the accompanying person will be asked to maintain social distancing and to wear a mask. The dental provider will be wearing appropriate PPE, which will include a face mask and a shield, as well as a waterproof gown. Infection risks will be minimized by reducing aerosol generating procedures, such as the use of SDF and ART to manage caries, and hand scaling for periodontal maintenance. If aerosols need to be generated, then the addition of extraoral high suction units can be employed to reduce the risk of aerosol-induced contamination.

Residents with dementia will have difficulties with tele-triage and the new protocols related to COVID-19. For instance, residents with dementia, who make up 48% of the LTCFs population [62], will react negatively to the use of face masks and shields by the clerical staff and dental providers (Fig. 10). This reaction can make providing dental treatment for these patients very disruptive. Many residents with hearing and vision problems will be unable to hear or lip read their dental provider if he/she is wearing a N95 respirator, a face mask, and a full-face shield [4].

Consequently, more older adults with dementia may need to be treated under general anesthesia (GA). The circumstances will depend on the patients' level of cognitive impairment, their disruptive behavior, and the type of dental care they need. Access to operating rooms for dental treatment under GA has been restricted in the past and has become extremely difficult due to COVID-19. A system for prioritization will need to be developed under these new conditions [75].

When dentists are allowed to reenter LTCFs to deliver elective dental care, they will need to use enhanced infection control precautions, such as inquiring if the

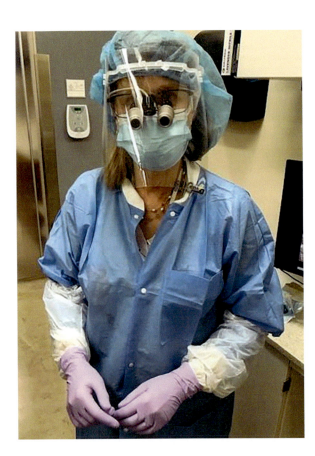

Fig. 10 Dentist wearing the appropriate PPE, which has evolved as a result of the COVID-19 pandemic

residents have had immunization for COVID-19 prior to the consultation. Additional measures should include improved decontamination of equipment and surfaces with 80% alcohol wipes. If aerosols need to be generated, the room being used should have the door closed, and the clinician will need to bring an extraoral high suction unit. Fogging protocols of the room should follow aerosol generating procedures, although this procedure has become controversial [3].

To support the required PPE and added equipment and supplies, reimbursement rates will need to be increased. Therefore, as a group the American Dental Association and other professional organizations will need to lobby third-party companies and government agencies to increase their reimbursement rates, if dental professionals are to safely care for these frail and functionally dependent older adults [3].

8 Conclusions

To be in compliance with OBRA-87, every LTCF should have a consultant dentist who has a contractual agreement with the facility to examine and treat all of the residents who consent to receive dental care. The consultant dentist should develop an oral health program for the institution together with the administrator, the director of nursing, and the medical director. Such a program should include:

1. Each resident should have a dentist of record included in their medical files.
2. An oral screening on or about the time of admission should be done by a dentist.
3. A yearly examination as required by the resident assessment instrument – minimum data set (RAI-MDS 2.0), either by a dentist or dental hygienist.
4. A yearly in-service for the nursing staff on an oral health topic, either by a dentist or dental hygienist.
5. All oral prosthesis should be marked with the resident's name or number.
6. There should be a customized written program of oral hygiene care for each resident, which includes:

    (a) The cleaning of teeth and/or dentures that should be performed daily, preferably by the resident, but if they are not competent, then by a staff member.
    (b) Modified or adapted toothbrushes for the resident's specific needs, if necessary.
    (c) An ultrasonic device for cleaning dentures.
    (d) The encouragement of residents to remove their dentures while sleeping, unless they are necessary to support a continuous positive airway pressure (CPAP) device.

7. If the resident requires treatment, then the treatment plan should follow the concepts of rational treatment planning, with the following priorities:

    (a) The highest priority is the relief of pain and the treatment of acute infection.

(b) Depending upon the life expectancy of the resident, dental treatment may be limited to emergency and maintenance procedures.
(c) Restoration of esthetics may be a valuable contribution to the emotional welfare of the family and the resident, even at the terminal phase of life.
(d) Restoration of function should be a priority taking into account what treatment is in the best interest of the residents after evaluating all their modifying factors.
(e) All other treatment is elective depending on the needs and expectations of the residents and their families.

References

1. Roberts AW, Ogunwole SU, Blackslee L, Rabe MA. The population over 65 years and older in the United States:2016. In: Bureau UC, editor. 2016.
2. Administration_for_Community_Living. 2018 Profile of Older Americans. In: Department_of_Health_and_Human_Services, editor. 2018. p. 1–20.
3. Harris-Kojetin L, Sengupta M, Park-Lee E, Valverde R, Caffrey C, Rome V, et al. Long-Term Care Providers and services users in the United States: data from the National Study of Long-Term Care Providers, 2013–2014. Vital & health statistics Series 3, Analytical and epidemiological studies. 2016(38):x–xii; 1–105.
4. Favreault M, Dey J. Long -term services and supports for older Americans: Risks and Financing.: ASPE Research Brief; 2016. Available from: https://aspe.hhs.gov/system/files/pdf/106211/ElderLTCrb-rev.pdf.
5. Kaye HS, Harrington C, LaPlante MP. Long-term care: who gets it, who provides it, who pays, and how much? Health Aff (Millwood). 2010;29(1):11–21.
6. Services CfMaM. Nursing Home Data Compendium 2015. Centers for Medicare and Medicaid Services; 2015. p. 251.
7. Berg R, Berkey DB, Tang JM, Baine C, Altman DS. Oral health status of older adults in Arizona: results from the Arizona Elder Study. Spec Care Dentist. 2000;20(6):226–33.
8. Choi JS, Yi YJ, Donnelly LR. Oral health of older residents in care and community dwellers: nursing implications. Int Nurs Rev. 2017;64(4):602–9.
9. Bush HM, Dickens NE, Henry RG, Durham L, Sallee N, Skelton J, et al. Oral health status of older adults in Kentucky: results from the Kentucky Elder Oral Health Survey. Spec Care Dentist. 2010;30(5):185–92.
10. Ettinger RL, Marchini L. Cohort differences among aging populations: an update. J Am Dent Assoc. 2020;151(7):519–26.
11. Dye BA, Weatherspoon DJ, Lopez Mitnik G. Tooth loss among older adults according to poverty status in the United States from 1999 through 2004 and 2009 through 2014. J Am Dent Assoc. 2019;150(1):9–23.e3.
12. Murray PE, Ede-Nichols D, Garcia-Godoy F. Oral health in Florida nursing homes. Int J Dent Hyg. 2006;4(4):198–203.
13. Benyamini Y, Leventhal H, Leventhal EA. Self-rated oral health as an independent predictor of self-rated general health, self-esteem and life satisfaction. Soc Sci Med. 2004;59(5):1109–16.
14. Ramsay SE, Whincup PH, Watt RG, Tsakos G, Papacosta AO, Lennon LT, et al. Burden of poor oral health in older age: findings from a population-based study of older British men. BMJ Open. 2015;5(12):e009476.
15. Yoneyama T, Yoshida M, Ohrui T, Mukaiyama H, Okamoto H, Hoshiba K, et al. Oral care reduces pneumonia in older patients in nursing homes. J Am Geriatr Soc. 2002;50(3):430–3.

16. Quagliarello V, Ginter S, Han L, Van Ness P, Allore H, Tinetti M. Modifiable risk factors for nursing home-acquired pneumonia. Clin Infect Dis. 2005;40(1):1–6.
17. Marchini L, Recker E, Hartshorn J, Cowen H, Lynch D, Drake D, et al. Iowa nursing facility oral hygiene (INFOH) intervention: a clinical and microbiological pilot randomized trial. Spec Care Dentist. 2018;38(6):345–55.
18. Preston AJ, Kearns A, Barber MW, Gosney MA. The knowledge of healthcare professionals regarding elderly persons' oral care. Br Dent J. 2006;201(5):293–5.
19. Ettinger RL, O'Toole C, Warren J, Levy S, Hand JS. Nursing directors' perceptions of the dental components of the Minimum Data Set (MDS) in nursing homes. Spec Care Dentist. 2000;20(1):23–7.
20. Thorne S, Kazanjian A, MacEntee M. Oral health in long-term care – the implications of organizational culture. J Aging Stud. 2001;15(3):271–83.
21. Ettinger RL, Miller-Eldridge J. An evaluation of dental programs and delivery systems for elderly isolated populations. Gerodontics. 1985;1(2):91–7.
22. Harris-Kojetin L, Sengupta M, Lendon J, Rome V, Valverde R, Caffrey C. Long-term care providers and services users in the United States, 2015–2016. Vital Health Stat. 2019;43(3):1–88.
23. Eskildsen M, Price T. Nursing home care in the USA. Geriatr Gerontol Int. 2009;9(1):1–6.
24. Grabowski DC, Angelelli JJ, Mor V. Medicaid payment and risk-adjusted nursing home quality measures. Health Aff (Millwood). 2004;23(5):243–52.
25. Buhr GT, Kuchibhatla M, Clipp EC. Caregivers' reasons for nursing home placement: clues for improving discussions with families prior to the transition. Gerontologist. 2006;46(1):52–61.
26. Dye BA, Fisher MA, Yellowitz JA, Fryar CD, Vargas CM. Receipt of dental care, dental status and workforce in U.S. nursing homes: 1997 National Nursing Home Survey. Spec Care Dentist. 2007;27(5):177–86.
27. Gift HC, Cherry-Peppers G, Oldakowski RJ. Oral health status and related behaviours of U.S. nursing home residents, 1995. Gerodontology. 1997;14(2):89–99.
28. Chen X, Shuman SK, Hodges JS, Gatewood LC, Xu J. Patterns of tooth loss in older adults with and without dementia: a retrospective study based on a Minnesota cohort. J Am Geriatr Soc. 2010;58(12):2300–7.
29. Caplan DJ, Ghazal TS, Cowen HJ, Oliveira DC. Dental status as a predictor of mortality among nursing facility residents in eastern Iowa. Gerodontology. 2017;34(2):257–63.
30. Turner MD. Hyposalivation and xerostomia: etiology, complications, and medical management. Dent Clin N Am. 2016;60(2):435–43.
31. Thomson WM. Dry mouth and older people. Aust Dent J. 2015;60(Suppl 1):54–63.
32. Tavares M, Lindefjeld Calabi KA, San Martin L. Systemic diseases and oral health. Dent Clin N Am. 2014;58(4):797–814.
33. Marchini L, Ettinger R, Hartshorn J. Personalized dental caries Management for Frail Older Adults and Persons with special needs. Dent Clin N Am. 2019;63(4):631–51.
34. De Visschere LM, Grooten L, Theuniers G, Vanobbergen JN. Oral hygiene of elderly people in long-term care institutions–a cross-sectional study. Gerodontology. 2006;23(4):195–204.
35. Monaghan NP, Morgan MZ. What proportion of dental care in care homes could be met by direct access to dental therapists or dental hygienists? Br Dent J. 2015;219(11):531–4. discussion 4
36. Marchini L, Ettinger RL. Coronavirus disease 2019 and dental care for older adults: new barriers require unique solutions. J Am Dent Assoc. 2020;151(12):881–4.
37. Willink A, Schoen C, Davis K. Dental care and Medicare beneficiaries: access gaps, cost burdens, and policy options. Health Aff (Millwood). 2016;35(12):2241–8.
38. Amerine C, Boyd L, Bowen DM, Neill K, Johnson T, Peterson T. Oral health champions in long-term care facilities-a pilot study. Spec Care Dentist. 2014;34(4):164–70.
39. Low LF, Fletcher J, Goodenough B, Jeon YH, Etherton-Beer C, MacAndrew M, et al. A systematic review of interventions to change staff care practices in order to improve resident outcomes in nursing homes. PLoS One. 2015;10(11):e0140711.

40. Zuluaga DJ, Ferreira J, Montoya JA, Willumsen T. Oral health in institutionalised elderly people in Oslo, Norway and its relationship with dependence and cognitive impairment. Gerodontology. 2012;29(2):e420–6.
41. Katsoulis J, Schimmel M, Avrampou M, Stuck AE, Mericske-Stern R. Oral and general health status in patients treated in a dental consultation clinic of a geriatric ward in Bern, Switzerland. Gerodontology. 2012;29(2):e602–10.
42. Lindroos EK, Saarela RKT, Suominen MH, Muurinen S, Soini H, Kautiainen H, et al. Burden of oral symptoms and its associations with nutrition, well-being, and survival among nursing home residents. J Am Med Dir Assoc. 2019;20(5):537–43.
43. Georg D. Improving the oral health of older adults with dementia/cognitive impairment living in a residential aged care facility. Int J Evid Based Healthc. 2006;4(1):54–61.
44. Sanz M, Ceriello A, Buysschaert M, Chapple I, Demmer RT, Graziani F, et al. Scientific evidence on the links between periodontal diseases and diabetes: consensus report and guidelines of the joint workshop on periodontal diseases and diabetes by the International Diabetes Federation and the European Federation of Periodontology. J Clin Periodontol. 2018;45(2):138–49.
45. Lockhart PB, Bolger AF, Papapanou PN, Osinbowale O, Trevisan M, Levison ME, et al. Periodontal disease and atherosclerotic vascular disease: does the evidence support an independent association?: a scientific statement from the American Heart Association. Circulation. 2012;125(20):2520–44.
46. van der Maarel-Wierink CD, Vanobbergen JN, Bronkhorst EM, Schols JM, de Baat C. Oral health care and aspiration pneumonia in frail older people: a systematic literature review. Gerodontology. 2013;30(1):3–9.
47. Shay K, Scannapieco FA, Terpenning MS, Smith BJ, Taylor GW. Nosocomial pneumonia and oral health. Spec Care Dentist. 2005;25(4):179–87.
48. Marchini L, Ettinger RL. COVID-19 pandemics and oral health care for older adults. Spec Care Dentist. 2020;40(3):329–31.
49. Marchini L, Ettinger R. COVID-19 and geriatric dentistry: what will be the new-normal? Braz Dent Sci. 2020;23(2):1–7.
50. Nunez B, Chalmers J, Warren J, Ettinger RL, Qian F. Opinions on the provision of dental care in Iowa nursing homes. Spec Care Dentist. 2011;31(1):33–40.
51. Cunha-Jr AP, dos Santos MBF, Santos JFF, Marchini L. Dentists' perceptions and barriers to provide oral care for dependent elderly at home, long-term care institutions or hospitals. Braz J Oral Sci. 2019;17:e18223. 1677–3225.
52. Hopcraft MS, Morgan MV, Satur JG, Wright FA. Dental service provision in Victorian residential aged care facilities. Aust Dent J. 2008;53(3):239–45.
53. Rucker R, Barlow PB, Hartshorn J, Kaufman L, Smith B, Kossioni A, et al. Dual institution validation of an ageism scale for dental students. Spec Care Dentist. 2019;39(1):28–33.
54. Kutner M, Greenberg E, Jin Y, Paulsen C. Health Literacy of America's adults: results from the 2003 National Assessment of Adult Literacy. NCES 2006-4832006. 76 p.
55. Dolim SJ. Is your dental office accessible to people with disabilities? J Calif Dent Assoc. 2013;41(9):695–8.
56. Ettinger RL, Marchini L, Hartshorn J. Consideration in planning dental treatment for older adults. Dent Clin North Am. 2021;65(2):361–76.
57. Ettinger RL, Chalmers J. Oral health care programmes for homebound people, nursing home residents and elderly inpatients. In: Holm-Pederson P, Walls AWG, Ship JA, editors. Textbook of geriatric dentistry. 1. Chichester: Wiley; 2015. p. 327–34.
58. Chalmers JM. Behavior management and communication strategies for dental professionals when caring for patients with dementia. Spec Care Dentist. 2000;20(4):147–54.
59. De Visschere LM, van der Putten GJ, Vanobbergen JN, Schols JM, de Baat C, Dutch Association of Nursing Home Physicians. An oral health care guideline for institutionalised older people. Gerodontology. 2011;28(4):307–10.

60. Zhou F, Yu T, Du R, Fan G, Liu Y, Liu Z, et al. Clinical course and risk factors for mortality of adult inpatients with COVID-19 in Wuhan, China: a retrospective cohort study. Lancet. 2020;395(10229):1054–62.
61. Shahid Z, Kalayanamitra R, McClafferty B, Kepko D, Ramgobin D, Patel R, et al. COVID-19 and older adults: what we know. J Am Geriatr Soc. 2020;68(5):926–9.
62. American Geriatrics Society (AGS) policy brief: COVID-19 and nursing homes. J Am Geriatr Soc. 2020;68(5):908–11.
63. McMichael TM, Clark S, Pogosjans S, Kay M, Lewis J, Baer A, et al. COVID-19 in a long-term care facility – King County, Washington, February 27-March 9, 2020. MMWR Morb Mortal Wkly Rep. 2020;69(12):339–42.
64. Hawes C, Mor V, Phillips CD, Fries BE, Morris JN, Steele-Friedlob E, et al. The OBRA-87 nursing home regulations and implementation of the resident assessment instrument: effects on process quality. J Am Geriatr Soc. 1997;45(8):977–85.
65. Thai PH, Shuman SK, Davidson GB. Nurses' dental assessments and subsequent care in Minnesota nursing homes. Spec Care Dentist. 1997;17(1):13–8.
66. Mezey M, Mitty E, Burger SG, McCallion P. Healthcare professional training: a comparison of geriatric competencies. J Am Geriatr Soc. 2008;56(9):1724–9.
67. Kossioni AE, Marchini L, Childs C. Dental participation in geriatric interprofessional education courses: a systematic review. Eur J Dent Educ. 2018;22(3):E530–E41.
68. Atchison KA, Weintraub JA. Integrating oral health and primary care in the changing health care landscape. N C Med J. 2017;78(6):406–9.
69. Fulmer T, Hyer K, Flaherty E, Mezey M, Whitelaw N, Jacobs MO, et al. Geriatric interdisciplinary team training program: evaluation results. J Aging Health. 2005;17(4):443–70.
70. Position statement on interdisciplinary team training in geriatrics: an essential component of quality health care for older adults. J Am Geriatr Soc. 2014;62(5):961–5.
71. Lewis A, Wallace J, Deutsch A, King P. Improving the oral health of frail and functionally dependent elderly. Aust Dent J. 2015;60(Suppl 1):95–105.
72. Ettinger R, Goettsche Z, Qian F. Pre-doctoral teaching of geriatric dentistry in US dental schools. J Dent Educ. 2017;81(8):921–8.
73. Queyroux A, Saricassapian B, Herzog D, Müller K, Herafa I, Ducoux D, et al. Accuracy of Teledentistry for diagnosing dental pathology using direct examination as a gold standard: results of the Tel-e-dent study of older adults living in nursing homes. J Am Med Dir Assoc. 2017;18(6):528–32.
74. Telles-Araujo GT, Caminha RDG, Kallás MS, Santos P. Teledentistry support in COVID-19 oral care. Clinics (Sao Paulo). 2020;75:e2030.
75. Royal_College_of_Surgeons_England. Recommendations for special care dentistry during COVID-19 pandemic. London: Royal College of Surgeons; 2020.

Oral Health of the Palliative and Hospice Patient

Valerie Hart, Dominique Tosi, and Khin Zaw

The World Health Organization defines palliative medicine as specialized medical care for people living with a serious illness. It focuses on providing comfort and quality of life through the comprehensive assessment and treatment of physical, psychosocial, and spiritual needs [1]. Oral healthcare represents an essential aspect in the management of patients with serious and advanced life-threatening conditions. As a result, oral healthcare professionals become indispensable members of palliative care and hospice interprofessional teams [2]. The purpose of this chapter is to review the concepts of palliative care and hospice in the context of dental practice. We will review the definitions of palliative care and hospice, focus on specific oral healthcare issues arising during the care of patients with palliative care and hospice needs, review key ethical concepts at the end of life, and discuss the role of oral healthcare professionals as members of the palliative care team.

Research shows that older adults with serious illness and those with life-limiting conditions at the end of life have a high prevalence of oral problems that results from the direct effects of the underlying disorders and the adverse effects of the recommended therapies for these conditions [3, 4]. Oral diseases including mucositis, xerostomia, oral candidiasis, and oral pain, can have significant local and

---

V. Hart
University of Miami/Jackson Health System, Miami, FL, USA

D. Tosi
Department of Medical Education, University of Miami Miller School of Medicine, Miami VA Healthcare System Geriatric Research, Education and Clinical Center (GRECC), Miami, FL, USA

K. Zaw (✉)
Palliative Medicine Program, Miami VA Healthcare System, Miami, FL, USA

Division of Geriatrics and Palliative Medicine, University of Miami Miller School of Medicine, Miami, FL, USA
e-mail: kzaw@med.miami.edu

© The Author(s), under exclusive license to Springer Nature Switzerland AG 2022
C.-M. Hogue, J. G. Ruiz (eds.), *Oral Health and Aging*,
https://doi.org/10.1007/978-3-030-85993-0_11

systemic consequences and substantially compromise the quality of life of individuals with serious illness. The early identification and treatment of oral conditions among older adults with palliative care and hospice needs could minimize pain and suffering [3]. However, there are important barriers to overcome when managing these patients. Evidence reveals that about 40% of palliative patients at one point during their illness may lose the ability to communicate their symptoms [5]. This may contribute to the underreporting and underestimation of oral conditions, which may result in the failure of healthcare professionals to properly address them [6]. Regular assessments may help identify oral conditions and facilitate the implementation of appropriate and timely interventions. As we will review during this chapter, caregivers play a critical role during clinical encounters when patients with palliative care and hospice needs are unable to communicate.

1 The Concepts of Palliative Care and Hospice

Palliative care and hospice are part of a continuum of healthcare for patients with serious illnesses. Palliative care can be provided at any time during the trajectory of any serious illness, while hospice care is offered for patients at the end of life. In the next sections, we address each of these concepts, highlighting the main commonalities and differences between both concepts (Fig. 1).

1.1 Palliative Care

Palliative care focuses on anticipating, preventing, diagnosing, and treating symptoms experienced by patients with serious illnesses. Moreover, palliative care professionals play an essential role in assisting patients and their families in making important healthcare decisions. Palliative care becomes a resource for anyone living with a serious illness, and it is appropriate at any stage of the illness. Palliative care can be provided along with the delivery of curative treatments [1, 3]. A centerpiece

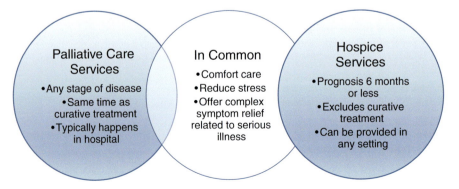

Fig. 1 Differences and similarities between palliative care and hospice

of the palliative care approach is the interprofessional team that provides comfort care while maintaining optimal function and well-being [7]. The team often consists of palliative care physicians, nurses, dietitians, social workers, and chaplains.

The delivery of palliative care early in the course of a life-limiting illness can improve the quality of life for patients; decrease overall healthcare utilization, including hospitalization [8]; shorten hospital stays; and reduce the need for non-beneficial therapies [9]. The palliative care approach does not aim to hasten or postpone death. Research shows that palliative care increases hospice care use and improves patients' quality of life and even survival [10]. In terms of healthcare utilization, palliative care interventions can significantly reduce total healthcare costs in patients with advanced cancers [8, 11]. Each year, an estimated 40 million people need palliative care. Unfortunately, despite the potential benefits of palliative care approaches for patients with serious illness, only about 14% of people, who need palliative care worldwide, currently receive it [1].

Worldwide, efforts are underway to expand palliative care services for patients in need. The 2014 World Health Assembly passed a resolution appealing to member countries to incorporate palliative care services into their respective healthcare systems [12]. Furthermore, two more important developments at the global policy level are worth mentioning. First, in 2000, palliative care was included in the United Nations' International Covenant on Economic, Social, and Cultural Rights, which states: "States are under the obligation to respect the right to health by, inter alia, refraining from denying or limiting equal access for all persons… to preventive, curative, and palliative health services." Second, essential medicines for palliative care were included into the 18th World Health Organization (WHO) essential medicines list in 2013 [13].

1.2 Hospice

As curative interventions no longer achieve the patient's care goals, patients may begin the transition to hospice care. Hospice care is defined as comfort care for patients facing a terminal illness [14]. Patients qualify for hospice care when their physicians estimate that the patient's prognosis for survival is 6 months or less if the disease runs its course. As with palliative care, hospice provides comprehensive comfort care as well as family support. Unlike palliative care, hospice no longer focuses on cure. Increasingly, people with serious illnesses that no longer respond to curative interventions are choosing hospice care as an alternative at the end of life. Hospice can be provided in any setting—home, nursing home, assisted living facility, or inpatient hospital. In the USA, hospice services are covered by government insurance such as Medicare or Medicaid, as well as most private healthcare insurance. Medicare and many private insurance plans cover the cost of palliative care. This coverage is different from the hospice care benefit [14]. In other high-income countries such as Australia, palliative and hospice services are funded by Medicare [15], whereas in Canada, palliative care is provided free of change to eligible patients [16]. An example of a middle-income country, Colombia, has a palliative care law requiring that palliative care be offered to all patients with cancer [17].

Table 1 Karnofsky Performance Scale Index [22]

Able to carry on normal activity and to work; no special care needed	*[100]* Normal no complains; no evidence of disease *[90]* Able to carry on normal activity; minor signs or symptons of disease *[80]* Normal activity with effort; some signs or symptons of disease
Unable to work; able to live at home and care for most personal needs; varying amount of assistance needed	*[70]* Cares for self; unable to carry a normal activity or to do active work *[60]* Requires occasional assistance but is able to care most of his personal needs *[50]* Requires considerable assistance and frequent medical care
Unable to care for self; requires equivalent of institutional or hospital care; disease may be progressing rapidly	*[40]* Disabled; requires special care and assistance *[30]* Severely disabled; hospital admission is indicated althought death not imminent *[20]* Very sick; hospital admission necessary; active supportive treatment necessary *[10]* Moribund; fatal processes progressing rapidly *[0]* Dead

Table 2 Palliative Performance Scale (PPS)

%	Ambulation	Activity level evidence of disease	Self-care	Intake	Level of consciousness
100	Full	Normal, no disease	Full	Normal	Full
90	Full	Normal, some disease		Normal	
80	Full	Normal with effort, some disease		Normal or reduced	
70	Reduced	Can't do normal job or work with effort, some disease		Normal or reduced	
60	Reduced	Can't do hobbies or housework significant disease	Occasional assistance needed	Normal or reduced	Full or confusion
50	Mainly sit/lie	Can't do any work, extensive disease	Considerable assistance needed	Normal or reduced	Full or confusion
40	Mainly in bed	Unable to do any work, extensive disease	Mainly assistance	Normal or reduced	Full or drowsy or confusion
30	Bed bound	Unable to do any work, extensive disease	Total care	Reduced	Full or drowsy or confusion
20		Unable to do any work, extensive disease		Minimal	
10		Unable to do any work, extensive disease		Mouth care only	Drowsy or coma
0	Death	–	–	–	–

In the USA, hospice eligibility requires that a physician certifies the patient has less than 6 months to live if the disease follows its usual course [18–20]. Accurate prognostic information is important for patients, families, and physicians, i.e., it can help physicians decide whether to initiate or continue anticancer therapies [21], facilitate transitions to hospice care, enable appropriate advance care planning, and ensure end-of-life shared decision-making. Clinicians may use performance status measures defined as global assessments of the patient's level of function. The Eastern Cooperative Oncology Group (ECOG) scale and the Karnofsky performance status (KPS) [22, 23] are two widely used methods to assess the functional status of patients with serious illnesses [24]. The Palliative Performance Scale (PPS) (Table 2) [25] is another tool to assess functional performance. It also helps determine progression toward the end of life. PPS ratings directly correlates with short-term prognosis for terminally ill patients with or without cancer. The ECOG is a scale extensively used in oncology settings to assess disease progression, assess the disease impact on activities of daily living, and determine appropriate treatments and prognosis. It describes the patient's level of functioning in terms of their ability to care for themselves, activities of daily living, and physical function. Researchers worldwide use the ECOG performance status when planning trials to study new treatment strategies. The ECOG assists physicians in monitoring the patient's level of functioning during treatment and determine disease progression. Like the ECOG, KPS (Table 1) classifies a patient according to their levels of functional impairment, compares the effectiveness of therapies, and assesses patient prognosis. The lower the Karnofsky score, the worse the survival for most serious illnesses [26]. It is generally accepted that a KPS or PPS score of 50 or less indicate that the patient may have a prognosis of 6 months or less for survival [25].

2 The Role of the Dental Care Professional in Palliative Care and Hospice

The World Congress of 2015 adopted the Tokyo Declaration on Dental Care and Oral Health for Healthy Longevity, with the main goal of collecting scientific evidence on the contribution of oral healthcare and formulate policies based on such evidence [27]. Oral health is a key indicator of overall health, well-being, and quality of life. The Global Burden of Disease Study 2017 estimated that oral diseases affect 3.5 billion people worldwide [28]. Unfortunately, there is insufficient data to assess the extent of oral health problems in patients with severe and life-limiting illness. This is likely because of an underestimation of oral conditions in many patients with serious illness receiving palliative care or hospice services.

Although not often considered standing members of core palliative care or hospice teams, dentists and other healthcare professionals play important roles in the care of these patients [3]. Dental professionals provide needed expertise to assess and manage the oral healthcare needs of individuals with serious and life-limiting illness, improving symptom management and promoting oral self-care in close collaboration with members of the core interprofessional team. Palliative oral care focuses on strategies for maintaining patients' quality of life and comfort. In palliative care, oral healthcare goals include adequate pain control, avoidance of infection, and prevention of and prompt removal of dental plaque, calculus, or food debris. The interprofessional team works in close collaboration with dental healthcare professionals, patients, and families to prevent and treat problems as they arise. The basic principle of oral palliative care is focused primarily on the principle that good oral hygiene is critical for oral integrity. Dentists may mitigate oral complications by performing regular oral prophylaxis and providing necessary preventive, corrective, and restorative dental treatments. These interventions may serve to alleviate oral symptoms, reduce their risk for mouth sores, denture sores, periodontal disease, and oral infections. Early and accurate clinical diagnosis of oral conditions in palliative patients must be instituted to minimize pain and suffering.

Although most palliative care patients may have compromised oral health, they seldom receive adequate and timely oral care services [29]. The reasons for these deficiencies are various [30]. Traditionally healthcare providers in palliative care have focused on general healthcare often overlooking oral needs. Other contributory factors are lack of dental insurance [31], high dental treatment costs, not understanding the importance of oral health [32], lack of access to dental care services, and lack of specialized dental training in palliative care and hospice [3]. Another common problem is that dental care professionals are not often included in core palliative care teams [33, 34]. Solutions to these problems may require a repertoire of strategies. Proposed solutions include promoting bedside oral healthcare for older adults with serious illness and symptom management through an enhanced collaboration between interprofessional team members, regular mouth care, and early identification of dental problems to minimize pain and complications. Finally, this interprofessional collaboration could also help dentists understand their patients' prognoses, better address when and how to implement palliative treatment, and how to minimize futile and potentially harmful dental treatments with the goal of improving quality of care [35].

3 The Oral Assessment of the Older Adult with Palliative Care and Hospice Needs

An adequate assessment is the first step to establish the patients' baseline oral health status. The assessment may determine the existence of any oral conditions requiring additional evaluation and treatment by a dental health professional. In institutionalized patients, examination of the mouth should be done daily for early detection and treatment of oral problems [36]. Multiple oral health assessment instruments have been developed. A meta-analysis compared several of these instruments and concluded that three instruments – the Brief Oral Health Status Examination Tool (BOHSE), the Oral Health Assessment Tool (OHAT), and the Dental Health Registration (DHR) – are valid and reliable assessment tools to assess the oral health of nursing home residents [36]. For community dwelling patients, if they are unable to perform self-care, much of their oral care is provided by family members or home health aides who provide care at home. We were not able to find research describing training or screening tools recommended for the assessment of oral health in palliative care patients in community settings. Therefore, it would be advisable to adapt some of the previously described instruments for use in community-dwelling settings.

Trained nursing personnel can use the BOHSE and the OHAT to assess the oral health of nursing home residents. Both tools serve as screening instruments that would trigger appropriate and timely referrals to dentists for additional evaluation and treatment. The DHR evaluates plaque formation as a measure of dental hygiene without the need of special equipment, which may not be widely available in long-term care facilities. The BOHSE consists of 10 items that reflect the status of oral health and function, including lips, tongue, tissue inside the cheek, floor and roof of mouth, gums, saliva, condition of natural teeth, condition of artificial teeth, pairs of teeth in chewing position, and oral cleanliness. The final score is the sum of the scores from the 10 categories and can range from 0 (very healthy) to 20 (very unhealthy) [37]. The OHAT is a modified version of the BOHSE consisting of eight areas: lips, tongue, gums/tissues, saliva, natural teeth, dentures, oral cleanliness, and dental pain. The final score can range from 0 (very healthy) to 16 (very unhealthy) and is obtained from the sum of the scores of the abovementioned eight areas, which are rated on a 0–2 scale: 0, healthy; 1, oral changes; and 2, unhealthy [38]. The DHR is a quick and easy to use assessment tool that nursing personnel can implement with dentate patients. It registers the presence or absence of plaque on teeth and can serve to monitor changes over time. The scale is scored from 1 to 4: 0, continue as usual; 1, check for deterioration and pay attention to difficult areas; and 2–4, dental hygiene needs to improve [39]. These tools have been validated in cognitively intact and cognitively impaired nursing home residents. However, there are no studies that have specifically validated these instruments in patients receiving palliative care or hospice. There is a need for more research that validates the use of these instruments in patients with palliative care and hospice needs in noninstitutional settings.

4 Risk Factors of Poor Oral Health

4.1 Poor Oral Hygiene

Poor oral hygiene is associated with physical, psychological, and social consequences for patients with palliative care needs. Unfortunately, poor oral hygiene is common in this population [40–43]. Healthcare professionals should regularly encourage their patients to participate in daily oral self-care activities. When unable, because of cognitive or functional impairment, caregivers should assist patients with these tasks. Risk factors for poor oral hygiene include patient and caregivers' educational level and lack of awareness of the importance of routine oral care to prevent complications [29]. Many patients may not have the means or ability to visit a dentist or dental hygienist in a timely manner due to limited transportation, lack of dental insurance, and/or economic constraints. For a more in-depth discussion on the topic of health disparities, please refer to chapter "Health Disparities in Oral Health".

4.2 Polypharmacy

Drugs are by far the most common cause of xerostomia, dysgeusia, and stomatitis [44]. Many medications can cause dry mouth including among the most frequent offending medications those with anticholinergic activity, including many antiemetics, antihistamines, antipsychotics, tricyclic antidepressants, antispasmodics, and bronchodilators. Other frequent culprits include several types of antihypertensives, diuretics, benzodiazepines, and opioids [44, 45]. Dysgeusia, the altered perception of taste, is associated with several medications use to treat serious illness, including antineoplastics (bleomycin, carboplatin, cisplatin, cyclophosphamide, doxorubicin, 5-fluorouracil, gemcitabine, levamisole, and methotrexate), psychotropics, opioids, antimicrobials, and antihypertensives [46]. A thorough medication review may identify responsible medications. If possible, deprescribing the suspected medications should be attempted as the initial approach to improve symptoms. For a more in-depth discussion on the topic of xerostomia, please refer to chapter "Xerostomia and Hyposalivation".

4.3 Functional Impairment and Frailty

Evidence suggests that functional impairment and frailty are associated with worse dental health [47]. In many patients with serious or terminally illness, traditional oral hygiene practices may not be feasible due to declining health and poor physical function [48, 49]. Many palliative patients are disabled, weak, cognitively impaired, and often institutionalized. Unfortunately, oral health procedures are frequently given low priority when compared to other care tasks performed by nursing staff and caregivers [50]. This can stem from inadequate training, limited time availability due to other competing needs, or the unpleasantness of the task [51]. Patients who need help with oral hygiene have twice as many cases of dental caries or retained roots than those who are independent [5]. Individualized oral hygiene care plans that incorporate caregivers, caregiver training programs, shorter intervals between dental evaluations, the use of fluoride, and management of xerostomia constitute adequate interventions [5].

4.4 Cognitive Impairment

Compared with patients with intact cognition, individuals with cognitive impairment have poorer oral hygiene, more gingivitis, more decayed root surfaces, a higher plaque index, higher number of decayed coronal surfaces, higher number of filled root surfaces, and more missing teeth [5, 52]. In community-dwelling patients with cognitive impairment, the risk of dental caries increases due to diminished oral hygiene, insufficient caregiver support, and lack of regular dental care [5]. Patients with severe cognitive impairment often require the assistance of a caregiver to perform oral care. These patients may also become uncooperative and even resist care with oral hygiene routines [53]. Strategies to improve patients' cooperation include allowing patients to determine the location of the examination, explaining the steps of the procedure, allowing rest periods during the examination, and including caregivers that the patient knows and trusts [37]. For a more in-depth discussion on the topic of dementia, please refer to chapter "The 3 Ds: Dementia, Delirium and Depression in Oral Health".

5 Common Oral Health Conditions in Palliative and Hospice

5.1 Swallowing Disorders and Aspiration

Dysphagia or difficulty swallowing is often present in patients with advanced physical and mental illness. Dysphagia frequently leads to aspiration, which can result in aspiration pneumonitis, pneumonia, and even death. Additionally, it can lead to dehydration, malnutrition, caregiver burden, and poor quality of life [54]. In many palliative patients with dysphagia, a joint decision between the palliative medicine team and patients or surrogates may be to allow patients to continue eating despite their risk of aspiration. In these cases, the goal is to provide pleasure, socialization, and nutrition. Different approaches are used to manage swallowing impairment and may include diet modifications, such as thickening liquids and pureeing solids, keeping an upright head position during meals, and exercise programs targeted to strengthening muscles involved in swallowing such as functional dysphagia therapy [55]. For a more in-depth discussion on the topic of swallowing disorders, please refer to chapter "Swallowing, Dysphagia, and Aspiration Pneumonia".

5.2 Cancer Treatment and Oral Mucositis/Stomatitis

Mucositis is the inflammation of the mucous membranes lining the digestive tract. It is caused by the loss of epithelial cells and release of proinflammatory substances frequently associated with radiotherapy of the head and neck, with or without chemotherapy [56]. Stomatitis is the inflammation of the mucous lining of the mouth structures [57]. Clinical manifestations can vary from erythema to necrosis or deep ulceration of the mucosa [58]. Mucositis causes severe discomfort and pain which can be debilitating and lead to intolerance of normal diets, sometimes to the point where patients may need gastrostomy tubes to provide supplemental nutrition and hydration [56]. It is important that patients with planned radiation therapy to the head and neck undergo a comprehensive, baseline oral/dental exam including radiographs. Providers should educate patients on maintaining good oral hygiene and avoiding caustic and drying agents that could further exacerbate their symptoms [59]. Most treatments for mucositis are limited to palliation and treatment of pain (see Orofacial Pain section). Providers should have a low threshold to obtain cultures for suspected infections, including fungal and viral, as they may not present typically, go unrecognized, and lead to bacterial superinfections.

5.3 Problems with Saliva

Xerostomia or dry mouth is quite common in palliative and hospice patients with some studies reporting a prevalence as high as 70%. It can be objective or subjective, depending on the presence of signs of dry mouth such as frothing, stringing of saliva or glazing of the oral mucosa [45, 60, 61]. There are several causes of xerostomia, including drug induced, irradiation, salivary gland diseases, infections, and dehydration [44, 45]. Xerostomia can cause discomfort and pain, difficulty eating and swallowing, problems with dentures, altered taste of food, difficulty speaking, increased risk of infections and dental caries, halitosis, nutritional impairment, and decreased quality of life [45, 60]. The main pillars of the treatment of xerostomia are treating the underlying causes, symptomatic treatments, and treatment of associated complications [62]. Any causal agents should be eliminated, if possible. Other treatment modalities consist of saliva substitutes, stimulation of residual gland function with sugar-free candy or chewing gum, and cholinergic agonists (pilocarpine and cevimeline). Staff should educate and encourage patients to maintain good oral hygiene, including the use of alcohol-free antimicrobial mouthwashes [45]. For a more in-depth discussion on the topic of xerostomia, please refer to chapter "Xerostomia and Hyposalivation".

Sialorrhea or excess salivation is usually caused by overproduction or excessive secretion of saliva [63, 64]. Sialorrhea usually represents a side effect of medications, vitamin deficiencies, gastroesophageal reflux, or poor oral clearance of saliva secondary to dysphagia. The most common causes of dysphagia associated with sialorrhea are underlying neurologic and neuromuscular diseases such as Parkinson's disease, and amyotrophic lateral sclerosis (ALS), and malignancies such as head a neck cancers. The excess saliva can then spill over the bottom lip leading to drooling, which in turn can cause rashes, skin irritation and breakdown, and poor quality of life. Sialorrhea can also result in aspiration, choking, poor oxygenation, and the onset of pneumonias [65]. Management of sialorrhea can be non-pharmacologic or pharmacologic. Non-pharmacologic modalities include orthodontic procedures, functional dysphagia therapy, use of cough assistance devices, and suction devices [63, 64]. Pharmacologic agents may include glycopyrrolate, scopolamine, atropine, and benztropine. These medications are anticholinergic and an expected adverse effect is xerostomia. Botulinum toxin injections into the salivary glands have also demonstrated positive effects [65].

5.4 Dysgeusia

Dysgeusia or distortion of the sense of taste is frequently seen in palliative patients [49, 66–68]. Dysgeusia can lead to the loss of eating pleasure, anorexia, nutritional deficiencies, and decreased quality of life [69]. Most affected are patients with head and neck cancers treated with chemotherapy and radiation. Dysgeusia can also be caused by infections, zinc deficiency, hypothyroidism, Cushing's syndrome, liver disease, sequelae from ENT operations, and some medications like psychotropics, opioids, and antihypertensives (Table 4). In cases of chemotherapy and radiation to the head and neck, taste disturbances are caused by damage to the taste buds or salivary dysfunction. Other causes may include an underlying infection which may require antimicrobial therapy. Providers should routinely ask about these symptoms as patients may not volunteer the information. Management of taste disturbances includes treatment of the underlying cause, dietary therapies focusing on foods that have pleasurable tastes and are culturally appropriate, avoiding unpalatable foods, and providing food enhancers. Zinc therapy is also recommended as its deficiency has been associated with dysgeusia [46].

5.5 Orofacial Pain

Causes or orofacial pain are various (Table 3). Orofacial pain is often encountered in palliative patients with a reported prevalence ranging from 4% to 67% (Table 3). Like in any other patient, individuals with serious and terminal illness may also complain of pain originating from common dental conditions, including dental caries, abscesses, pulpal pain, and periodontal disease. Lesions of the oral mucosa may also include aphthous stomatitis, herpes simplex, candidiasis, blistering conditions, traumatic lesions, and radiation- or chemotherapy-induced mucositis [70]. Pain is usually located around the tooth or lesion. This type of pain can lead to anorexia as chewing and temperature changes usually increase pain. Periodontal and pulpal pain disorders are managed by dental practitioners. Musculoskeletal pain disorders such as temporomandibular disorders (TMD) are usually secondary to pain of the muscles of mastication, the temporomandibular joints (TMJ), and/or associated ligaments and tendons. Pain is usually felt in the preauricular areas and can lead to restricted mouth opening and pain with eating or talking. Management usually includes

Table 3 Causes of oral pain

System	Sources of pain
Dentoalveolar/oral mucosal	Dental Periodontal Pulpal Salivary gland disease Oral mucosal disease Maxillary sinusitis Cancer
Musculoskeletal	Temporomandibular disorders

Neurovascular	*Primary headache*
	  Migraine
	  Tension-type headache
	  Temporal arteritis
	  Trigeminal autonomic cephalalgias

	Neuropathic pain
	  Trigeminal neuralgia/trigeminal neuropathic pain
	  Glossopharyngeal neuralgia
	  Postherpetic neuralgia
	  Burning mouth

	Other
	  Central stroke pain
	  Chronic idiopathic facial pain
	  Atypical odontalgia

Modified from: Orofacial Pain (Book) Zakrzewska, Joanna [70]

Table 4 Prevalence of oral health problems in different studies

Study	Population type/size	Oral pain (%)	Xerostomia (%)	Dysgeusia (%)
Oneschuk et al. 2000 [43]	Patients with advanced cancer ($n = 99$)	16	88	
Davies et al., 2001 [62]	Inpatient or outpatient palliative advanced cancer patients ($n = 120$)	–	78	–
Alt-Epping et al. 2012 [66]	Palliative care inpatients ($n = 101$)	4	83	68
Wilberg et al. 2012 [67]	Palliative care cancer inpatients ($n = 99$)	67	78	68
Van Lancker et al. 2016 [68]	Older patients receiving palliative cancer care ($n = 400$)	17.3	77	35
Özalp et al. 2017 [99]	Palliative care clinic ($n = 170$)	–	87.6	–
Magnani et al. 2019 [49]	Hospice patients ($n = 75$)	14.7	74.9	49.3

exercise programs, pain medications, and intraoral splint therapy. It is important to include a psychosocial evaluation of these patients, since depression and anxiety can be associated to TMD. Cognitive behavioral strategies can lead to better outcomes in patients with TMD and depression or anxiety [70]. Neuropathic pain is felt in structures that follow a nerve distribution but may not show any clinical evidence of pathology. The pain is usually described as tingling, burning, pins and needles, and electrical and may be associated with anesthesia, paresthesia, dysesthesia, hyperesthesia, or hypoesthesia. Trigeminal neuralgia, postherpetic neuralgia, and burning mouth syndrome are examples of this type of pain. Neurovascular pain includes migraines, temporal arteritis, and tension headaches. Neuropathic and neurovascular pain disorders are managed medically with therapies directed to the underlying pathophysiology [70]. In patients with cancer receiving palliative care, pain can be the consequence of a primary, systemic, or metastatic cancer affecting peripheral and/or central nervous systems [71]. Three of the most common pain presentations of patients with intracranial tumors who come to the dental office are symptoms of TMD, trigeminal neuralgia, and persistent idiopathic facial pain [72]. Pain can be secondary to metastatic lesions to the mandible, the TMJ, and other areas of the head and face. In systemic cancers like lymphoma, leukemia, and myeloma, pain can result from tumor infiltration of bone, gingiva, and tissues proximal to teeth [72].

Pharmacologic management of orofacial pain includes the use of NSAIDs. However, dentists should be aware of the significant risks associated with the use of these medications in older adults. When used chronically, NSAIDS can cause hypertension, worsening of kidney function, and gastric irritation. Topical analgesics can be used in different forms: injections of lidocaine for trigeminal neuralgia or lidocaine patches for neuropathic pain [70]. Liquid anesthetic administered intraorally may be beneficial in oral mucosal lesions. Corticosteroids can be applied topically or injected directly into the TMJ. However, these medications should be reserved for cases of acute trauma, severe limitations of mouth opening, or as a brief therapeutic trial [70]. Antidepressants, including tricyclic, selective serotonin reuptake inhibitors (SSRI), and serotonin noradrenaline reuptake inhibitors (SNRI), are an important part of the management of neuropathic pain. Opioids should be reserved for patients with malignant pain and those with nonmalignant pain for whom more conservative measures have failed or who are at high risks of adverse effects from the use of other medications, including NSAIDs.

5.6 Oral Infections

The oral cavity is colonized by a stable microbiota ("microbial homeostasis"). Biofilm is a layer of microorganisms that covers the teeth, the gingival crevice, and the dorsum of the tongue. Multiple mechanisms help to maintain the normal commensal flora and prevent infections. The *oral mucosa* serves as a physical barrier to invading organisms, and in many areas, a biofilm cannot establish due to the rapid turnover of the surface cells. Oral infections occur in patients with damage to the oral mucosa. *Commensal flora* prevents the colonization of pathogenic organisms by competing for space and nutrients. Commensal organisms can be affected by the use of antibiotics, salivary disfunction, and a high carbohydrate diet, which leads to a decrease in the pH of the oral cavity favoring the growth of pathogenic microorganisms that cause dental caries. *Saliva* has many different actions and salivary gland dysfunction can lead to an increased prevalence of oral and systemic infections. The *immune system* in the mouth includes innate immunity, consisting of phagocytes and complement, and acquired immunity consisting of humoral (immunoglobulins including secretory IgA, and serum IgG, IgM, and IgA) and cellular immunity that includes T cells. The components of the immune system reach the mouth through the gingival crevicular fluid, which is a serum transudate that passes into the gingival crevice from the systemic circulation. Immunodeficiency causes changes of the oral microflora that may lead to an increased prevalence of oral infections [36]. Infections affecting the mouth can be bacterial, viral, and fungal.

5.7 Halitosis

Halitosis is defined as offensive odors emanating from the mouth, nose, sinuses, or pharynx. Pathologic halitosis can be a symptom of regional pathology such as periodontal disease or systemic pathologies such as esophagitis, pyloric stenosis, uremia, diabetes ketosis, or neoplasms. Xerostomia (discussed above) can also contribute to halitosis [73]. Halitosis can have psychological and social effects in patients with serious and terminal illness [46].

6 Oral Health at the End of Life: Dying with Dignity

The Institute of Medicine defines as a good death "one that is free from avoidable distress and suffering for patients, families, and caregivers; in general, in accord with patients' and families' wishes and reasonably consistent with clinical, cultural, and ethical standards" [74]. Oral healthcare professionals have a responsibility to address oral symptoms at the end of life with the goal of improving or maintaining patients' comfort and quality of life.

Hospice patients have a high prevalence of oral problems associated with their serious and terminal illnesses [3, 4, 75]. Evidence shows that 40% of palliative patients suffer from oral conditions for a prolonged period. The loss of the patients' ability to communicate their oral health needs may further contribute to the underreporting of oral conditions among terminally ill patients. The early identification and treatment of these oral conditions by dentists will minimize patients' pain and suffering. Table 5 shows an example of strategies aimed at maintaining and treating oral health for patients at the end of life.

7 Ethical Considerations at the End of Life

Clinicians play a pivotal role both in defining and executing the medical care plan and in providing continuity of care as goals evolve and change over time [76]. Practitioners often initiate discussions about life-sustaining treatments, educate

Oral Health of the Palliative and Hospice Patient

Table 5 The Scottish palliative care guidelines for the management of oral care of patients nearing the end of life [100]

Include mouth care in the patient's care plan
Encourage family members to participate in mouth care activities with guidance and support from the team
If possible, change or stop medications that are causing dry mouth
Conduct mouth care as often as necessary to maintain a clean mouth
In patients who are conscious, the mouth can be moistened every 30 minutes with water from a water spray or dropper or ice chips can be placed in the mouth
In unconscious patients, moisten the mouth frequently, when possible, with water from a water spray, dropper, or sponge stick or ice chips placed in the mouth
Water-soluble lubricant should be applied to prevent cracking of the lips
Use a room humidifier or air-conditioning when the weather is dry and hot
Ensure help is offered to clean teeth or dentures
Manage oral pain symptomatically, using analgesics via a suitable route
Most importantly, stop treatment of the underlying cause of oral pain when the burden of treatment outweighs the benefits

patients and families, help families deliberate care options, and make recommendations about treatment plans. As part of this role, the hospice team is responsible for guaranteeing that the patient's wishes are documented and supported by the appropriate medical orders [76, 77]. Oral health professionals may contribute to this conversation by sharing their expert opinion on best practices for adequate oral health maintenance and treatment. The focus of the following sections is on ethical issues at the end of life. For a more in-depth discussion on the topic of ethics, please refer to the chapter "Ethical Considerations".

7.1 *Withholding and Withdrawal of Life Support*

The withholding and withdrawal of life-sustaining therapies are considered by most experts ethical, moral, and medically appropriate decisions when the treatment no longer fulfills the patient's goals. Although withdrawal and withholding of life support are considered ethically equivalent, the reality is that most clinicians and patients may not feel so. The experience of withholding as compared to withdrawal therapy has been examined in two large questionnaire-based surveys, one from North America and the other from Europe [78, 79]. In the North American study, 61% of physicians reported being more distressed at the prospect of the withdrawal of therapy than they were about withholding treatments. Similarly, a European survey [78], showed that physicians were more willing to withhold treatment than they were about the withdrawal of the same therapies. Healthcare professionals are under no obligation to offer ineffective treatments, i.e., treatments that no longer offer benefits to the patient. Acceptable clinical practices on withdrawal or withholding of treatments depend on an understanding of medical, ethical, cultural, and religious issues. There is a need to individualize goals of care discussions considering the preferences, beliefs, values, and cultural background of both the patient and their families [76]. A strong consensus is that the withdrawal or withholding of life supporting treatments is seen as a decision that allows the disease to run its natural course, rather than a decision to hasten death.

7.2 Shared Decision-Making (SDM)

Shared decision-making is a structured method that incorporates clinical evidence as well as patient values and preferences into medical decision-making. Clinicians should periodically revisit treatment preferences as goals evolve and change over time in patients with serious and life-limiting illnesses. Shared decision-making is supported by evidence from 86 randomized trials showing that participation in SDM fosters patients and family's knowledge of their conditions, increases patients' confidence in their decisions, makes patients more active participants in their care, and, in many situations, leads patients to select more conservative treatment options [80]. Achieving shared decision-making depends on building a good relationship between clinicians and patients so that information is shared, and patients are supported in the deliberation and expression of their preferences and views. To accomplish these tasks, there is a proposed model based on choice, option, and decision talk. The model has three steps: (a) introducing choice; (b) describing options, often by integrating the use of patient decision support; and (c) helping patients explore preferences and make decisions. This model rests on supporting a process of deliberation and understanding that clinicians must respect the patients' preferences [80, 81].

7.3 Informed Consent

Informed consent has become the mainstay for protecting patients' legal rights and guiding the ethical practice of medicine [82]. The higher standard of informed consent further protects patients' rights to autonomy, self-determination, and inviolability. The ethical principle of informed consent seeks to respect patient autonomy by ensuring that treatments are directed toward the ends desired by the patient. Informed consent involves providing patients with accurate and adequate information about the risks, benefits, and alternatives of a treatment in a manner that is free from coercion. Unfortunately, research evidence shows that patients remember little of the information disclosed during the informed consent process [83–86] and that their level of comprehension is often overestimated [87, 88]. Comprehension is related to factors such as patient age, education, intelligence [86], cognitive function, locus of control, and anxiety [82, 83, 89]. These problems are exacerbated in older adults at the end of life when the prevalence of terminal delirium is high, impairing the patient's ability to actively participate in the decision-making process. In this

7.4 Decision-Making Capacity

As we have seen in the previous section, active participation in the medical decision-making process requires that patients retain the ability to understand the benefits and risks of, and the alternatives to, a proposed treatment or intervention (including the option of no treatment). Patients have medical decision-making capacity if they can demonstrate an understanding of the situation, appreciation of the consequences of their decision, reasoning in their thought process for the decision, and the ability to communicate their wishes. Physicians will often be called to determine the patient capacity to give consent for treatment. During the process, the physician making these determinations will consider four elements: Patients must be able to (1) demonstrate understanding of the benefits and risks of, and the alternatives to, a proposed treatment or intervention (including no treatment); (2) demonstrate appreciation of those benefits, risks, and alternatives; (3) show reasoning, or the ability to compare benefits and risks in making a decision; and (4) communicate their choice [90, 91]. If the patient is unable to meet the capacity criteria, the healthcare team will have to rely on appointed or designated surrogate decision-makers.

7.5 Advance Care Planning (ACP) and Advance Directives (AD)

Advance care planning is the communication process that supports adults at any age or stage of health in understanding and sharing their personal values, life goals, and preferences regarding future medical care [92]. The objective of ACP is to ensure that patients make treatment decisions in anticipation of the onset of serious illness so that clinicians can provide care that is consistent with such goals [93]. Advance directives, on the other hand, are documentation of the patients' goals and values reflecting the results of advance care planning discussions [94–97]. ACP may or may not include completion of an advance directive (AD). Advance directives may state how treatment decisions should be made on their behalf in the event they lose the capacity to make such decisions in the future. There are various kinds of ADs, but the most recognized in the United States are the Living Will (LW) and the Durable Power of Attorney for Health Care (DPAHC). LWs document patient preferences for life-sustaining treatments and resuscitation. DPAHCs (also known as "Health Care Proxy Designations") document their choice of a surrogate decision-maker. It is a signed legal document authorizing another person to make medical decisions on the patient's behalf in the event the patient loses decisional capacity [98]. Most recently, the Physician Orders for Life-Sustaining Treatment (POLST) have become a valuable addition to the arsenal of available advance directives [89]. A key advantage of POLST advance directives is that these documents serve as a set of actionable and transferable medical orders that direct medical care consistent with patients' goals of care at the end of life. Dental professionals will need to be aware of their patients' preferences as they may be caring for patients with serious and life-limiting illness who may have lost their ability to participate in shared decision-making.

8 Conclusions

Oral health professionals have an opportunity to make significant contributions to palliative care by addressing oral symptoms of patients with serious and terminal illness and thereby contribute to improving and maintaining their comfort and quality of life. Palliative dentistry is necessary in the management of patients with advanced life-threatening diseases or conditions. Dentists and other oral health care professionals may be able to alleviate some of the common oral problems faced by these individuals. Oral health care professionals may offer these patients preventive, corrective, and restorative dental treatments. Educating healthcare team members on the important role of dental care providers in palliative care teams is essential for achieving patients' comfort and well-being. Advance care planning and completion of advance directives may serve to foster a process of shared decision-making that aims to preserve patients' autonomy.

References

1. Fact sheets palliative care [Internet] 2020. Available from: https://www.who.int/news-room/fact-sheets/detail/palliative-care
2. De Rossi SS, Slaughter YA. Oral changes in older patients: a clinician's guide. Quintessence Int. 2007;38(9):773–80.
3. Saini R, Marawar P, Shete S, Saini S, Mani A. Dental expression and role in palliative treatment. Indian J Palliat Care. 2009;15(1):26–9.
4. Ohno T, Morita T, Tamura F, Hirano H, Watanabe Y, Kikutani T. The need and availability of dental services for terminally ill cancer patients: a nationwide survey in Japan. Support Care Cancer. 2016;24(1):19–22.
5. Chen X, Chen H, Douglas C, Preisser JS, Shuman SK. Dental treatment intensity in frail older adults in the last year of life. J Am Dent Assoc. 2013;144(11):1234–42.
6. Venkatasalu MR, Murang ZR, Ramasamy DTR, Dhaliwal JS. Oral health problems among palliative and terminally ill patients: an integrated systematic review. BMC Oral Health. 2020;20(1):79.
7. Rome RB, Luminais HH, Bourgeois DA, Blais CM. The role of palliative care at the end of life. Ochsner J. 2011;11(4):348–52.
8. Morrison RS, Dietrich J, Ladwig S, Quill T, Sacco J, Tangeman J, et al. Palliative care consultation teams cut hospital costs for Medicaid beneficiaries. Health Aff (Millwood). 2011;30(3):454–63.

9. Norton SA, Hogan LA, Holloway RG, Temkin-Greener H, Buckley MJ, Quill TE. Proactive palliative care in the medical intensive care unit: effects on length of stay for selected high-risk patients. Crit Care Med. 2007;35(6):1530–5.
10. Temel JS, Greer JA, Muzikansky A, Gallagher ER, Admane S, Jackson VA, et al. Early palliative care for patients with metastatic non–small-cell lung cancer. N Engl J Med. 2010;363(8):733–42.
11. Lim T, Nam SH, Kim MS, Yoon KS, Kim BS. Comparison of medical expenditure according to types of hospice care in patients with terminal cancer. Am J Hosp Palliat Care. 2013;30(1):50–2.
12. World Health Organization. Strengthening of palliative care as a component of comprehensive care throughout the life course. J Pain Palliat Care Pharmacother. 2014;28(2):130–4.
13. Powell RA, Mwangi-Powell FN, Radbruch L, Yamey G, Krakauer EL, Spence D, et al. Putting palliative care on the global health agenda. Lancet Oncol. 2015;16(2):131–3.
14. Aging NNIo. What are palliative care and hospice care? NIH national institute on aging 2021. Available from: https://www.nia.nih.gov/health/what-are-palliative-care-and-hospice-care
15. Roosa TR, Elias M, Ana D, Wharton GA. International health care system profiles Australia 2020.
16. Ministry of Health MoL-TC. Palliative and end-of-life care 2021.
17. Knaul FM, LeBaron VT, Calderon M, Arreola-Ornelas H, Bhadelia A, Krakauer EL, et al. Developing palliative care capacity in Colombia and Mexico. J Clin Oncol. 2014;32(31_suppl):103.
18. Health AG. What does palliative care cost? 2019.
19. CHPCA. Fact sheet: hospice palliative care in Canada 2020.
20. CMS TCfMMS. Hospice 2021.
21. Jang RW, Caraiscos VB, Swami N, Banerjee S, Mak E, Kaya E, et al. Simple prognostic model for patients with advanced cancer based on performance status. J Oncol Pract. 2014;10(5):e335–e41.
22. Schag CC, Heinrich RL, Ganz PA. Karnofsky performance status revisited: reliability, validity, and guidelines. J Clin Oncol. 1984;2(3):187–93.
23. Péus D, Newcomb N, Hofer S. Appraisal of the karnofsky performance status and proposal of a simple algorithmic system for its evaluation. BMC Med Inform Decis Mak. 2013;13:72.
24. Azam F, Latif MF, Farooq A, Tirmazy SH, AlShahrani S, Bashir S, et al. Performance status assessment by using ECOG (eastern cooperative oncology group) score for cancer patients by oncology healthcare professionals. Case Rep Oncol. 2019;12(3):728–36.
25. Anderson F, Downing GM, Hill J, Casorso L, Lerch N. Palliative performance scale (PPS): a new tool. J Palliat Care. 1996;12(1):5–11.
26. Crooks V, Waller S, Smith T, Hahn TJ. The use of the karnofsky performance scale in determining outcomes and risk in geriatric outpatients. J Gerontol. 1991;46(4):M139–44.
27. World Tokyo C. Dental care and oral health for healthy longevity in an ageing society 2015.
28. WHO. Oral health 2017.
29. Kvalheim SF, Strand GV, Husebø BS, Marthinussen MC. End-of-life palliative oral care in Norwegian health institutions. An exploratory study. Gerodontology. 2016;33(4):522–9.
30. Hawley P. Barriers to access to palliative care. Palliat Care. 2017;10:1178224216688887.
31. Patrick DL, Lee RSY, Nucci M, Grembowski D, Jolles CZ, Milgrom P. Reducing oral health disparities: a focus on social and cultural determinants. BMC Oral Health. 2006;6(Suppl 1):S4–S.
32. Singh A, Gambhir RS, Singh S, Kapoor V, Singh J. Oral health: how much do you know? A study on knowledge, attitude and practices of patients visiting a North Indian dental school. Eur J Dent. 2014;8(1):63–7.
33. Wiseman MA. Palliative care dentistry. Gerodontology. 2000;17(1):49–51.
34. D'Souza V. Perceived oral care needs of terminally ill adults – a qualitative investigation 2019.
35. American Dental Association. The ADA principles of ethics and code of conduct. Counc Ethics Bylaws Judicial Aff. 2021:1–23.

36. Davies A. Finlay I. Oral assessment. Oxford University Press; 2011. p. 1–250.
37. Kayser-Jones J, Bird WF, Paul SM, Long L, Schell ES. An instrument to assess the oral health status of nursing home residents. The Gerontologist. 1995;35(6):814–24.
38. Chalmers J, Johnson V, Tang JH-C, Titler MG. Evidence-based protocol: oral hygiene care for functionally dependent and cognitively impaired older adults. J Gerontol Nurs. 2004;30(11):5–12.
39. Fjeld KG, Eide H, Mowe M, Hove LH, Willumsen T. Dental hygiene registration: development, and reliability and validity testing of an assessment scale designed for nurses in institutions. J Clin Nurs. 2017;26(13–14):1845–53.
40. Chen X, Clark JJ, Preisser JS, Naorungroj S, Shuman SK. Dental caries in older adults in the last year of life. J Am Geriatr Soc. 2013;61(8):1345–50.
41. Wiseman M. The treatment of oral problems in the palliative patient. J Can Dent Assoc. 2006;72(5):453–8.
42. Ettinger RL. The role of the dentist in geriatric palliative care. J Am Geriatr Soc. 2012;60(2):367–8.
43. Oneschuk D, Hanson J, Bruera E. A survey of mouth pain and dryness in patients with advanced cancer. Support Care Cancer. 2000;8(5):372–6.
44. Scully C. Drug effects on salivary glands: dry mouth. Wiley; 2003. p. 165–76.
45. Eveson JW. Xerostomia. Wiley; 2008. p. 85–91.
46. Davies A. Finlay I. Taste disturbance. Oxford University Press; 2011. p. 115–22.
47. Österberg T, Mellström D, Sundh V. Dental health and functional ageing. Community Dent Oral Epidemiol. 1990;18(6):313–8.
48. MacEntee MI, Donnelly LR. Oral health and the frailty syndrome. Periodontology. 2016;72(1):135–41.
49. Magnani C, Mastroianni C, Giannarelli D, Stefanelli MC, Di Cienzo V, Valerioti T, et al. Oral hygiene care in patients with advanced disease: an essential measure to improve oral cavity conditions and symptom management. Am J Hosp Palliat Care. 2019;36(9):815–9.
50. Fitzgerald R, Gallagher J. Oral health in end-of-life patients: a rapid review. Spec Care Dentist. 2018;38(5):291–8.
51. Gil-Montoya JA, de Mello ALF, Cardenas CB, Lopez IG. Oral health protocol for the dependent institutionalized elderly. Geriatr Nurs. 2006;27(2):95–101.
52. Wu B, Plassman B, Crout R, Kao E, Boone M, Caplan D, et al. P2-173: cognitive impairment and oral health in older adults. Alzheimers Dement. 2011;7(4S_Part_10):S368.
53. Kambhu PP, Levy SM. Oral hygiene care levels in Iowa intermediate care facilities. Spec Care Dentist. 1993;13(5):209–14.
54. Rogus-Pulia N, Wirth R, Sloane PD. Editorial dysphagia in frail older persons: making the most of current knowledge. J Am Med Dir Assoc. 2018;19(9):736–40.
55. Krekeler BN, Broadfoot CK, Johnson S, Connor NP, Rogus-Pulia N. Patient adherence to dysphagia recommendations: a systematic review. New York: Springer; 2018. p. 173–84.
56. Sonis ST. Oral mucositis. Wiley; 2011. p. 607–12.
57. Knight J, Carter AY, Frey RJ. Stomatitis. In: Longe JL, editor. The gale encyclopedia of medicine. 6th ed. Farmington Hills: Gale; 2020. p. 4898–900.
58. Trotti A, Byhardt R, Stetz J, Gwede C, Corn B, Fu K, et al. Common toxicity criteria: version 2.0. An improved reference for grading the acute effects of cancer treatment: impact on radiotherapy. Int J Radiat Oncol Biol Phys. 2000;47(1):13–47.
59. Rodríguez-Caballero A, Torres-Lagares D, Robles-García M, Pachón-Ibáñez J, González-Padilla D, Gutiérrez-Pérez JL. Cancer treatment-induced oral mucositis: a critical review. Int J Oral Maxillofac Surg. 2012;41(2):225–38.
60. Sweeney MP, Bagg J, Baxter WP, Aitchison TC. Oral disease in terminally ill cancer patients with xerostomia. Oral Oncol. 1998;34(2):123–6.
61. Sweeney MP, Bagg J. The mouth and palliative care. Am J Hosp Palliat Care. 2000;17(2):118–24.
62. Davies AN, Broadley K, Beighton D. Xerostomia in patients with advanced cancer. J Pain Symptom Manag. 2001;22(4):820–5.

63. Paine CC, Snider JW. When saliva becomes a problem: the challenges and palliative care for patients with sialorrhea. AME Publishing Company; 2020. p. 1333–9.
64. Wolff A, Joshi RK, Ekström J, Aframian D, Pedersen AML, Proctor G, et al. A guide to medications inducing salivary gland dysfunction, xerostomia, and subjective sialorrhea: a systematic review sponsored by the world workshop on oral medicine VI. Drugs R&D. 2017;17(1):1–28.
65. Davies A. Finlay I. Salivary gland dysfunction. Oxford University Press; 2011. p. 97–110.
66. Alt-Epping B, Nejad RK, Jung K, Gross U, Nauck F. Symptoms of the oral cavity and their association with local microbiological and clinical findings–a prospective survey in palliative care. Support Care Cancer. 2012;20(3):531–7.
67. Wilberg P, Hjermstad MJ, Ottesen S, Herlofson BB. Oral health is an important issue in end-of-life cancer care. Support Care Cancer. 2012;20(12):3115–22.
68. Van Lancker A, Beeckman D, Verhaeghe S, Van Den Noortgate N, Van Hecke A. Symptom clustering in hospitalised older palliative cancer patients: a cross-sectional study. Int J Nurs Stud. 2016;61:72–81.
69. Bloise R, Davis MP. Dysgeusia #304. J Palliat Med. 2016;19(4):462–3.
70. Zakrzewska JM. Orofacial pain. Rev Pain. 2011;5(1):1.
71. Epstein JB, Elad S, Eliav E, Jurevic R, Benoliel R. Orofacial pain in cancer: part II--clinical perspectives and management. J Dent Res. 2007;86(6):506–18.
72. Romero-Reyes M, Salvemini D. Cancer and orofacial pain. Med Oral Patol Oral Cir Bucal. 2016;21(6):e665–e71.
73. Sushma N, Glenn TC. Halitosis: a breath of fresh air. Clin Infect Dis. 1997;25:S218–S9.
74. Gustafson DH. A good death. J Med Internet Res. 2007;9(1):e6.
75. Venkatasalu MR, Murang ZR, Husaini HA, Idris DR, Dhaliwal JS. Why oral palliative care takes a backseat? A national focus group study on experiences of palliative doctors, nurses and dentists. Nurs Open. 2020;7(5):1330–7.
76. Manalo MFC. End-of-life decisions about withholding or withdrawing therapy: medical, ethical, and religio-cultural considerations. Palliat Care. 2013;7:1–5.
77. Emanuel LL, Ferris FD. Education for physicians on end-of-life care Participant's handbook, module 11, withholding, withdrawing therapy EPEC project. The Robert Wood Johnson Foundation; 1999.
78. Levin PD, Sprung CL. Withdrawing and withholding life-sustaining therapies are not the same. Crit Care. 2005;9(3):230–2.
79. Chung GS, Yoon JD, Rasinski KA, Curlin FA. US physicians' opinions about distinctions between withdrawing and withholding life-sustaining treatment. J Relig Health. 2016;55(5):1596–606.
80. Elwyn G, Frosch D, Thomson R, Joseph-Williams N, Lloyd A, Kinnersley P, et al. Shared decision making: a model for clinical practice. J Gen Intern Med. 2012;27(10):1361–7.
81. Bae J-M. Shared decision making: relevant concepts and facilitating strategies. Epidemiol Health. 2017;39:e2017048.
82. Hall DE, Prochazka AV, Fink AS. Informed consent for clinical treatment. CMAJ. 2012;184(5):533–40.
83. Lloyd A, Hayes P, Bell PR, Naylor AR. The role of risk and benefit perception in informed consent for surgery. Med Decis Mak. 2001;21(2):141–9.
84. Leeb D, Bowers DG Jr, Lynch JB. Observations on the myth of "informed consent". Plast Reconstr Surg. 1976;58(3):280–2.
85. Hutson MM, Blaha JD. Patients' recall of preoperative instruction for informed consent for an operation. J Bone Joint Surg Am. 1991;73(2):160–2.
86. Lavelle-Jones C, Byrne DJ, Rice P, Cuschieri A. Factors affecting quality of informed consent. BMJ. 1993;306(6882):885–90.
87. Lashley M, Talley W, Lands LC, Keyserlingk EW. Informed proxy consent: communication between pediatric surgeons and surrogates about surgery. Pediatrics. 2000;105(3 Pt 1):591–7.
88. Tait AR, Voepel-Lewis T, Malviya S. Do they understand? (part II): assent of children participating in clinical anesthesia and surgery research. Anesthesiology. 2003;98(3):609–14.

89. Mariano J, Min LC. Chapter 4 – Assessment. In: Naeim A, Reuben DB, Ganz PA, editors. Management of cancer in the older patient. Philadelphia: W.B. Saunders; 2012. p. 39–50.
90. H-CDA U. National conference of commissioners on uniform state laws 1993.
91. American Bar Association. Assessment of older adults with diminished capacity: a handbook for psychologists apa.org2018. Available from: http://www.apa.org/pi/aging/programs/assessment/capacity-psychologist-handbook.pdf
92. Sudore RL, Lum HD, You JJ, Hanson LC, Meier DE, Pantilat SZ, et al. Defining advance care planning for adults: a consensus definition from a multidisciplinary Delphi panel. J Pain Symptom Manag. 2017;53(5):821–32, e1.
93. Sudore RL, Fried TR. Redefining the "planning" in advance care planning: preparing for end-of-life decision making. Ann Intern Med. 2010;153(4):256–61.
94. Doukas DJ, McCullough LB. The values history. The evaluation of the patient's values and advance directives. J Fam Pract. 1991;32(2):145–53.
95. Hawkins NA, Ditto PH, Danks JH, Smucker WD. Micromanaging death: process preferences, values, and goals in end-of-life medical decision making. The Gerontologist. 2005;45(1):107–17.
96. Schonwetter RS, Walker RM, Solomon M, Indurkhya A, Robinson BE. Life values, resuscitation preferences, and the applicability of living wills in an older population. J Am Geriatr Soc. 1996;44(8):954–8.
97. Pearlman RA, Starks H, Cain KC, Cole WG. Improvements in advance care planning in the veterans affairs system: results of a multifaceted intervention. Arch Intern Med. 2005;165(6):667–74.
98. Sabatino CP. The evolution of health care advance planning law and policy. Milbank Q. 2010;88(2):211–39.
99. Özalp GŞ, Uysal N, Oğuz G, Koçak N, Karaca Ş, Kadıoğulları N. Identification of symptom clusters in cancer patients at palliative care clinic. Asia Pac J Oncol Nurs. 2017;4(3):259–64.
100. NHSScotland. Mouth care 2018 2020. Available from: https://www.palliativecareguidelines.scot.nhs.uk/guidelines/symptom-control/Mouth-Care.aspx

Ethical Considerations in Geriatric Dentistry

Carlos S. Smith

1   What Is Ethics?

Ethics has long been defined as a branch of philosophy and theology that involves systematizing, defending, and recommending concepts of right and wrong behavior. The American College of Dentists defines ethics as studying systematically what is right and good with respect to character and conduct [1]. In short, ethics is about choices. The choosing to act or to not act. Ethical issues faced by dentists and members of the dental team (dental hygienists, dental therapists, dental assistants, and dental office administrative staff) are ever-evolving, both increasing in number and in the complexity of factors needing to be reviewed, considered, and addressed [2]. Ethics affect every decision made in the dental office and are inextricably linked to the daily decisions of overall dental practice. The pursuit of embodying the best of dental ethics and ethical decision-making is both an individual and collective matter.

What one dentist chooses to do or not do has implications and consequences not only for that individual but also for the profession as a whole. What dentist hasn't heard the inevitable phrase, "I hate dentists," upon entering an operatory and greeting a new patient. Often regarded as simple patient anxiety, it is worth noting that a previous dental provider, although not expressly causing the dental anxiety/trauma, certainly could have had a role in shaping or exacerbating such patient anxiety in a prior encounter. A previous dentist's choosing to act or not to act could have heavily influenced the patient's view of both that dentist specifically, but also the patient's view of dentists generally and the profession as a whole. Research has shown that the skills, attitudes, and philosophies of various dentists that persons may have encountered in their life spans can affect their oral health status [3].

C. S. Smith (✉)
Department of Dental Public Health and Policy, VCU School of Dentistry, Richmond, VA, USA
e-mail: cssmith2@vcu.edu

2 Providing Care for the Geriatric Patient

The US Census Bureau projects that by 2030, more than 20% of the population will be 65 years or older compared with 13% in 2010 [4]. While the geriatric population is ever-growing, the typical older patient is no longer simply a denture wearer. Particularly, as the geriatric population booms, this generation of seniors is often more educated, is more financially well-off, and has a history of routine dental care utilization [5]. Yet typical socioeconomic barriers to access to care remain. Along with continued advancement in dental treatments and more complex treatment planning options, today's geriatric patient has increasingly retained their natural teeth; thus, a larger number of older people will be seeking dental care in the upcoming years [6]. The retention of teeth also presents a challenge for both patient self-care and oral professional care to maintain the dentition for a whole lifetime [7]. Oral health status in older adults also reflects the cumulative outcomes of oral health behaviors, diseases, and their treatments during a life span [7].

The dental needs of older adults are also changing and growing. "The management of older patients requires not only an understanding of the medical and dental aspects of aging, but also many other factors such as ambulation, independent living, socialization, and sensory function. Many barriers may interfere with providing older patients with dental care, including heightened dental complexity, multiple medical conditions, diminished functional status, loss of independence, uninformed attitudes about dental care in old age, and limited finances."[7] Dental practice specific to geriatric patient care raises specific ethical issues due to the evolving dental needs of older adults. While ethical dilemmas have been vastly studied, taught, and applied, all dentist-patient interactions do not necessarily give rise to an ethical dilemma. However, every dentist-patient, or even dentist-team member, interaction does have within it an ethical dimension.

3 Informed Consent and the Geriatric Patient

One of the most well-known ethical aspects of dental practice is obtaining informed consent. However, despite its common practice, it is also one of the most leniently applied and understood concepts with significant ethical underpinnings. While widely minimized to a signature of understanding and approval, informed consent is of particular interest and concern among an aging patient population. Obtaining informed consent is in all reality more than a simple conversation. It is a communication between patients and their healthcare providers with a goal to ensure full understanding of the clinical procedures that will be performed [6]. The informed consent process should include a discussion of the expected risks, benefits, and alternatives that are available to them and an opportunity to ask questions, discuss their choices, and have time to reflect and provide a clear indication of their eventual decision [6]. The literature suggests that informed consent should include five basic elements or domains: capacity, information, comprehension, voluntariness, and a final decision or choice [6].

Capacity to consent refers to the patient's ability to understand the purpose, implication, and consequences of treatment [2]. Capacity is an issue of the patient's physical and cognitive ability to fully participate in the informed consent process [6]. Within the geriatric patient population, there are those who suffer limited capacity to make decisions for themselves, including cognitive impairments as a result of mental illness, stroke, dementia, delirium, or other related issues [8]. It has long been established that Alzheimer's patients present "unique caregiving problems because of troublesome symptoms including impaired memory, disorientation, poor judgment, inappropriate, unpredictable, or dangerous behaviors, incontinence, and the need for constant surveillance" [8]. For a more in-depth discussion on the topic of cognitive impairment, please refer to Chapter "The 3 Ds: Dementia, Delirium and Depression in Oral Health".

One of the most significant ethical challenges within the issue of informed consent and geriatric dentistry is the fact that capacity to participate in the informed consent process may fluctuate over time. There is also very little standardization of how capacity is accessed and if it is appropriate in the dental clinical setting for that to be a chairside assessment and/or decision. It is also possible that ageism, the holding of negative stereotypes and beliefs regarding older adults, may influence dentist, patient, or even caregiver understandings and actions [8]. "The decision not to treat a condition or illness made on age considerations alone, or the seeking of advice from adult children without first talking with the older patient are, in many instances, examples of ageist behaviors" [8]. Dentists, dental team members, and even caregivers must be careful as many decisions may relate to providing or withholding treatment, especially when a patient may verbally or behaviorally refuse care. An ultimate decision must be made whether or not to override refusal. The role of the caregiver or family member is sometimes a burden of care, and professional altruism and empathy are necessary. For example, if a patient resists riding in the car to make an office visit, planning longer treatment sessions, which limit the need for multiple visits, will reduce caregiver burden substantially. Some cognitively impaired patients have better mental function and less disruptive behaviors at one time of day as opposed to others. For these patients, flexibility in scheduling visits during their "good" time (e.g., only morning visits) will reduce stress for the family caregiver, to say nothing of the dentist [8].

The specific question of declining capacity necessitates both a means for assessing capacity and methodologies for ensuring a patient with declining capacity is able to have autonomy in their treatment care decisions before capacity has indeed declined. While not particularly common in dental care settings, in medical care the advance directive is a customary means of predetermining a patient's wishes in the event they can no longer consent for themselves. Medicine also has options such as DNR or do not resuscitate orders. On the surface, DNRs may seem to have little relevance to clinical dental care not seemingly surrounding a matter of life or death. However, at their simplest understanding, a DNR order is a decision to not render treatment. Likely occurring much more frequently than clinicians care to admit, the decision to treat or not to treat health problems, including those related to the oral cavity, is made based largely upon the goal of maintaining function and comfort of older patients [8].

Although capacity assessment tools exist, most are not used in everyday healthcare practice, and many are considered time-consuming and insufficient at determining if patients really have the capacity to consent [6]. Some suggest the practicality, efficiency, acceptability, affordability, and sustainability of capacity assessment tools in dentistry makes their useage highly unlikely [6]. In the past, researchers have suggested that dental professionals ask the patient, "who would you like me to consult regarding your treatment if something should happen to you and you are no longer able to express your wishes" [8]. The patient's response is subsequently documented in the dental record. While this seems simple and satisfying on its surface, like most decisions with ethical implications, simplicity and experiences within ethical dimensions often present with more than what meets the eye. Thus, assessing a patient's ability to provide consent can be challenging for dentists under a variety of circumstances, including when capacity is affected by mental health status or is transient. With decisions of capacity and informed consent having legal and regulatory implications, the research is inconclusive as to the extent to which dental practitioners should become involved in legally declaring a patient capable or incapable [6].

Best practices within a dental care setting have yet to be clearly established; however, the literature recommends a medical referral for capacity evaluation if the dentist is unsure of the patient's ability to consent for treatment [9]. Accounting for older patients, in dental care settings, often declining additional information about treatment procedures, some scholars suggest geriatric patients should have 24 hours before any routine dental procedure to process the information provided in the consent forms [10]. Dentist and dental team members must be attuned to nonverbal cues from patients such as visible confusion and inconsistencies in the patient's behavior, and if the patient's decision-making capacity appears questionable, immediately involve family members or caregivers in the decision-making process [6].

Worth noting is the concept of geriatric assent, meaning agreement of someone not able to give legal consent to participate in the activity. Accounting for many of the same aforementioned challenges with informed consent and declining capacity, even garnering assent can be challenging. The geriatric assent process still involves the accumulating burden over time on caregivers who may choose to "shortcut" communication for the sake of decisional efficiency and expediency [11]. Despite office productivity goals and maximized efficiency, dentists and dental team members are ethically bound to promote assent, even when consent is unattainable or inconclusive. Promoting assent is a more proactive procedure than merely arranging for incompetent patients to passively abide by decisions for which they have had little or no input [11].

4 Elder Abuse, Evolving Technologies, and Changing Models of Care Delivery

Elder abuse is a multifaceted and pervasive public health issue, which includes physical, sexual, and emotional abuse, financial exploitation, and neglect (caregiver neglect and self-neglect) [12]. It is estimated that only a fraction of elder abuse cases actually come to the attention of adult protective services [13]. Two-thirds of physical abuse cases result in injuries to the head, neck, and/or mouth—areas visible to oral healthcare providers during examination and treatment [14, 15]. Dentists, dental hygienists, dental therapists, dental assistants, and all dental team members are in a unique position to detect elder abuse and neglect.

As the practice of dentistry advances technologically, there arises an increased need to garner an ethical perspective as it relates to new and evolving treatment modalities. With the overwhelming increases and availability of both implants and digital dentistry, appropriating an ethical lens is necessary. Scholars have formulated an ethical framework for "responsibly practiced implantology" [16]. Among issues noted are supposed prevalence in potential placement of implants as a rationale for tooth extraction. This concept is specifically guarded against in that there is concerted effort in retaining natural dentition. "The mere option of replacing the tooth with an implant should not be the leading factor in the decision of whether or not to extract a tooth" [17].

Dental caries is still clearly a public health problem for many older Americans, such as those of lower socioeconomic status, with dementia, who are homebound, and who are institutionalized [5]. Studies have shown that the perceived need of dental care is reduced as functional dependency increases, and dental care use concurrently decreases, especially in those older adults who are institutionalized [18, 19]. Adequate access to dental care does not exist for many United States nursing home residents [18]. The dental treatment geriatric patients seek and ultimately receive is directly dependent on their self-perceived need, their financial ability to pay for that care, and issues such as transportation and documentation, rather than the normative need detected during an oral examination by a dentist [19]. It has been established that the majority of dental care for older adults takes place in private practices [5]. For functionally independent and older adults with frailty, minor modifications in office design or flow to allow for age-related changes allows private practitioners to treat this population [20].

Providing dental care for institutionalized geriatric patients presents both challenges and opportunities. With much emphasis on interprofessional and collaborative care, geriatric health and specifically oral health present a great opportunity for evolving models of care delivery. Although the geriatric population is increasing, institutionalization and nursing home utilization are declining, and there is a greater desire among seniors and their families to age in place [21]. One of the most significant developments in geriatric care is the shift to a model of care based in community living often termed adult day-care centers. The current generation of older adults wants to age in place, and they do not want to be institutionalized. Models, such as the Programs of All-inclusive Care for the Elders (PACE), have been gaining traction [21, 22]. Ethical duty and obligation implores that dentists and dental team members strive to be part of the interprofessional teams that care for older adults in these new models of care. The PACE is a managed care organization that provides comprehensive medical and social services to a population of frail, community-dwelling older adults, most of whom are dually eligible, having Medicare and Medicaid benefits, US government-based forms of healthcare insurance for the poor and older adults, respectively [23]. The PACE actually has its origins with the work of a public health dentist and social worker in San Francisco in the 1970s who recognized a need for long-term care services that kept individuals in the community while maintaining a good quality of life [24, 25]. Effectiveness of a dental program in long-term care has been found to be contingent on dental care, routine and continual oral hygiene, and assessment [24]. In particular, they found routine oral hygiene and assessment were most important to a program's success and that simply providing dental services is insufficient to having an effective dental program [21].

PACE programs readily offer dental services, which often include partnering with a community dentist [26]. This can and often includes providing dental services on-site, affording more significant interaction between dental professionals and other members of the patient care team [27]. Physically including dentistry within PACE programs sites could allow community dentists to shadow, network, and refer complex, medically compromised geriatric patients. There are also advanced dental education programs or general practice residency programs who have partnered with hospitals that are connected to PACE facilities and programs [28]. Dental schools may also seek partnerships with local PACE programs to expose students to a model of collaborative team-based care in geriatrics [27].

Researchers have suggested that similar programs that care for the growing population of older adults who prefer to remain in the community should place an emphasis on routine oral hygiene care and should not make providing on-site dental care a sole focus of their programs. In addition, programs should have a coordinated system of referral to dentists. The proposed model suggests the important role that nurses and an interprofessional team can play as communicators and facilitators in this process. Lastly, a communal gathering location, such as the PACE center, is necessary to ensure a common location where members regularly congregate and health providers and nurses have access to individuals. This is where older adults can receive routine medical and dental assessments and obtain preventive home care products, such as fluoridated toothpaste and toothbrushes [21]. Opportunities abound for ethical practice among dentists and dental team members to forge creative partnerships for delivering collaborative care.

5 Barriers to Care: An Ethical Lens on Medical Mistrust and the History of Racism in Healthcare

Geriatric patients of certain demographic backgrounds and cultural identities may invoke yet another ethical dimension of care, namely, medical mistrust and the history of racism within healthcare delivery systems. Particularly in the United States, where denial of healthcare and even basic human rights were once fully legal, remnants of those historic atrocities still unfortunately remain. Particularly at a time when a patient's zip code (US postal codes) is the best predictor of health outcomes

[29], dentists and dental team members must wrestle with the long-lasting effects of structural racism within healthcare. This remains true particularly in geriatric populations who are of the age to have been born prior to, lived in, or were raised during legal American segregation. Many studies have shown that there are substantial racial differences in trust in healthcare providers and healthcare systems. African Americans were significantly more likely than Whites to report low trust in healthcare providers in this study [30, 31]. Even after controlling for sociodemographic, prior healthcare experiences, and structural characteristics of care, African American race had a significant effect on low trust in healthcare. However, different factors were associated with low trust among African Americans and Whites. Among African Americans, the source of medical care had a significant independent association with low trust, whereas among Whites, the number of annual healthcare visits was associated significantly with low trust. It is possible that different factors were associated with low trust among African Americans and Whites because of differences in healthcare experiences and sources of medical care between these populations" [30]. It has been suggested that among African Americans, previous experiences with healthcare providers and sources of medical care may be more important sources of distrust in healthcare providers than sociodemographic characteristics.

With the ever-evolving discoveries and medical mistrust that continued to be revealed, what once was merely folklore in nature has come to modern light as ethical lapses of monumental proportions. The research and subsequent book and movie detailing the origin of the commonly used HeLa cells underpins much of the practice of modern medicine in the United States. These "HeLa cells" originated from the flesh and blood of an African American woman named Henrietta Lacks. Her cells were taken for scientific purposes without any consent or foreknowledge from her, nor her family and loved ones. These cells were used for decades, even to this day. They have been involved in key discoveries in many fields including cancer, immunology, and infectious disease [32]. Even most recently, they have been used in research to develop vaccines aimed at combating the COVID-19 pandemic [33]. Yet another ethical abuse destined for the big screen involves the story of the first heart transplant in the segregated southern United States in 1968. This also involved the lack of informed consent to obtain the heart and kidneys of a black patient, Bruce Tucker, for the purposes of performing organ transplants for other recipients [34]. Actions such as these, and their subsequent lack of ethical and moral behavior, have direct linkages to communal mistrust, and some may argue an earned distrust, in healthcare, healthcare professionals, and healthcare delivery systems [35]. These historic ethical lapses are often in the memories and minds of minority geriatric patients that themselves have been participants, positively or negatively, within old institutions of segregation and overt racism.

While racism may or may not remain as overt within healthcare today, racial biases undoubtedly remain [36]. In fact, perceived racism particularly with older minority patients has been found to be a possible contributor to health disparities [37]. Within dentistry, healthcare providers' racial bias is also evident. Dentists' decision-making has been impacted by the race of the patient, resulting in a greater likelihood of extractions (less root canal therapy recommendations) for Black patients presenting with a broken-down tooth and symptoms of irreversible pulpitis [38]. Showing that treatment planning decisions may indeed be subject to and/or influenced by racial bias. It is an ethical duty for dentists and dental team members to be self-aware, hopefully reducing the impact potential biases can have on the treatment and care patients receive. For a more in-depth discussion on the topic of health disparities, please refer to Chapter "Health Disparities in Oral Health".

All decisions that healthcare providers make are affected by their own cultural background as well as the background of the persons for whom the decisions are made [39]. Different ethnic groups have varied attitudes toward seeking help, proposing ideal solutions to problems, and even considering who is part of the family [40]. Often the most vulnerable and susceptible populations to disease have the most historic impediments to healthcare access [41]. Overall, while untreated dental caries in older Americans significantly has decreased, health disparities and inequities remain with higher prevalence of untreated dental caries in older African Americans and Hispanics Americans, those with lower incomes and less education and current or former smokers [5, 42]. Greater retention of teeth predisposes many older adults to a continual risk of both new and recurrent coronal and root caries and extends the risk for developing gingivitis and periodontal diseases [43]. This is particularly true of vulnerable populations most directly affected by a lack of access to oral healthcare. A barrier to care, in need of ethical exploration is also the issue of language. While not often seen as an ethical dilemma in its purest sense, the issue of language and potential language barriers that may exist between dental providers and patients is an ever-present ethical dimension. Though the number of Spanish-speaking providers in the United States is on the rise, studies have shown an increased presence of periodontal disease in Spanish-speaking older adults of Mexican ancestry despite having regular dental care at home [44]. While access to care issues are multivariate in nature, the ethical lens must also remain a consideration.

6 The COVID-19 Global Pandemic and the Geriatric Patient: An Ethical Lens

Patients with pneumonia of unknown cause were reported in Wuhan, China, in December, 2019 [45]. Later named, COVID-19, the virus quickly spread across the global landscape, in short order being declared a pandemic by the World Health Organization [46]. "Due to the rapid spread of COVID-19, the risk of it causing significant fatality and the stress it poses for health care workers and its potential to overwhelm the capacity of health care systems resulted in many countries adopting measures to restrict human mobility, in an attempt to limit the spread of the disease" [47]. Dental care providers were required to halt all nonemergency treatment procedures due to the concern that many dental procedures may produce aerosols and facilitate COVID-19 spread [48]. Older patients were thought to be highly susceptible, and one of the hardest hit populations were residents of long-term care facilities or geriatric patients who are institutionalized [49]. The earliest outbreak of COVID-19 in the United States was in a long-term care facility in the state of Washington, USA, which had a high fatality rate [50].

In addition to affecting long-term care facilities in unknown proportions, it has been established that PACE programs within the United States are on trend with the aging population's desire to age in place and even chose home-based care. This trend and choice, along with forced social distancing restrictions, has only increased with the effects of COVID-19 on long-term care and home care industries catering to older adults [23]. The COVID-19 pandemic has further exacerbated problems accessing oral healthcare for those populations already most at risk for oral disease. The pausing of care, while appropriate for some populations, may have seen a worsening of dental caries, periodontal disease, or even pathology for older populations. The soaring positivity rates of the virus has resulted in disruptions in the delivery of maintenance dental treatments for many geriatric patients who were forced to take indefinite hiatus in their oral care.

The COVID-19 pandemic has laid bare many of the healthcare inequities and disparities that have long gone unnoticed by the masses leading to a full mainstream understanding and public conversation [51]. Connecting to the history of medical mistrust by minority US populations, barriers to greater participation of Black people in COVID-19 trials still exist as well as the hesitancy in taking advantage of vaccine administration that are now widely available in most high-income countries [52–54]. Although the COVID-19 pandemic presents an additional ethical hurdle for geriatric patients and their dental providers, like other disruptions before, innovation is birthed. Greater acceptance for teledentistry, a move away from live patient board exams, and even an expansion of dental and dental hygiene scopes of practice to include vaccine administration are just a few of the many positive disrupters by which the COVID-19 pandemic has challenged the status quo [55–57].

7 Ethical Decision-Making: Principles and Embracing Narrative Ethics

Ethical decision-making for dentists can be relatively straightforward and simple or can delve into quite a complex process of weighing out options and various stakeholder viewpoints. Due to the ever-evolving complex nature of dentistry and dental practice, several models of ethical decision-making have been developed and utilized over time. Most models involve contemplation of ethical principles and include multiple considerations [1]. Professions, including dentistry, are largely defined as such in part because of self-governed and developed codes of ethics. A code of ethics defines the moral boundaries within which professional services may be ethically provided. Many dental organizations have codes of ethical conduct for guidance of dentists in their practice. The American Dental Association (ADA) has five guiding and fundamental principles which are the following: patient autonomy, non-maleficence, beneficence, justice, and veracity (Fig. 1).

Many models and frameworks exist to aid healthcare practitioners in managing ethical challenges that arise during clinical care. The most classical understanding of dental ethics and ethical decision-making stems from the classic work of Ozar's Central Values of Dental Practice. These values are delineated as follows: (a) the patient's life and general health, (b) the patient's oral health, (c) the patient's autonomy, (d) the dentist's preferred patterns of practice, (e) esthetic values, and (f) efficiency in the use of resources [58]. Also widely used is the Four Box Model derived from Jonsen, Siegler, and Winslade, in which ethical problems are analyzed in the context of four domains: medical indications, patient preferences, quality of life, and contextual features (i.e., social, economic, legal, and administrative) [59]. Each topic can be approached through a set of specific questions with the goal of identifying the various circumstances of a given case and linking them to their underlying ethical principle [60].

One of the most recent developments in dental ethics has been the use of narrative ethics as a model for ethical decision-making. Narrative ethics is a different way of thinking about teaching ethics. While principle-based ethics is useful, it can tend to put ideas into specified boxes and silos. Narrative ethics enables one to deconstruct cases in a broader sense with the ethical choices made more easily subject to reflection and evaluation [61]. It also helps one think about an ethical scenario as a story, helping to better empathize with other persons' thoughts and feelings and enabling more thoughtful decision-making. Some critique put forth concerning narrative ethics has been the lack of appeal to rules, principles, or other ethical constructs [62].

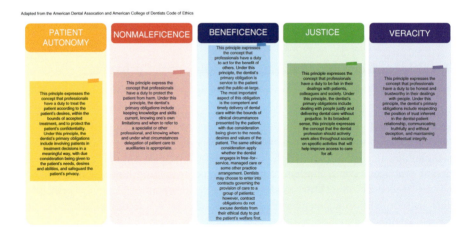

Fig. 1 Principles of dental ethics

Roucka and More have developed a specific narrative dental ethics decision-making model rubric and framework relying on both narrative and story as well incorporating consideration of classic healthcare ethical principles (Fig. 2 and Table 1). Their model includes the following: identifying the stakeholders, asking if harm was done to anyone and by whom, rating (4 being excellent 1 being poor) the outcome from the perspective of each stakeholder, inquiry of how the story makes one feel, determining if the circumstances give the perception of an optimal outcome, identifying flaws one may identify (breach of principles, procedural and/or ethical), and lastly, an attempt at rewriting the story to make the scenario such that an optimal outcome is perceived by all stakeholders [63].

The narrative dental ethics decision-making model allows for building of empathy, inspires self-reflection, encourages memory through emotional connection, and aids in illustrating various points of view. A narrative dental ethics approach also reminds the user that ethics and ethical decision-making are not conducted in a vacuum. Dentists bring their varying life experiences and perspectives to the proverbial ethical decision-making table. This would include, but not limited to, personal experience and upbringing, religious beliefs or the lack thereof, professional training and experiences, practice locations, patient expectations, social customs, societal norms, and more. These various life experiences and perspectives shape dentists understanding and well-being, ultimately affecting patient outcomes. Most assuredly, open consideration of ethical issues leads to improved quality of decisions [8], ultimately yielding a better life for geriatric patients and increased satisfaction and altruism for dentists and the dental care team.

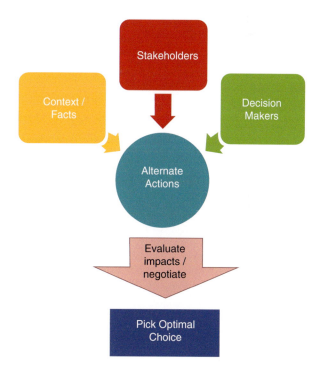

Fig. 2 The process of narrative ethics

Table 1 Roucka/More Narrative Ethics Rubric

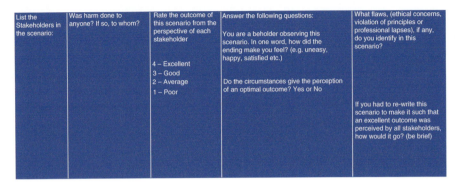

8 Conclusions

Providing care for the geriatric dental patient highlights numerous ethical issues, some applicable across the patient demographic but some highly specialized for elder care. Understanding and fully applying informed consent, particularly in the age of rising dementia and declining capacity; elder abuse, evolving technologies and changing models of care delivery; medical mistrust and history of racism in healthcare; and the effects of the global COVID 19 pandemic are all issues best seen through an ethical lens. Although a myriad of frameworks exist for ethical decision-making, the use of narrative ethics for dentists and dental team members offers much promise.

References

1. American College of Dentists. Ethics handbook for dentists: an introduction to ethics, Professionalism, and Ethical Decision Making. Uince Orchard Boulevard Gaithersburg, Maryland. USA, 2002 (Revised 2016);3.
2. Kaur S, Singh R. Ethics in dentistry. Ann Geriatr Educ Med Sci. 2018;5:7–10.
3. Ettinger RL. Restoring the aging dentition: repair of replacement. Int Dent J. 1990;40:275–82.
4. Ortman JM, Velkoff VA, Hogan HH. An aging nation: the older population in the United States. Washington, DC: US Census Bureau; 2014.
5. Chalmers JM. Ettinger RL. Public health issues in geriatric dentistry in the United States. Dent Clin N Am. 2008;52(2):423–46, vii-viii. https://doi.org/10.1016/j.cden.2007.12.004. PMID: 18329452
6. Mukherjee A, Livinski AA, Millum J, Chamut S, Boroumand S, Iafolla TJ, Adesanya MR, Dye BA. Informed consent in dental care and research for the older adult population: a systematic review. J Am Dent Assoc. 2017;148(4):211–220. https://doi.org/10.1016/j.adaj.2016.11.019. Epub 2017 Jan 5. PMID: 28065430; PMCID: PMC5376239
7. Issrani R, Ammanagi R, Keluskar V. Geriatric dentistry--meet the need. Gerodontology. 2012;29(2):e1–5. https://doi.org/10.1111/j.1741-2358.2010.00423.x. PMID: 22612827
8. Wetle T. Ethical issues in geriatric dentistry. Gerodontology. 1987;6:73–8. https://doi.org/10.1111/j.1741-2358.1987.tb00392.x

9. Van TT, Chiodo LK, Paunovich ED. Informed consent and the cognitively impaired geriatric dental patient. Tex Dent J. 2009;126(7):582–9. PubMed: 19753812
10. Rubinos Lopez E, Rodriguez Vazquez LM, Varela Centelles A, et al. Impact of the systematic use of the informed consent form at public dental care units in Galicia (Spain). Med Oral Patol Oral Cir Bucal. 2008;13(6):E380–4. PubMed: 18521058
11. Molinari V, McCullough LB, Coverdale JH, Workman R. Principles and practice of geriatric assent. Aging Ment Health. 2006;10(1):48–54. https://doi.org/10.1080/13607860500307829.
12. Dong X, Chen R, Chang E-S, Simon M. Elder abuse and psychological well-being: a systematic review and implications for research and policy - a mini review. Gerontology. 2013;59:132–42. https://doi.org/10.1159/000341652.
13. Acierno R, Hernandez MA, Amstadter AB, Resnick HS, Steve K, Muzzy W, Kilpatrick DG. Prevalence and correlates of emotional, physical, sexual, and financial abuse and potential neglect in the United States: the National Elder Mistreatment Study. Am J Public Health. 2010;100:292–7.
14. Wiseman M. The role of dentist in recognizing elder abuse. J Can Dent Assoc. 2008;74(8):715–20.
15. Gironda MW, Lefever KH, Anderson EA. Dental students' knowledge about elder abuse and neglect and the reporting responsibilities of dentists. J Dent Educ. 2010;74(8):824–9.
16. Gross D, Gross K. Schmidt M Ethical dilemmas of dental implantology: ready for aftercare? Quintessence Int. 2018;49(5):367–75. https://doi.org/10.3290/j.qi.a40050. PMID: 29532813
17. Levin L. Ethical issues in replacing a periodontally involved tooth with dental implants: thoughts, beliefs, and evidence. Ethics Biol Eng Med Int J. 2011;2:187–94.
18. Dolan TA, Atchison K. Huynh TN Access to dental care among older adults in the United States. J Dent Educ. 2005;69(9):961–74.
19. Kiyak HA. Reichmuth M Barriers to and enablers of older adults' use of dental services. J Dent Educ. 2005;69(9):975–86.
20. Ettinger RL. Management of elderly patients in the private practice system. Int Dent J. 1993;43(1):29–40.
21. Oishi MM, Gluch JI, Collins RJ, Bunin GR, Sidorov I, Dimitrova B, Cacchione PZ. An oral health baseline of need at a predominantly African American Program of All-Inclusive Care for the Elderly (PACE): opportunities for dental-nursing collaboration. Geriatr Nurs. 2019;40(4):353–9. https://doi.org/10.1016/j.gerinurse.2018.12.014. Epub 2019 Mar 14. PMID: 30878281
22. Gonzalez L. Will for-profits keep up the Pace in the United States? The future of the program of all-inclusive care for the elderly and implications for other programs serving medically vulnerable populations. Int J Health Serv. 2020;5:20731420963946. https://doi.org/10.1177/0020731420963946. Epub ahead of print. PMID: 33019864.
23. Stefanacci R, Buffa A. Full-risk population health programs for older adults like PACE benefit from COVID-19. Popul Health Manag. 2020; https://doi.org/10.1089/pop.2020.0228. Epub ahead of print. PMID: 33017282
24. Hirth V, Baskins J, Dever-Bumba M. Program of all-inclusive care (PACE): past, present, and future. J Am Med Dir Assoc. 2009;10:155–60.
25. Thorne S, Kazanjian A, MacEntee M. Oral health in long term care: the implications of organisational culture. J Aging Stud. 2001;15:271.
26. Mezey M, Mitty E. Burger SG Nursing homes as a clinical site for training geriatric health care professionals. J Am Med Dir Assoc. 2009;10(3):196–203.
27. Matthew M. Interdisciplinary education and health care in geriatric dental medicine. Dent Clin N Am. 2021;65(2):377–91. ISSN 0011-8532, ISBN 9780323778442, https://doi.org/10.1016/j.cden.2020.11.001
28. Centers for Medicare and Medicaid Services. Regulations and guidance Available at: https://www.cms.gov/Regulations-and-Guidance/Guidance/Manuals/Downloads/pace111c06.pdf Accessed 14 Jan 2021.
29. Krieger N, Waterman P, Chen JT, Soobader MJ, Subramanian SV, Carson R. Zip code caveat: bias due to spatiotemporal mismatches between zip codes and us census–defined geographic areas—the public health disparities geocoding project. Am J Public Health. 2002;92(7):1100–2.

30. Halbert CH, Armstrong K, Gandy OH Jr, Shaker L. Racial differences in trust in health care providers. Arch Intern Med. 2006;166(8):896–901.
31. Boulware LE, Cooper LA, Ratner LE, LaVeist TA, Powe NR. Race and trust in the health care system. Public Health Rep. 2003;118(4):358–65.
32. Sodeke SO, Powell LR. Paying tribute to Henrietta Lacks at Tuskegee University and at the Virginia Henrietta Lacks Commission, Richmond, Virginia. J Health Care Poor Underserved. 2019;30(4S):1–11. https://doi.org/10.1353/hpu.2019.0109.
33. Zhou P, Yang XL, Wang XG, et al. A pneumonia outbreak associated with a new coronavirus of probable bat origin. Nature. 2020;579:270–3. https://doi.org/10.1038/s41586-020-2012-7
34. Jones C. The organ thieves : the shocking story of the first heart transplant in the segregated South / Chip Jones. First gallery books hardcover edition. New York: Gallery Books/Jeter Publishing; 2020. Print.
35. Lee SSJ, Cho MK, Kraft SA, et al. "I don't want to be Henrietta Lacks": diverse patient perspectives on donating biospecimens for precision medicine research. Genet Med. 2019;21:107–13. https://doi.org/10.1038/s41436-018-0032-6
36. Johnson TJ, Ellison AM, Dalembert G, et al. Implicit Bias in Pediatric Academic Medicine. J Natl Med Assoc. 2017;109(3):156–63. https://doi.org/10.1016/j.jnma.2017.03.003.
37. Rhee TG, Marottoli RA, Van Ness PH, Levy BR. Impact of perceived racism on healthcare access among older minority adults. Am J Prev Med. 2019;56(4):580–5. ISSN 0749-3797, https://doi.org/10.1016/j.amepre.2018.10.010
38. Patel N, Patel S, Cotti E, Bardini G, Mannocci F. Unconscious racial bias may affect dentists' clinical decisions on tooth restorability: a randomized clinical trial. JDR Clin Trans Res. 2019;4(1):19–28. https://doi.org/10.1177/2380084418812886. Epub 2018 Nov 16. PMID: 30931761
39. Yeo G. Background. In: Yeo G, Gallagher-Thompson D, editors. Ethnicity and the dementias. Washington DC: Taylor & Francis; 1996. p. 123–135.
40. McGoldrick M. Ethnicity and family therapy: an overview. In: McGoldrick M, Pearce JK, Giordano J, editors. Ethnicity and family therapy. New York: The Guilford Press; 1982. p. 3–30.
41. Dye BA, Tan S, Smith V, Lewis BG, Barker LK, Thornton-Evans G, Eke PI, Beltrán-Aguilar ED, Horowitz AM, Li CH. Vital Health Stat. 2007;11(248):1–92.
42. Griffin SO, Jones JA, Brunson D, Griffin PM, Bailey WD. Burden of oral disease among older adults and implications for public health priorities. Am J Public Health. 2012;102(3):411–8. https://doi.org/10.2105/AJPH.2011.300362.
43. Ship J. Oral health in the elderlydwhat's missing? Oral Surg Oral Med Oral Pathol Oral Radiol Endod. 2004;98(6):625–6.
44. Garcia D, Tarima S, Glasman L, Cassidy LD, Meurer J, Okunseri C. Latino acculturation and periodontitis status among Mexican-origin adults in the United States: NHANES 2009-2012. Fam Community Health. 2017;40(2):112–20. https://doi.org/10.1097/FCH.0000000000000142.
45. Zhu N, Zhang D, Wang W, et al. A novel coronavirus from patients with pneumonia in China, 2019. N Engl J Med. 2020;382(8):727–33.
46. Cucinotta D, Vanelli M. WHO declares COVID-19 a pandemic. Acta Biomed. 2020;91(1):157–60.
47. Marchini L, Ettinger RL. COVID-19 pandemics and oral health care for older adults. Spec Care Dentist. 2020;40(3):329–31. https://doi.org/10.1111/scd.12465.
48. American Dental Association . ADA interim guidance for minimizing risk of COVID-19 transmission. 2020. https://www.ada.org/~/media/CPS/Files/COVID/ADA_COVID_Int_Guidance_Treat_Pts.pdf. Accessed 15 Dec 2020.
49. Lundberg A, Hillebrecht AL, McKenna G, Srinivasan M. COVID-19: impacts on oral healthcare delivery in dependent older adults. Gerodontology. 2020; https://doi.org/10.1111/ger.12509. Epub ahead of print. PMID: 33169864

50. American Geriatrics Society. American Geriatrics Society (AGS) policy brief: COVID-19 and nursing homes. J Am Geriatr Soc. 2020; https://doi.org/10.1111/jgs.16477.
51. Chowkwanyun M, Reed AL. Racial health disparities and Covid-19—caution and context. N Engl J Med. 2020;383:201–3.
52. Warren RC, Forrow L, Hodge DA, Truog RD. Trustworthiness before trust – Covid-19 vaccine trials and the black community. N Engl J Med. 2020,383(22):e121. https://doi.org/10.1056/NEJMp2030033.
53. Vergara RJD, Sarmiento PJD, Lagman JDN. Building public trust: a response to COVID-19 vaccine hesitancy predicament [published online ahead of print, 2021 Jan 18]. J Public Health (Oxf). 2021:fdaa282. https://doi.org/10.1093/pubmed/fdaa282.
54. Razai MS, Osama T, McKechnie DGJ, Majeed A. Covid-19 vaccine hesitancy among ethnic minority groups. BMJ. 2021;372:n513. https://doi.org/10.1136/bmj.n513.
55. Giudice A, Barone S, Muraca D, Averta F, Diodati F, Antonelli A, Fortunato L. Can Teledentistry improve the monitoring of patients during the Covid-19 dissemination? A descriptive pilot study. Int J Environ Res Public Health. 2020;17(10):3399. https://doi.org/10.3390/ijerph17103399. PMID: 32414126; PMCID: PMC7277372
56. Iyer P, Aziz K, Ojcius DM. Impact of COVID-19 on dental education in the United States. J Dent Educ. 2020;84(6):718–22.
57. Ridpath H. My experience as a foundation dentist administering the flu vaccine. Br Dent J. 2021;230:197. https://doi.org/10.1038/s41415-021-2766-9
58. Ozar DT, et al. Dental ethics at chairside: professional obligations and practical applications. 3rd ed. Georgetown University Press; 2018. JSTOR, www.jstor.org/stable/j.ctvvngwh. Accessed 21 Feb 2021.
59. Jonsen AR, Siegler M, Winslade WJ. Clinical ethics: a practical approach to ethical decisions in clinical medicine. 6th ed. New York: McGraw-Hill; 2006.
60. Sokol DK. The "four quadrants" approach to clinical ethics case analysis; an application and review. J Med Ethics. 2008;34(7):513–6.
61. Brody H, Clark M. Narrative ethics: a narrative. Hast Cent Rep. 2014;44(1):S7–S11.
62. Lagay F. Virtual Mentor. 2014;16(8):622–5. https://doi.org/10.1001/virtualmentor.2014.16.8.jdsc1-1408.
63. Roucka TM, More F, Smith CS, Aguirre O. Special ethics course – the power of stories - examining ethics through a narrative approach, The American College of Dentists (ACD) Annual Meeting, Virtual, October 2020.

Health Disparities in Oral Health

Cherae M. Farmer-Dixon, Machelle Fleming Thompson, and Joyce A. Barbour

1 The Older Adult Population

The United States has become increasingly diverse. In addition, the adult population is living longer and therefore growing. According to the 2010 US Census as reported by the Centers for Disease Control and Prevention (CDC), approximately 36% of the population belongs to a racial or ethnic minority group. In addition, it is projected that by 2060, people 65 and older will reach 98 million and comprise 24% of the population. The older population will represent just over one in five US residents by the end of 2060, up from one in seven in 2012. The increase in the number of the "oldest old" will be even more dramatic—those 85 and older are projected to more than triple from 5.9 million to 18.2 million, reaching 4.3 percent of the total population [1].

It is projected that between 2015 and 2060 the number of African American older adults in the United States will nearly triple, and the number of Hispanic older adults will more than quintuple, while the number of Whites will less than double. Specifically, it is estimated that the White population will expand from 37.4 million in 2015 to 55.2 million in 2060; Hispanics will expand from 3.7 million to 19.9 million; African Americans will expand from 4.2 million to 11.4 million; and other Non-Hispanics (Asians, Native Americans, Alaska Natives, and multicultural populations) will expand from 2.4 to 10.3 million [2]. With older adults living longer and the United Stated becoming more diverse, there is a potential for greater healthcare needs of this population.

C. M. Farmer-Dixon (✉) · M. F. Thompson · J. A. Barbour
Meharry Medical College, Nashville, TN, USA
e-mail: cdixon@mmc.edu; mfthompson@mmc.edu; jbarbour@mmc.edu

© The Author(s), under exclusive license to Springer Nature Switzerland AG 2022
C.-M. Hogue, J. G. Ruiz (eds.), *Oral Health and Aging*,
https://doi.org/10.1007/978-3-030-85993-0_13

2 Oral Health in American and the Older Adult Population

The 2000 US Surgeon General's Report marked a historical landmark by including oral health in America. The major message of this report was that oral health is essential to the overall health and well-being of all Americans and can be achieved by all Americans. This report was a call to action to health professionals to design programs that promote oral health and prevent disease. While many challenges have been overcome, not all Americans are achieving the same degree of oral healthcare. Despite the safe and effective means of maintaining oral health that have benefited most Americans over the past half century, many still experience needless pain and suffering, complications that devastate overall health and well-being, and financial and social costs that diminish the quality of life and burden American society. What amounts to "a silent epidemic" of oral diseases is affecting the most vulnerable citizens—poor children, older adults, and many members of racial and ethnic minority groups [3].

The report underscores that oral health is far more than just healthy teeth and that it is integral to general health. It encompasses all components of the oral cavity and head and neck regions. Oral soft tissue lesions, chronic oral-facial pain conditions, oral and pharyngeal (throat) cancers, birth defects such as cleft lip and palate, and scores of other diseases and disorders that affect the oral, dental, and craniofacial tissues must be considered in assessing the oral health status. Simply stated, one cannot be classified as healthy without oral health. Therefore, oral health and general health should not be interpreted as separate entities. Oral health is a critical component of health and must be included in the provision of healthcare and the design of community programs.

Oral health and disease have been associated with systemic diseases such as cardiovascular disease, immune disorders, microbial infections, and cancers. New research is pointing to the associations between chronic oral infections and heart and lung diseases, stroke, low birth weight, and premature births. Associations between gum (periodontal) disease and diabetes have also long been noted [4].

The 2020 US Surgeon Generals' Report will continue the initial work and focus of the 2000 Report. It will evaluate oral health and the interaction between oral health and general health throughout the life span, considering advances in science, healthcare integration, and social influences to articulate promising new directions for improving oral health and oral health equity across communities [5].

The nation's oral health has greatly improved since the 1960s [6]. Water fluoridation has played a significant role in improving the oral health status in America, and more emphasis has been placed on dental care prevention. As a result, over the last several decades, there has been a decline in caries levels and tooth loss. However, as the older adult population is living longer, they potentially may experience changes and problems in their oral health such as tooth decay, tooth loss, gum (periodontal) disease, dry mouth (xerostomia), chronic disease, and oral cancer and precancer conditions. These problems may cause pain, problems with chewing and

Health Disparities in Oral Health

eating, and difficulty with smiling and communication, as well as have an impact on the longevity of life.

Nearly all adults (96%) aged 65 years or older have had a cavity; one in five have untreated tooth decay [7]. Total tooth loss is experienced in nearly one in five of adults aged 65 or older. Complete tooth loss is twice as prevalent among adults aged 75 and older (26%) compared with adults aged 65–74 (13%) [7]. A high percentage of older adults have gum (periodontal) disease. About two in three (68%) adults aged 65 years or older have gum (periodontal) disease [8]. The prevalence, however, varies among race and ethnic groups. For example, the oral health status of African Americans differs in comparison to other races/ethnicities. Forty-six (46%) percent of African American adults have decay as compared to twenty-seven (27%) percent of adults nationwide [9].

Most older Americans take both prescription and over-the-counter drugs; many of these medications can cause dry mouth (xerostomia). The reduced saliva flow increases the risk of cavities [8]. Cancers of the mouth (oral and pharyngeal cancers) are primarily diagnosed in older adults. The median age of diagnosis is 62 years [10]. In addition, African American men have a particularly high risk for this disease [11].

3 Social Determinants of Health

Social determinants of health (SDOH) are the conditions in the environments, where people are born, live, learn, work, play, worship, and age that affect a wide range of health, functioning, and quality-of-life outcomes and risks [12]. SDOH in older adults includes income, healthcare access, communities, and social support. The older adults impacted by factors relating to SDOH often find themselves experiencing financial hardships which creates a domino effect impacting healthcare, safe and affordable homes, and their ability to remain socially connected. People with steady employment are less likely to live in poverty and more likely to be healthy. Social determinants of health have disproportionately affected communities of color, particularly African American communities, for a long time. Research shows that systemic racism ensures that African American people are more likely to live in poorer neighborhoods with fewer social services, less access to healthy food, and a higher risk of exposure to environmental contaminants [13].

Older African Americans consistently have higher rates of major health problems than do non-Hispanic Whites. They also have the highest rates of functional limitations. While the gap in disease and disability rates diminishes with control studies for Black–White population differences in wealth and other socioeconomic characteristics, most studies continue to find that race has an independent effect on poor health. Older Hispanics clearly are disadvantaged socioeconomically, having very high rates of diabetes and obesity, and engaging less in exercise than non-Hispanic Whites. In addition, hypertension is at least as prevalent among Mexican American older adults as it is among the general older adult population.

Race affects the health of minorities throughout their life course through both perceived and structural mechanisms. Experiences of discrimination and implicit bias lead to increased stress, unhealthy adaptive behaviors, and historical trauma across all socioeconomic statuses [14].

4 Health Disparities Defined

The US government defines health disparity as "a particular type of health difference that is closely linked with social or economic disadvantage" [15]. "Healthy People 2020" expands this definition and defines a *health disparity* as "a particular type of health difference that is closely linked with social, economic, and/or environmental disadvantage. Health disparities adversely affect groups of people who have systematically experienced greater obstacles to health based on their racial or ethnic group; religion; socioeconomic status; gender; age; mental health; cognitive, sensory, or physical disability; sexual orientation or gender identity; geographic location; or other characteristics historically linked to discrimination or exclusion" [16].

Health disparities across ethnic groups in the US society have been recognized for over 30 years. The federal government has established various entities in an effort to address health disparities in minority populations. In 1990, the National Institutes of Health (NIH) created the Office of Research on Minority Health (NIMHD, 2013). In 1993, Public Law 103-43, the Health Revitalization Act of 1993, established the Office of Research on Minority Health in the Office of the Director, NIH. In 2000, the National Center on Minority Health and Health Disparities was established by the passage of the Minority Health and Health Disparities Research and Education Act of 2000. The Institute of Medicine (IOM) of the National Academy of Sciences has released at least three reports examining health disparities in the United States (IOM, 2001, 2003, 2012). The 2003 IOM report defined health disparities as "racial or ethnic differences in the quality of healthcare that are not due to access-related factors, or clinical needs, preferences, and appropriateness of interventions." Despite this recognition and several studies identifying specific areas of disparity, differences in access to health services and quality treatment persist (IOM, 2012). More importantly, health disparities continue to exist and impact certain populations at a higher rate.

5 Health Disparities in Oral Health

Tooth retention is greater among nonpoor older adults. Older adults who are in poor and near poor poverty status levels show less tooth retention from 1994 to 2014 as indicated in the table below.

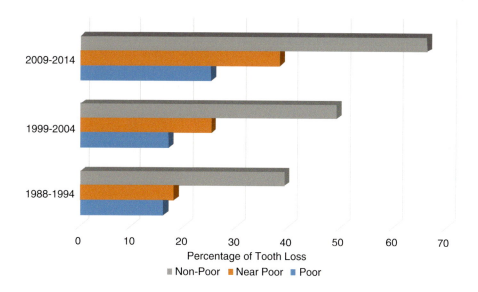

Health disparities significantly impact the oral and overall health of patients, and the older adult population is not exempt. Disparities in older adults vary across race, ethnicity, gender, and demographics. Certain populations have a higher prevalence for particular diseases, thus creating variations in health status and medical conditions. In addition, some minorities experience a disproportionate burden of preventable disease, death, and disability compared with non-minorities [17].

As adults age, oral health-related quality of life is negatively affected by tooth loss and tooth decay [18]. While improvements have helped to create a healthier society, studies have documented that the health and life expectancy of a patient can be associated with their dental health. It is estimated that over $45 billion is lost in productivity in the United States each year because of untreated oral disease [19]. In addition, nearly 18% of all working-age adults, and 29% of those with lower incomes, report that the appearance of their mouth and teeth affects their ability to interview for a job [20].

6 Dental Coverage

More people are unable to afford dental care than other types of healthcare [21]. In 2015, the percentage of people in the United States with no dental insurance was 29% overall and 62% for older adults [22]. The oral health for older adults is largely neglected by health policy makers. Many older Americans do not have dental insurance because they lost their benefits upon retirement. In addition, Medicare is the primary source of health coverage for older adults, but the program does not cover routine dental care [23]. Studies have linked a patient's oral health status to chronic disease such as diabetes and heart disease. The average older adult who is retired lives on a fixed income. Surveys, particularly among minority older adults, indicate that dental services are sought more for emergency care versus preventive care due to the high costs for treatment. Many low-income adults do not have public dental insurance. Health services that are provided by states through the Medicaid program do not require that adult coverage be included. As a result, Medicaid programs' dental coverage varies widely from state to state. Many states that provide adult dental coverage through Medicaid programs have limited coverage for emergency services such as extractions. The Affordable Care Act, however, allowed for Medicaid expansion which permitted modifications that resulted in small increases in utilization among adults with public insurance. However, in many states, access is also a concern as many dentists do not accept Medicaid because of the low reimbursement rates. With the growing number of persons living longer with chronic diseases, some of which are linked to preventable oral health conditions such as gum (periodontal) disease, a multi-prong approach is needed. Firstly, policy makers must work to develop and pass legislation that will move from just emergency or optional care benefits to adding comprehensive oral and preventive care as an integral part of Medicaid and Medicare programs. Secondly, healthcare providers must continue in the quest to provide optimal care to older adults reducing tooth loss and the number living with gum (periodontal) disease.

7 Health Literacy

According to the World Health Organization (WHO) Health Policy 1998, "Oral health literacy implies the achievement of a level of knowledge, personal skills and confidence to take action to improve oral health by changing personal lifestyles and living conditions" [24].

Some of the greatest disparities in oral health literacy occur among racial and ethnic minority groups from different cultural backgrounds and those who do not speak English as a first language. Results from the National Assessment of Adult Literacy demonstrated that Hispanic adults have the lowest average oral health literacy scores of all racial/ethnic groups, followed by African American and then American Indian/Alaska Native adults [25]. People with low oral health literacy and limited English proficiency are twice as likely as individuals without these barriers to report poor oral health status. One study found that 74% of Spanish-speaking patients have less-than-adequate oral health literacy as compared to 7% of English-speaking patients. Cultural beliefs may also impact communication between patients and providers and affect a patient's ability to follow instructions [26].

Oral health literacy challenges may impact older adults more than other age groups. On average, adults age 65 and older have lower oral health literacy than adults under the age of 65. Low oral health literacy among older adults is associated with increased reports of poor physical functioning, pain, limitations of daily activities, and poor mental health status [27]. For a more in-depth discussion on this topic, please refer to the chapter "The Role of Oral Health Literacy and Shared Decision Making."

8 Living Conditions and Disabilities

It is well-documented that oral care to the older population living at home or in nursing homes, assisted living, or other care facilities is lacking. The older population living in nursing homes will include the medically compromised, physically and intellectually disabled. Older adults who have disabilities may experience challenges, such as limited manual dexterity that inhibits proper oral hygiene; masticatory challenges that negatively affect the oral flora and processing of food; or prescription medicines that impact the oral cavity. As the older population living in nursing home increases, the principles of dental health are becoming increasingly relevant for members of the dental team, medical team, health educators, social workers, and others. More than 1 million nursing home residents faced the greatest barriers to accessing dental care of any population group. Barriers to appropriate oral care in long-term care facilities include poorly organized processes and policies, a lower priority of dental care, care provider's lack of knowledge of oral care, and an adequate number of care providers (both dental and non-dental). Long-term care residences are also less likely to have access to comprehensive dental care. Impaired mobility, lack of ability, and motivation to perform oral care are identified as additional barriers [28–31].

According to multiple studies, not only is there an inadequate number of care providers both dental and non-dental but it is also how prepared they feel in providing oral care services. *The Caregivers' Perceived Comfort Regarding Oral Care Delivery: A Pilot Study* found 56% of caregivers did not feel comfortable providing appropriate oral care due to lack of experience, lack of training, and being uncomfortable with oral hygiene in general. One study showed that 80% of the non-dental caregivers reported that many of the older adults living in care facilities did not open their mouths, bite the toothbrush, or refused oral care completely. Also, the non-dental caregivers have many duties and stated they were too busy and would eliminate mouthcare as part of their patient's care. This further emphasizes that oral health is not a priority in the daily activities of non-dental caregivers.

The Commission on Dental Accreditation (CODA) standards for Predoctoral Dental Education Programs do not include a standard that specifically addresses the older adult population. There is however, a standard that states "Graduates must be competent in providing oral health care within the scope of general dentistry to patients in all stages of life," which allows dental schools to determine how to provide care to the older population. A study conducted by the American Dental Education Association (ADEA) showed fewer graduates who felt prepared to care for the older adult population despite the amount of content on geriatrics that was presented and considered appropriate [28–31].

9 Tooth Decay

Older Americans with the poorest oral health tend to be those who are economically disadvantaged, lack insurance, and are members of racial and ethnic minorities. They experience more tooth decay and tooth loss. Over 40% of low-income and non-Hispanic

Black adults have untreated tooth decay, which has a large impact on quality of life and productivity [32]. The CDC's Oral Health Surveillance Report: "Trends in Dental Caries and Sealants, Tooth Retention, and Edentulism, United States 1999–2004, 2011–2016" indicates that more than nine in ten older adults have had cavities and one in six have untreated cavities. Older non-Hispanic Black or Mexican American adults have 2–3 times the rate of untreated cavities as older non-Hispanic White adults. The report also noted the impact of educational level and tooth decay in older adults stating, "Older adults with less than a high school education have untreated cavities at nearly 3 times the rate of adults with at least some college education" [33]. For a more in-depth discussion on this topic, please refer to the chapter "Management of Caries in Older Adults."

10 Tooth Loss

Seventeen percent of older adults have lost all their teeth. Having missing teeth or wearing dentures can affect nutrition, because people without teeth or with dentures often prefer soft, easily chewed foods instead of foods such as fresh fruits and vegetables – which are basic elements of a healthy diet. Low-income older adults, those with less than a high school education, or those who are current smokers are more than three (3) times as likely to have lost all of their teeth as compared to adults with higher incomes, with more than a high school education, or who have never smoked. Additionally, often the loss of teeth leads to embarrassment and low self-esteem, which results in contributing to loneliness and social isolation [33].

According to the 2020 US Surgeon General's Preliminary Report, the percentage of adults 65 and older experiencing tooth loss has declined from 1988 to 2014 by 18%. However, disparities still remain among lower-income adults by 34%. This disproportionately affects some adults according to where they live.

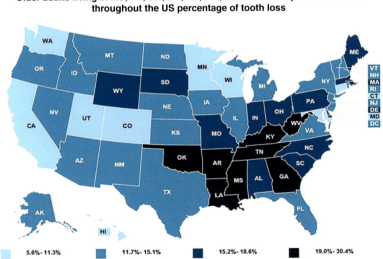

Source: Kaiser Family Foundation analysis of the Center for Disease Control and Prevention (CDC)'s Behavioral Risk Factor Surveillance System (BRFSS)2016 Survey Results

11 Gum Disease

Gum (periodontal) disease is a common oral disease among older adults. Recent data reported by the CDC indicated that 42% of adults have some form of gum disease. Among adults aged 65 and older, the rate of gum disease increases to 60%. Severe gum disease is most common among adults aged 65 or older, Mexican American, and non-Hispanic Black adults as compared to non-Hispanic Whites, and people who smoke [34]. Important to note however, is with proper diagnosis and treatment, the disease can be reversed. For a more in-depth discussion on this topic, please refer to the chapter "Management of Periodontal Disease in Older Adults."

12 Dry Mouth

Dry mouth or xerostomia is a condition in which the salivary glands in the mouth do not make enough saliva. The primary role of the saliva is to protect the oral tissue by keeping it moist. The reduction in salivary flow increases the risk of oral diseases and tooth decay as well the difficulty in eating, chewing, and communicating [8, 35]. And while dry mouth is not a normal part of aging, it is a common concern in the older adult population and is mostly related to adverse effects from medications (prescription and over the counter), dehydration, electrolyte and fluid balance, and changes in saliva. The greatest risks have been associated with drugs used for urinary incontinence, hypertension, and antidepressants [36]. For a more in-depth discussion on xerostomia, please refer to the chapter "Xerostomia and Hyposalivation".

13 Oral Cancer/Precancer

Cancers of the mouth and precancer lesions such as leukoplakia are more commonly seen in older adults. The average age for diagnosis is 62 years. A review of the literature suggests that tobacco use and alcohol consumption are high-risk factors in oral cancer and precancer. Men are twice as likely to experience head and neck cancers than women. The 5-year survival rate for oral pharyngeal (throat) cancers is lower among Black men (41%) than White men (62%) [37–39]. Tobacco use is the most important determinant of oral cancer and precancerous lesions, but excessive consumption of alcohol, diet, and personal hygiene can be contributing factors as well [39].

14 COVID-19

According to the CDC, older adults are at a higher risk for contracting the virus and requiring hospitalization. Also, documented is that eight out of ten COVID-19 deaths reported were in persons 65 years or older.

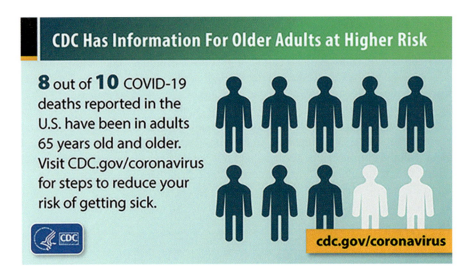

The CDC has also reported that the COVID-19 pandemic has disproportionately impacted populations with preexisting conditions, such as hypertension, cardiovascular disease, obesity, asthma, and cancer, many of whom are older adults and/or minorities. Minorities disproportionately have higher prevalence of many of these medical conditions. The percent of cases for racial and ethnic minority groups is higher than the percent of these populations within the total US population.

The US Census Bureau 2018 Community Survey compared the racial and ethnic disparities in COVID cases in comparison to the percent of the total US population:

Illnesses

- White people represent a majority of the US population (60%), followed by Hispanic or Latino people (18%), non-Hispanic Black people (12%), non-Hispanic Asian people (6%), non-Hispanic people who identify with more than one race (3%), American Indian or Alaska Native people (1%), and Native Hawaiian or other Pacific Islander people (less than 1%).
- White people represent 67% of COVID illnesses, followed by non-Hispanic Black people (12%), Hispanic or Latino people (11%), non-Hispanic Asian people (3%), and American Indian or Alaska Native people (1%). Among people aged less than 50 years, and notably among children aged less than 18 years, a noticeably higher percent of COVID-19 cases is among Hispanic or Latino people compared with the percent of the total US population.

Deaths

Like the data reported on COVID illnesses, COVID-related death indicates similar disparities. Data on race and ethnicity for more than 90% of people who died from COVID-19 reveal that the percent of Hispanic or Latino, non-Hispanic Black, and non-Hispanic American Indian or Alaska Native people who have died from COVID-19 is higher than the percent of these racial and ethnic groups among the total US population. This disparity is even greater when the percentages are age-standardized (adjusted for differences in the age distribution across racial and ethnic groups). Hispanic or Latino, non-Hispanic Black, and non-Hispanic American Indian or Alaska Native people also have a disproportionate burden of COVID-19 deaths among specific age groups across the life span – children, youth, adults, and older adults.

CDC COVID tracking data indicates that Black people represent 12% of the US population and 23% of COVID-related deaths; Hispanic or Latino people are 20% of the US population and 38% COVID related deaths; and American Indian or Alaska Native people are 1% of the US population and 3% of COVID related deaths.

15 Summary

As oral health continues to be recognized as an integral part of overall health, it is paramount that special attention be paid to the oral health of the older adult population. To ensure continued progress, efforts must continue that expand the current workforce, improve the ability of providers to communicate with their patients, and empower the older adult to communicate their understanding of their dental care.

Federal policy makers must design legislation that will fill the gap of insurance coverage for older adults by providing Medicare oral health coverage for all. If we are to improve the oral health of all older adults, we must not only recognize the health disparities and social determinants of health but also implement strategies for improvement.

References

1. Colby SL, Ortman JM. Projections of the size and composition of the US population: 2014 to 2060. Current population reports. Washington DC: US Census Bureau; 2015. p. 13. Report No.: P25-1143.
2. Fox-Grage W. American association of retired persons, the growing racial and ethnic diversity of older adults 2016. Available from: https://blog.aarp.org/thinkingpolicy/the-growing-racial-and-ethnic-diversity-of-older-adults
3. U.S. General Accounting Office (GAO). Oral health in low-income populations. GAO/HEHS-00-72 2000.
4. 2000 Surgeon General's Report on Oral Health in America | National Institute of Dental and Craniofacial Research (nih.gov).
5. Surgeon General's Report-Oral Health in America-APHA 2019 (nih.gov).
6. National Institute of Dental and Craniofacial Research. Oral health in America: a report of the surgeon general. National Institutes of Health, US Department of Health and Human Services; 2000.
7. Dye BA, Thornton-Evans G, Xianfen L, Iafolla TJ. Dental caries and tooth loss in adults in the united states, 2011–2012. NCHS Data Brief, no 197. Hyattsville, MD: National Center for Health Statistics; 2015.
8. Eke PI, Dye BA, Wei L, et al. Update on prevalence of periodontitis in adults in the United States: NHANES 2009 to 2012. J Periodontol. 2015;86(5):611–22. https://doi.org/10.1902/jop.2015.140520.

9. USDHHS, 2000a.
10. National Cancer Institute. Surveillance, Epidemiology, and End Results (SEER) Program. (N.D.) SEER stat fact sheets: oral cavity and pharynx cancer 2016.Available from: http://seer.cancer.gov/statfacts/html/oralcav.html
11. Are you at risk for oral cancer? What African American men need to know, National Institutes of Health. http://www.nidcr.nih.gov/oralhealth/Topics/OralCancer/AfricanAmericanMen/oral_exam_brochure.htm
12. Social Determinants of Health – Healthy People 2030 | health.gov
13. https://www.wellandgood.com/social-determinants-health/
14. Wallace SP. Equity and social determinants of health among older adults. Generations. 2014;38(4):6–11. www.jstor.org/stable/26556070. Accessed 18 Mar 2021.
15. Very Well Health. Health disparities: what they are and why they matter 2020. Available from: www.verywellhealth.com/health-disparities-4173220#
16. U.S. Department of Health and Human Services. The secretary's advisory committee on national health promotion and disease prevention objectives for 2020. Phase I report: recommendations for the framework and format of healthy people 2020 [Internet]. Section IV: advisory committee findings and recommendations [cited 2010 January 6]. Available from: http://www.healthypeople.gov/sites/default/files/PhaseI_0.pdf
17. Centers for Disease Control and Prevention. Minority health. minority health determines the health of the nation 2020. https://www.cdc.gob/minorityhealth/index.html#:~:text+Minority%20Health%20Determines%20Health,racial%20or%20ethnic%20minority%20group
18. Thomas WM. Epidemiology of oral health conditions in older people. Gerodontology. 2014;31(Suppl 1):9–16. https://doi.org/10.1111/ger.12085.
19. Naavaal S, Kelekar U. School hours lost due to acute/unplanned dental care. Health Behav Policy Rev. 2018;5(2):66–73. https://doi.org/10.14485/HBPR.5.2.7.
20. Righolt AJ, Jevdjevic M, Marcenes W, Listl S. Global-, regional-, and country-level economic impacts of dental diseases in 2015. J Dent Res 2018; 97(5):501–507. https://doi.org/10.1177/0022034517750572.
21. Braveman P, Gottlieb L. The social determinants of health: it's time to consider the causes of the causes. Public Health Rep. 2014;129(suppl 2):19–31. https://doi.org/10.1177/00333549141291S206.
22. Vujicic M, Buchmueller T, Klein R. Dental care presents the highest level of financial barriers, compared to other types of health care services. Health Aff. 2016;35(12):2176–82. https://doi.org/10.1377/hlthaff.2016.0800.
23. Griffin SO, Jones JA, Brunson D, Griffin PM, Bailey WD. Burden of oral disease among older adults and implications for public health priorities. Am J Public Health. 2012;102(3):411–8. https://doi.org/10.2105/AJPH.2011.300362.
24. Happy People 2020.
25. Cho YI, Lee SY, Arozullah AM, Crittenden KS. Effects of health literacy on health status and health service utilization amongst the elderly. Soc Sci Med. 2008;66(8):1809–16.
26. Sentell T, Braun KL. Low health literacy, limited English proficiency, and health status in Asians, Latinos, and other racial/ethnic groups in California. J Health Commun. 2012;17(Suppl 3):82–99. https://doi.org/10.1080/10810730.2012.712621.
27. Brice JH, Travers D, Cowden CS, Young MD, Sanhueza A, Dunston Y. Health literacy among Spanish-speaking patients in the emergency department. J Natl Med Assoc. 2008;100(11):1326–32.
28. Jobman KJ, Weber-Gasparoni K, Ettinger RLQ, F. The care givers' perceived comfort regarding oral care delivery: a pilot study. Spec Care Dentist. 2012;32(3):91.
29. Lowe O, Rossopoulos E. Assessment of the oral health status of elderly population living in residential care facilities. Annals of Dentistry and Oral Health; 2018.
30. Dounis G, Ditmyer MM, McClain MA, Cappelli DP, Mobley CC. Preparing the dental workforce for oral disease prevention in an aging population. J Dent Educ. 2010;74(10):1092.

31. Szabo KB, Boyd LD, LaSpina LM. Educational preparedness to provide care for older adults in alternative practice settings: perceptions of dental hygiene practitioners. J Dent Hyg. 2018;92(6):16–22.
32. Center for Health Care Strategies. Medicaid adult dental benefits: an overview 2019. Available from: https://www.chcs.org/resource/medicaid-adult-dental-benefitsoverview/
33. Centers for Disease Control and Prevention. Oral health surveillance report. trends in dental caries and sealants, tooth retention, and edentulism, United States, 1999–2004 to 2011–2016. US Dept of Health and Human Services; 2019.
34. Eke PI, Thornton-Evans GO, Wei L, Borgnakke WS, Dye BA, Genco RJ. Periodontitis in US adults: national health and nutrition examination survey 2009. J Am Dent Assoc. 2018;149(7):576–88, e576. https://doi.org/10.1016/j.adaj.2018.04.023.
35. Kumar B. The composition, function and role of saliva in maintain oral health: a review. Int J Contemp Dent Med Rev. 2017;2017:011217. https://doi.org/10.15713/ins.ijcdmr.121.
36. Tan ECK. Medication that cause dry mouth as an adverse effect in older people: a systemic review and metaanalysis. J Am Geriatr Soc. 2018;66(1):77–84.
37. American Cancer Society. Cancer facts and figures 2017. Available from: https://www.cancer.org/research/cancer-facts-statistics/all-cancer-facts-figures/cancerfacts-figures-2017.html
38. Centers for Disease Control and Prevention. United States Cancer Statistics Working Group. United States cancer statistics: data visualizations. Accessed Jan 2020. Available from: https://gis.cdc.gov/Cancer/USCS/DataViz.html
39. Peterson PE. Oral health and quality of life of older people – the need for public health action. Oral Health Prev Dent. 2018;16:113–24. https://doi.org/10.3290/j.ohpd.a40309.

Frailty and Oral Health

Jorge G. Ruiz and Christie-Michele Hogue

1 Physical Frailty

Frailty is a geriatric syndrome characterized by individual's vulnerability to stressors resulting from physiological reserve losses across multiple body systems [1, 2]. Frailty is common in older adults. A meta-analysis of population studies around the world has shown that the prevalence of frailty ranges between 12% and 24% of people over 50 years [3]. The syndrome is even more common in institutionalized populations and homebound. As a multisystemic disorder, frailty is bound to also involve oral health structures and functions. Frailty is associated with the aging process, but their exact pathophysiological mechanisms are incompletely understood. Investigators have proposed various causes and mechanistic pathways leading to the onset of frailty. Among the proposed mechanisms are age-related changes in the immune system or immunosenescence, defined as the deterioration of the immune response with aging [4], and inflammaging, a state of low-grade chronic inflammation [5]. In addition to the effects of reduced inactivity and nutritional intake, and associated anabolic resistance, these immune system changes may cause sarcopenia, the age-related loss of muscle mass, function, and strength, which may represent a key precursor to the development of frailty [6, 7]. Impairment of

---

J. G. Ruiz (✉)
Miami VA Healthcare System, Geriatric Research, Education and Clinical Center (GRECC), Miami, FL, USA

Division of Geriatrics and Palliative Medicine, University of Miami Miller School of Medicine, Miami, FL, USA
e-mail: j.ruiz@med.miami.edu

C.-M. Hogue
Department of Dental Services - VA Healthcare System, Division of Geriatrics and Gerontology, Emory University School of Medicine, Emory University School of Medicine, Atlanta, GA, USA

physiological stress responses may also contribute to the onset of frailty, and improvement in these mechanisms may improve resilience [8]. Independent risk factors for the onset of frailty include among others, older age, African-American race, Hispanic ethnicity [9], lower education, lower socioeconomic status, obesity, poor functional status, inactivity [10], medical and psychological multimorbidity [11], and polypharmacy [12–14]. Frailty is associated with a higher risk of adverse health-care outcomes including disability [15, 16], morbidity [11, 17], surgical complications including impaired wound healing and infections [18], increased health-care utilization [19], and mortality [20, 21]. There is an association between frailty and cognitive impairment with as much as half of all older adults with frailty suffering from cognitive impairment. For a more in-depth discussion on the topic of dementia, please refer to chapter "The 3 Ds: Dementia, Delirium and Depression in Oral Health."

2 Recognizing Frailty

There are currently two major conceptualizations of frailty: the frailty phenotype, which requires the presence of three or more of five components, weight loss, exhaustion, weakness, slowness, and low physical activity [2], and the deficit accumulation model, which combines symptoms, diseases, conditions, disability, and diagnostic tests into a score called the frailty index (FI) [22]. We will refer to both conceptualizations as they often complement each other when approaching older adults with oral pathology. It is important to distinguish frailty from multimorbidity, defined as the presence of two or more chronic conditions, and disability, the need for assistance with activities of daily living (ADLs). Although frailty may often coexist with these two conditions, frailty is a dynamic state of vulnerability that may predispose individuals to both multimorbidity and disability. The recognition of frailty may take the form of questionnaires or scales administered in health-care settings. Several reliable and valid self-report questionnaires have been developed for the evaluation of frailty in diverse care settings. They vary in the number of items included, whether administered face-to-face or self-completed during a clinical encounter or delivered by mail [23, 24]. The FRAIL scale is an example of a validated questionnaire based on the frailty phenotype and deficit accumulation models that consists of five questions assessing fatigue, resistance, ambulation, illnesses, and loss of weight (Table 1). The frail score ranges from 0 to 5 (i.e., 1 point for each component; 0 = best to 5 = worst) and patients are assigned into three categories: robust (0 points), prefrail (1–2 points), and frail (3–5 points) [25]. Physical performance assessments may include the timed get up and go test, the 6-minute walk test, the short physical performance battery (SPPB), or the measurement of handgrip strength. These assessments may not be practical for most dental health professionals, who may not have the time to administer these instruments to older individuals. Most recently, automated tools have assisted clinicians in identifying older persons with frailty. In comparison to the administration of time-consuming

Table 1 The FRAIL scale

Criteria	Question	Scoring
*F*atigue	How much of the time during the past 4 weeks did you feel tired?	1 = All of the time; 2 = most of the time; 3 = some of the time; 4 = a little of the time; and 5 = none of the time ≥ 3 = 0 points ≤ 2 = 1 point
*R*esistance	Do you have any difficulty walking up ten steps without resting and without using aids	No = 0 points Yes = 1 point
*A*mbulation	Do you have any difficulty walking several hundred yards alone without aids?	No = 0 points Yes = 1 point
*I*llnesses	Did a doctor ever tell you that you have (illness)?	0–4 = 0 points 5–11 = 1 point
*L*oss of weight	How much do you weigh with your clothes on but without shoes (current weight)?; 1 year ago, how much did you weigh without your shoes and with your clothes on?	<5% = 0 points $\geq$5% loss of weight = 1 point

From Ref. [25]

questionnaires which are subject to interrater variability, automated screenings can have a significant impact on early detection and the subsequent implementation of evidence-based interventions for frailty in primary care settings.

3 Evidence-Based Strategies to Manage Frailty

Evidence-based treatments for frailty include among others multicomponent exercise and physical activity programs, the Mediterranean and high protein diet, and the use of vitamin D for those individuals that are deficient [26]. An umbrella systematic review of seven systematic reviews including 58 relevant trials and involving 6927 participants summarized the evidence of the efficacy of exercise at improving physical function in older adults with frailty. Most of the included trials examined mobility, physical performance, gait speed, muscle strength, and balance. The overall conclusion of the review was that an optimal combination of intensity, duration, and frequency of exercise interventions may lead to improvements in physical function in these patients. Multicomponent interventions should be performed up to three times per week for 45–60 minutes per exercise session with a gradual increase from moderate- to high-intensity exercise. The exercise programs may last for at least 2 months but preferably for 6 months [27]. Adherence to a Mediterranean-style diet is associated with a lower risk for mortality, cognitive decline, and dementia. Whether adherence to a Mediterranean-style diet protects against the onset of age-related frailty is not known. A meta-analysis of longitudinal analyses showed that higher adherence to a Mediterranean-style diet was associated with lower odds of developing frailty compared with those with lower adherence

[28]. Another meta-analysis of ten studies, seven cross-sectional, and three longitudinal studies including 50,284 older adults from three different continents demonstrated that a high protein intake was negatively associated with frailty status in older adults [29]. Whether providing protein supplements prevent the development of frailty or ameliorates the burden of frailty is not settled as randomized controlled trials have not been completed. A systematic review of a seven studies (17,815 participants) revealed that a low level of vitamin D was significantly associated with the onset of frailty [30]. The use of vitamin D supplements is recommended only in those individuals with documented deficiency. The evidence on other interventions is small or mixed. For a more complete review, please refer to recent comprehensive reviews [26, 31].

4 The Concept of "Oral Frailty"

In 2018, Japanese investigators introduced the concept of oral frailty, defined as a reversible, age-related, decline in oral function [32]. The six key criteria for the diagnosis of this condition include impaired masticatory function, decreased articulatory oral motor skills (oral diadochokinesis), difficulties eating tough food, swallowing difficulty, low tongue pressure, and having less than 20 teeth (Table 2). One or two of the six criteria define oral prefrailty whereas more than three criteria define oral frailty [32]. The evaluation of oral frailty relies on a combination of subjective and objective instrumented oral assessments which may not be feasible for most practicing dental professionals. An 8-item oral frailty checklist represents a more practical alternative to assess oral frailty in clinical settings [34]. The concept of oral frailty does not enjoy wide acceptance outside of Japan. Recent research suggests that oral frailty was not only associated with physical frailty but that it may be a predictor of physical frailty in cohort studies [32, 35]. The research also revealed that oral frailty was associated with poor nutritional status [34, 36]. However, there are no controlled trials that look at whether treating oral frailty improves clinical outcomes in those with frailty or prevent the development of frailty in older adults. In much the same way we would not call age-related or acquired changes in the

Table 2 Oral frailty

Oral condition	Measurement
Number of remaining teeth (<20)	Oral exam
Chewing ability	Color-changing chewing gum
Oral diadochokinesis	Repetitive articulation of syllables as quickly as possible
Tongue pressure	Balloon probe and manometer
Difficulties eating tough foods	Single question about difficulties eating tough foods compared to 6 months ago (yes/no)
Difficulties in swallowing	Two questions about choking with liquids and experiencing dry mouth (yes/no)

From Refs. [32, 33]

heart, liver, or kidneys, cardiac frailty, liver frailty, or renal frailty, respectively, it would not be advisable to call the age-related changes in oral function, oral frailty. Adding the noun "frailty" to any organ or system dysfunction risks confusion and defies the growing body of evidence that demonstrates the multisystemic nature of physical frailty [2, 37, 38]. The term "oral hypofunction" was proposed by major dental societies [39] and represents a preferable term when referring to oral health issues in the assessment and management of older adults with frailty. Still, the clustered criteria have merit and demonstrates a good scientific basis.

5 Frailty and Oral Health: A Bidirectional Relationship

The suggestion of a bidirectional relationship between oral hypofunction and frailty is plausible and credible. The multisystemic involvement that characterizes frailty may lead to structural and functional alterations which may impair the individual's inability to respond to external stressors. Older adults may in turn become weak, tired, and functionally and cognitively impaired. These deficits may translate into a reduction in the individuals' performance of self-care oral behaviors (toothbrushing, flossing, diet, etc.) aimed at achieving adequate oral health promotion and prevention of poor dental outcomes. However, the evidence in this regard is practically nonexistent. Studying older adults who had recently become frail and were adherent to health oral behaviors at baseline would be a reasonable step. Seeing how frailty contributes to future deterioration of self-care behaviors in turn leading to poor oral health-care outcomes in these patients may confirm the independent role of frailty. On the other hand, most of the research evidence comes from cross-sectional and longitudinal studies showing that baseline oral hypofunction is longitudinally associated with the onset of frailty. Chronic impairment of masticatory and swallowing functions may result in reduced oral intake, reduced protein intake, anorexia of aging, impaired oral health, and loss of acuity in taste, smell, and sight, consequently contributing to muscle catabolism and eventually sarcopenia. A cause of sarcopenia is a low intake of dietary protein which has been associated with a loss of body muscle mass, function, and strength [40]. In fact, epidemiological studies have shown that protein intake has been inversely associated with frailty [41]. Whether interventions aimed at correcting these apparently reversible deficits in oral hypofunction would alter the course of the condition and interrupt the development of frailty is unknown.

6 Practical Considerations for Oral Health-Care Professionals

The dental professional plays a very important role in the recognition and management of older adults with frailty. As we have seen, oral health professionals will often care for older adults with frailty and related oral hypofunction. As reviewed earlier in this chapter, the older individual may have developed frailty as a result of untreated or unrecognized oral health conditions. On the other hand, the dental professional may face an older person who does not seem to be appropriately responding to the oral plan of care. The management of older adults with frailty should be part of joint team effort that includes dentist, primary care clinicians, and other professionals. In long-term care settings, interprofessional teams may also include in addition to dental professionals an expanded team of physicians, pharmacists, nurses, dieticians, speech pathologists, and occupational and physical therapists. As recommended by experts, the first step of any overall strategy is the recognition of physical frailty [26]. The complex needs and findings in these patients demand that a team approach be a key component of the approach for these patients. However, many older adults may present to the dental office with frailty that may have gone unrecognized in primary care settings. We suggest that given the high prevalence of frailty in community settings, a quick approach may involve the use of self-administered questionnaires such as the FRAIL scale [25]. The FRAIL scale can be mailed to the patients in anticipation of dental appointments, or the patient or caregiver may complete it in the office waiting areas. Frailty assessment can assist in gathering essential clinical information that can be incorporated into the patients' dental care plan [42]. Prompt notification of primary care clinicians will ensure adequate follow-up for these individuals. Table 3 describes interventions aimed at specific aspects of frailty in patients with oral health needs. We categorized these interventions into those addressing oral hypofunction and those related to physical frailty. For those patients lacking access to regular dental care, physicians may incorporate oral screenings as a part of the patient's overall workup. If these clinicians identify an oral health condition, they may initiate a referral to a dentist when appropriate. As discussed in chapters "Health Disparities and Oral Health" and "Barriers to Access to Dental Care," not all older adults would have routine access to adequate dental care. For the oral health professional, recommendations may include particular attention to the prescription of medications, closer follow-up, modified diets, exercise and physical activity, and oral health promotion activities.

7 Future Research

More research is needed into the bidirectional relationship of frailty and oral hypofunction. As we have seen in this chapter, the associations between oral hypofunction and physical frailty have not been explored exhaustively. Existing and future prospective cohort studies may incorporate assessments of oral hypofunction into the overall evaluation of older adults without frailty at baseline. These longitudinal studies may further clarify how oral hypofunction may contribute to the development of incident frailty in older individuals. We need randomized controlled trials of lifestyle interventions aimed at improving oral hypofunction and how these approaches may lower the incidence or ameliorate the burden of frailty. Investigators may study whether progression to frailty in those older persons without evidence of

Table 3 Specific interventions for older adults with oral health needs and frailty

Features	Intervention
Oral hypofunction ("oral frailty")	
Impaired masticatory function	Extend number of masticatory cycles (duration of oral food management); xerostomia treatment; address tooth losses; orthodontist evaluation [43]
Oral diadochokinesis	Pronunciation and singing exercises; speech pathology evaluation [39, 44]
Difficulties eating tough food	Choose foods that are soft and palatable (i.e., soft mechanical diets); minced textures; cut food in small pieces [45, 46]
Swallowing difficulty	Adaptive eating aids; mealtime supervision for safe eating; proper techniques for safe eating assistance; texture-modified foods; speech pathology evaluation
Low tongue pressure	Tongue resistance training; jaw opening exercises; self-exercise of oral function; Shaker exercise; referral to speech pathology for tongue-strengthening protocols [39, 47–49]
Less than 20 teeth	Dental implants; removable dentures; prosthodontic rehabilitation; dietetic evaluation [50]
Physical frailty	
Weakness	Adapted eating utensils; resistance exercise training; assistance with meals; dietetic evaluation [51]
Slow walking speed	Allow more time for patients in the office; arrange special transportation; physical therapy evaluation [52]
Self-reported exhaustion	Extend duration of food management; frequent, small meals [51]
Unintentional weight loss	Mediterranean, high protein diets; protein-caloric supplements; dietetic evaluation [53, 54]
Low physical activity	Multicomponent exercise program [26, 27]

oral pathology at baseline may lead over time to declines in the performance of oral self-care activities that may in turn cause impairment of oral structures and function. The other areas are how to adapt lifestyle and therapeutic approaches to the needs of older adults with frailty with special consideration to the role of caregivers.

8 Conclusions

This chapter reviewed the concept of physical frailty in the context of oral health care for older adults. Frailty, a state of vulnerability to stressors resulting from physiological reserve losses across multiple body systems, is common in older adults and is associated with poor health-care outcomes. The concept of oral hypofunction ("oral frailty") is still in evolution but there is evidence of its predictive ability for physical frailty. Oral health professionals will often encounter patients with frailty in their practices and thereby play a vital role in their evaluation and management. Recognizing frailty is the first step. Primary care clinicians may have already identified older adults with frailty. However, most patient may go unrecognized in which case the use of simple self-administered instruments such as the FRAIL scale may assist oral health professionals in the identification of these patients. Information about the patients' frailty status can then be incorporated into the dental care plan. Oral health professionals may implement several general and specific strategies aimed at preventing the development frailty or mitigating its future complications.

References

1. Clegg A, et al. Frailty in elderly people. Lancet. 2013;381(9868):752–62.
2. Fried LP, et al. Frailty in older adults: evidence for a phenotype. J Gerontol A Biol Sci Med Sci. 2001;56(3):M146–56.
3. O'Caoimh R, et al. Prevalence of frailty in 62 countries across the world: a systematic review and meta-analysis of population-level studies. Age Ageing. 2020;50(1):219.
4. Gruver AL, Hudson LL, Sempowski GD. Immunosenescence of ageing. J Pathol. 2007;211(2):144–56.
5. Ferrucci L, Fabbri E. Inflammageing: chronic inflammation in ageing, cardiovascular disease, and frailty. Nat Rev Cardiol. 2018;15(9):505–22.
6. von Haehling S, Morley JE, Anker SD. An overview of sarcopenia: facts and numbers on prevalence and clinical impact. J Cachexia Sarcopenia Muscle. 2010;1(2):129–33.
7. Cruz-Jentoft AJ, et al. Nutrition, frailty, and sarcopenia. Aging Clin Exp Res. 2017;29(1):43–8.
8. Walston J, et al. Moving frailty toward clinical practice: NIA intramural frailty science symposium summary. J Am Geriatr Soc. 2019;67(8):1559–64.
9. Espinoza SE, Hazuda HP. Frailty in older Mexican-American and European-American adults: is there an ethnic disparity? J Am Geriatr Soc. 2008;56(9):1744–9.
10. Feng Z, et al. Risk factors and protective factors associated with incident or increase of frailty among community-dwelling older adults: a systematic review of longitudinal studies. PLoS One. 2017;12(6):e0178383.
11. Vetrano DL, et al. Frailty and multimorbidity: a systematic review and meta-analysis. J Gerontol A Biol Sci Med Sci. 2019;74(5):659–66.
12. Veronese N, et al. Frailty is associated with an increased risk of incident type 2 diabetes in the elderly. J Am Med Dir Assoc. 2016;17(10):902–7.
13. Jamsen KM, et al. Effects of changes in number of medications and drug burden index exposure on transitions between frailty states and death: the Concord health and ageing in men project cohort study. J Am Geriatr Soc. 2016;64(1):89–95.
14. Herr M, et al. Frailty, polypharmacy, and potentially inappropriate medications in old people: findings in a representative sample of the French population. Eur J Clin Pharmacol. 2017;73(9):1165–72.
15. Covinsky KE, et al. The last 2 years of life: functional trajectories of frail older people. J Am Geriatr Soc. 2003;51(4):492–8.
16. Topinkova E. Aging, disability and frailty. Ann Nutr Metab. 2008;52(Suppl 1):6–11.
17. Gobbens RJ, et al. Determinants of frailty. J Am Med Dir Assoc. 2010;11(5):356–64.
18. Panayi AC, et al. Impact of frailty on outcomes in surgical patients: a systematic review and meta-analysis. Am J Surg. 2019;218(2):393–400.
19. Zylberglait Lisigurski M, et al. Healthcare utilization by frail, community-dwelling older veterans: a 1-year follow-up study. South Med J. 2017;110(11):699–704.
20. Mitnitski AB, et al. The mortality rate as a function of accumulated deficits in a frailty index. Mech Ageing Dev. 2002;123(11):1457–60.

21. Romero-Ortuno R, Kenny RA. The frailty index in Europeans: association with age and mortality. Age Ageing. 2012;41(5):684–9.
22. Rockwood K, Mitnitski A. Frailty in relation to the accumulation of deficits. J Gerontol A Biol Sci Med Sci. 2007;62(7):722–7.
23. Clegg A, Rogers L, Young J. Diagnostic test accuracy of simple instruments for identifying frailty in community-dwelling older people: a systematic review. Age Ageing. 2015;44(1):148–52.
24. Buta BJ, et al. Frailty assessment instruments: systematic characterization of the uses and contexts of highly-cited instruments. Ageing Res Rev. 2016;26:53–61.
25. Morley JE, Malmstrom TK, Miller DK. A simple frailty questionnaire (FRAIL) predicts outcomes in middle aged African Americans. J Nutr Health Aging. 2012;16(7):601–8.
26. Ruiz JG, et al. Screening for and managing the person with frailty in primary care: ICFSR consensus guidelines. J Nutr Health Aging. 2020;24(9):920–7.
27. Jadczak AD, et al. Effectiveness of exercise interventions on physical function in community-dwelling frail older people: an umbrella review of systematic reviews. JBI Database System Rev Implement Rep. 2018;16(3):752–75.
28. Kojima G, et al. Adherence to Mediterranean diet reduces incident frailty risk: systematic review and meta-analysis. J Am Geriatr Soc. 2018;66(4):783–8.
29. Coelho-Junior HJ, et al. Low protein intake is associated with frailty in older adults: a systematic review and meta-analysis of observational studies. Nutrients. 2018;10(9):1334.
30. Zhou J, et al. Association of vitamin D deficiency and frailty: a systematic review and meta-analysis. Maturitas. 2016;94:70–6.
31. Travers J, et al. Delaying and reversing frailty: a systematic review of primary care interventions. Br J Gen Pract. 2019;69(678):e61–9.
32. Tanaka T, et al. Oral frailty as a risk factor for physical frailty and mortality in community-dwelling elderly. J Gerontol A Biol Sci Med Sci. 2018;73(12):1661–7.
33. Ohara Y, et al. Association of eating alone with oral frailty among community-dwelling older adults in Japan. Arch Gerontol Geriatr. 2020;87:104014.
34. Nomura Y, et al. Nutritional status and oral frailty: a community based study. Nutrients. 2020;12(9):2886.
35. Hakeem FF, Bernabe E, Sabbah W. Association between oral health and frailty: a systematic review of longitudinal studies. Gerodontology. 2019;36(3):205–15.
36. Iwasaki M, et al. Association between Oral Frailty and Nutritional Status among Community-Dwelling Older Adults: the Takashimadaira Study. J Nutr Health Aging. 2020;24(9):1003–10.
37. Fried LP. Conference on the physiologic basis of frailty. April 28, 1992, Baltimore, Maryland, U.S.A. Introduction. Aging (Milano). 1992;4(3):251–2.
38. Fried LP, et al. Untangling the concepts of disability, frailty, and comorbidity: implications for improved targeting and care. J Gerontol A Biol Sci Med Sci. 2004;59(3):255–63.
39. Minakuchi S, et al. Oral hypofunction in the older population: position paper of the Japanese Society of Gerodontology in 2016. Gerodontology. 2018;35(4):317–24.
40. Beasley JM, Shikany JM, Thomson CA. The role of dietary protein intake in the prevention of sarcopenia of aging. Nutr Clin Pract. 2013;28(6):684–90.
41. Beasley JM, et al. Protein intake and incident frailty in the Women's Health Initiative observational study. J Am Geriatr Soc. 2010;58(6):1063–71.
42. van der Putten GJ, et al. Poor oral health, a potential new geriatric syndrome. Gerodontology. 2014;31(Suppl 1):17–24.
43. Peyron MA, et al. Oral declines and mastication deficiencies cause alteration of food bolus properties. Food Funct. 2018;9(2):1112–22.
44. Sakayori T, et al. Evaluation of a Japanese "Prevention of long-term care" project for the improvement in oral function in the high-risk elderly. Geriatr Gerontol Int. 2013;13(2):451–7.
45. Keller H, et al. Issues associated with the use of modified texture foods. J Nutr Health Aging. 2012;16(3):195–200.

46. Aguilera JM, Park DJ. Texture-modified foods for the elderly: status, technology and opportunities. Trends Food Sci Technol. 2016;57:156–64.
47. Park JS, et al. Effects of resistive jaw opening exercise in stroke patients with dysphagia: a double- blind, randomized controlled study. J Back Musculoskelet Rehabil. 2020;33(3):507–13.
48. Cho YS, et al. Effects of bedside self-exercise on oropharyngeal swallowing function in stroke patients with dysphagia: a pilot study. J Phys Ther Sci. 2017;29(10):1815–6.
49. Shiraishi A, Wakabayashi H, Yoshimura Y. Oral management in rehabilitation medicine: oral frailty, oral sarcopenia, and hospital-associated oral problems. J Nutr Health Aging. 2020;24(4):1–6.
50. Kossioni AE. The association of poor oral health parameters with malnutrition in older adults: a review considering the potential implications for cognitive impairment. Nutrients. 2018;10(11):1709.
51. Roberts HC, et al. The challenge of managing undernutrition in older people with frailty. Nutrients. 2019;11(4):808.
52. de Vries NM, et al. Patient-centred physical therapy is (cost-) effective in increasing physical activity and reducing frailty in older adults with mobility problems: a randomized controlled trial with 6 months follow-up. J Cachexia Sarcopenia Muscle. 2016;7(4):422–35.
53. Wells JL, Dumbrell AC. Nutrition and aging: assessment and treatment of compromised nutritional status in frail elderly patients. Clin Interv Aging. 2006;1(1):67–79.
54. Fougere B, Morley JE. Editorial: weight loss is a major cause of frailty. J Nutr Health Aging. 2017;21(9):933–5.

The Role of Oral Health Literacy and Shared Decision Making

Marlena Fernandez, Christie-Michele Hogue, and Jorge G. Ruiz

Mrs. Geneva Williams is a 69-year-old African American woman referred to an endodontist with the chief complaint of throbbing pain for the past 5 days associated with sensitivity and occasional pain in the right region of her lower posterior teeth. The pain kept her awake at night and was originating from the lower right side of her face with radiating pain to her right ear. On clinical examination, the patient had a defective occlusal amalgam restoration. A pulp test suggested irreversible pulpitis. Radiographically, the recurrent caries encroached the pulp. She has a history of well-controlled hypertension, osteoarthritis, and mild hypothyroidism. As a result of the oral pain, Mrs. Williams had modified her diet, eating predominantly soft foods, high in carbohydrates.

M. Fernandez
Miami VA Healthcare System, Geriatric Research, Education and Clinical Center (GRECC), Miami, FL, USA

C.-M. Hogue
Department of Dental Services - VA Healthcare System, Division of Geriatrics and Gerontology, Emory University School of Medicine, Emory University School of Medicine, Atlanta, GA, USA

J. G. Ruiz (✉)
Miami VA Healthcare System, Geriatric Research, Education and Clinical Center (GRECC), Miami, FL, USA

Division of Geriatrics and Palliative Medicine, University of Miami Miller School of Medicine, Miami, FL, USA
e-mail: j.ruiz@med.miami.edu

© The Author(s), under exclusive license to Springer Nature Switzerland AG 2022
C.-M. Hogue, J. G. Ruiz (eds.), *Oral Health and Aging*,
https://doi.org/10.1007/978-3-030-85993-0_15

1 Definitions

Health literacy is defined as the capacity to obtain, process, and use basic health information and services needed to make healthcare decisions [1]. It encompasses the skills of listening, reading, integrating, and evaluating health information, analyzing risks, and applying these skills to situations arising when receiving health care [2, 3]. Health literacy is a multidimensional process, including system demands and complexities as well as the skills and abilities of individuals. Health literacy is a dynamic concept that may change with the individual's mental or emotional state, illness, and life stressors [4]. Health literacy also consists of two essential and closely intertwined skills: numeracy and graphical literacy. Numeracy is a set of quantitative abilities needed by patients to comprehend, manage, and manipulate numerical expressions of probability about healthcare information [5, 6]. Lastly, graphical literacy constitutes the ability to comprehend basic graphical representations used to present quantitative health-related information, an increasingly important skill in the era of Internet-based health care [7, 8]. Health literacy may be a labile state, fluctuating with a patient's emotional state, health status, life stressors, or cognitive status, such as in patients with dementia or delirium [9]. In the field of oral health care, oral health literacy (OHL) has emerged as an extension of the overarching concept of health literacy. OHL is the degree to which individuals can obtain, understand, and process oral health information and services necessary for appropriate decisions as they relate to their oral health [10]. Health literacy, specifically as it relates to oral health, is a complex and multifaceted concept, the definition of which is constantly evolving.

Mrs. Williams had completed a high school education and had retired from her job as a postal worker 7 years ago. She reported these symptoms to her dentist who then recommended she seeks further evaluation by an endodontist. Mrs. Williams visited the endodontist who recommended root canal treatment. He explained the risks and benefits of the oral procedure going over multiple studies demonstrating its effectiveness. She told the dentist that she will want to discuss the issue with her older daughter. The endodontist explained that should she not get the procedure, her condition will continue to worsen, and she will have continued pain and possibly need an extraction. Upon returning home, Mrs. Williams told her oldest daughter that she will not undergo the proposed procedure. She is confused and reports "I didn't know other options were available, this was the only way to feel better." She is upset and wonders if she made the right choice.

2 Extent of the Problem

Investigators have reported a high prevalence of inadequate health literacy [11–13] and numeracy [14, 15] in older individuals. The reasons for this differential are various but among the most common are generational differences related to lower levels of educational achievement [16, 17]. However, age itself may not be an independent risk factor for inadequate health literacy. Factors that represent more important contributors to the higher levels of inadequate health literacy in older adults include multimorbidity, frailty, polypharmacy, and cognitive and sensory impairments [17]. Research shows that after controlling for cognitive ability, age is no longer associated with health literacy [11, 16, 18, 19]. Studies have also documented higher levels of inadequate health literacy and numeracy in minority older populations contributing to further healthcare disparities [11, 19–25].

Mrs. Williams' daughter convinces her mother to see the endodontist once again and promises to accompany her to the next appointment. One week later, both patient and daughter returned to the dental office. The endodontist had recently learned that inadequate health literacy is a serious and common problem in the older population, especially among minorities. He apologizes to Mrs. Williams stating that he may have been a little "too technical" in his explanation of the procedure. He obtains permission to ask her a question to assess her ability to understand health information. To the question "How confident are you filling out medical or dental forms by yourself?" Mrs. Williams replies that her daughter often helps her complete healthcare forms and that she usually accompanies her to medical appointments. However, this has become more difficult as her daughter had just started a new job.

3 Recognition

The identification of health literacy is the first step in the implementation of interventions aimed at mitigating the consequences associated with this problem. Researchers in diverse healthcare fields have developed several instruments to assess health literacy deficits. The most widely instruments are the Rapid Estimate of Adult Literacy in Medicine (REALM), the Test of Functional Health Literacy in Adults (TOFHLA), and the Newest Vital Sign (NVS). The REALM is a word recognition test that is highly dependent on the individual's educational level, and health knowledge and experience, or crystallized intelligence [26], potentially resulting in an underestimation of inadequate health literacy [27, 28]. The TOFHLA is a valid and reliable measure of health literacy that includes 67 items assessing reading comprehension of healthcare information and health numeracy. It takes 22 min to administer [29]. The TOFHLA is one of the commonly used instruments in the health literacy research literature. A shorter version, the S-TOFHLA, has eight items and takes 7–12 min to administer. It was significantly associated with knowledge about medical facts and clinical outcomes [30]. The Newest Vital Sign (NVS) is the most recent addition to the portfolio of health literacy assessment instruments [31]. It consists of a nutritional label and six associated questions. The cutoff for appropriate health literacy is four or more correct answers and it takes approximately 3 min to complete. The instrument is reliable and has demonstrated internal consistency [31]. The NVS and TOHFLA are strongly correlated with each other reflecting fluid intelligence and independence from the effects of education [27, 32]. A common advantage for both the NVS and S-TOFHLA is that these instruments not only assess reading ability and comprehension but also assess health numeracy [29, 33]. The advantages of the NVS as the preferred instrument to assess health literacy are its brevity and ability to discriminate among high scoring individuals [27].

Oral health investigators have developed or adapted existing health literacy instruments to focus on oral health information. Most of these new oral health literacy tools have used general health literacy instruments as reference standards for their validation. Table 1 shows some of the most common oral health literacy tools in English, organized in ascending order of administration time. The Two-Stage Rapid Estimate of Adult Literacy in Dentistry (TS-REALD) seems like a valid and reliable instrument that according to the authors takes only 1 min to administer. However, despite appearing as a rapid, simple, and practical measure of oral health literacy, the TS-REALD may not be ready for wider use in older populations. The TS-REALD was only validated in women, and the authors did not report the age of the study participants, limiting its applicability [34]. The Rapid Estimate of Adult Literacy in Dentistry-30 (REALD-30) is by far the most studied instrument in the oral health literature [35]. The REALD-30 is a reading comprehension instrument that consists of 30-word recognition items with increasing levels of difficulty [36]. A limitation of the REALD-30 is that it does not include assessments of numeracy, or graph literacy. Another disadvantage is that the REALD-30 may overestimate levels of adequate oral health literacy [37]. The Rapid Estimate of Adult Literacy in Medicine and Dentistry (REALM-D) represent an adaptation of the widely used REALM. As its predecessor instrument, it tests the individual's ability to recognize and pronounce medical and dental words as measures of comprehension [38]. The REALM-D seems relatively efficient and feasible, but the mean age of the participants in the original study suggests that during the validation study, the investigator did not enroll many older individuals [38, 39]. The Oral Health Literacy Instrument (OHLI) is another oral instrument testing reading comprehension and numeracy. However, the OHLI can be quite cumbersome and lengthy to administer [40]. The Test of Functional Health Literacy in Dentistry (TOFHLiD) is also a reading comprehension test adapted from the original TOFHLA. The TOFHLiD was originally validated with the parents of children receiving dental care and did not include anybody in the older age group [41]. Furthermore, this test takes the longest to administer making impractical as a health literacy screen for most dental practices.

Although useful for research purposes, most of the oral health literacy tools described earlier may not be feasible for implementation by busy dental practices. A group in the USA validated the single screening question "How confident are you filling out medical forms by yourself?" to assess patients for inadequate health literacy [42]. Although not yet validated in oral healthcare settings, it represents a practical, feasible, and ecologically valid approach to screen for inadequate health literacy in dental offices. The question could be conceivably be adapted to use "dental" instead of "medical" forms.

The Role of Oral Health Literacy and Shared Decision Making 267

Table 1 Properties of selected oral health literacy instruments (English) [35]

Instrument	Participants, type of test, number of items, and scoring	Participants in the validation	Reliability and validity	Time it takes to administer (minutes)	Country
Two-Stage Rapid Estimate of Adult Literacy in Dentistry (TS-REALD) [34]	11 items Score: possible range: 0–9 (raw score – transformed)	Adults: age not reported! (women)	Content validation Concurrent validity: newest vital Sign ($r = 0.51$), and REALD ($r = 0.96$) Reliability: Cronbach's $\alpha > 0.85$.	1	USA
Rapid Estimate of Adult Literacy in Dentistry-30 (REALD-30) [36]	Word recognition, 30 items Score: 0–30 (lowest to highest literacy)	Adults: mean age 44.7 years (SD = 14.6), age range not reported	Content validation Concurrent validity: REALM ($r = 0.86$) and TOHFLA ($r = 0.64$) Predictive validity: oral health related quality of life Reliability: Cronbach's $\alpha = 0.87$	5	USA
Rapid Estimate of Adult Literacy in Medicine and Dentistry (REALM-D) [38, 39]	Word recognition, 84 words Score: 0–84 (lowest to highest literacy)	Adults: 19–87 (mean age: 41 years)	Content validation Concurrent validity: REALM-66 ($r = 0.99$) Predictive validity: confidence filling out medical forms Reliability: Cronbach's $\alpha = 0.958$	5–7	USA
Oral Health Literacy Instrument (OHLI) [40]	57 items Score: possible range: 0–100 (0–59, inadequate HL; 60–74, marginal HL; and 75–100, adequate HL)	Adults 19–69 (mean age: 39 years)	Content validation Concurrent validity: TOFHLA ($r = 0.61$) and discriminate oral knowledge ($r = 0.57$). Reliability: Cronbach's $\alpha = 0.898$	20	Canada
Test of Functional Health Literacy in Dentistry (TOFHLiD) [41]	68 reading comprehension, 12 numeracy items Score: weighted score 0–100	Adults: 26–59 (median age: 35 years)	Content validation Concurrent validity: REALD-99 ($r = 0.82$) Reliability: Cronbach's $\alpha = 0.63$–0.86	30	USA

4 Consequences of Inadequate Health Literacy

Patients with inadequate health literacy suffer from poorer health status, unhealthy behaviors, and worse clinical outcomes than those individuals demonstrating adequate levels of health literacy. Research studies have documented poor knowledge of disease [43], poor patient-physician communication [44, 45], lower adherence to healthy behaviors [20], impaired self-management skills [46], worse self-perception of health status [47], disability [48], worse clinical outcomes [49–51], diminished ability to participate in shared decision-making [52], and higher healthcare utilization [47, 53]. Regarding oral health, studies have also shown poor oral healthcare outcomes. Using the REALD-20, a study showed that patients with higher OHL had two more teeth on average than those in the lowest score range. This same study also showed a significant association between lower plaque scores and higher REALD-20 scores before and after treatment [54]. The number of missing and filled teeth were significantly higher in those patients with inadequate literacy as compared with participants with adequate levels of health literacy. Limited OHL is also linked to the presence of biofilm in younger adults [55] and severe periodontitis [56]. In terms of healthcare utilization, having lower health literacy was associated with a twofold increase in missed dental appointments [56] and a higher number of emergency dental visits [55]. Others reported higher rates of dental anxiety in individuals with lower levels of OHL [10], dissatisfaction with their own oral health care [57], and impaired quality of life [55]. These studies show that there is an association between lack of OHL and dental outcomes.

The endodontist outlines the risks, benefits, and possible adverse outcomes of the root canal intervention. The dentist uses lay language and graphic illustrations to explain the root canal procedure to save the tooth. He also discusses alternatives to the root canal, including tooth extraction, natural remedies (eliminating processed sugars from her diet, eating high-quality protein and avoiding grains), and irrigating the tooth canal with a calcium hydroxide solution, and he also presents the option of no treatment, explaining this could lead to further recurrent infections. The endodontist wants to make sure that Mrs. Williams understood the procedure and alternatives, so he asks: "Ms. Geneva, I want to be sure that I did a good job explaining the root canal procedure. Would you mind please explaining back to me what we discussed?" After clarifying misunderstandings, the specialist is confident that Mrs. Williams had understood the benefits and burdens associated with the root canal as well as the alternatives he presented. After asking her daughter's opinion, Ms. Williams agrees to undergo the root canal. Together, they decide on a plan of care for her. She feels supported and confident in their joint decision.

5 Shared Decision-Making and Health Literacy in Dentistry

Shared decision-making (SDM) is the process by which patients and healthcare professionals make assessment and management healthcare decisions together, incorporating the best available evidence [58, 59]. SDM involves a bidirectional information flow between the clinician and the patient, patient knowledge of treatment options, and physician elicitation of patient preferences. Shared decision-making builds a dentist-patient partnership, working on the oral health problems at hand by laying out the available diagnostic and therapeutic options, including that of no treatment. During the process the dentist explains the benefits and risks, eliciting the patient's views and preferences on these options and agreeing on a joint course of action. SDM aims to empower patients to make better healthcare decisions [60–62]. Adequate levels of health literacy are a prerequisite for active participation in the decision-making process [63]. Unfortunately, individuals with inadequate health literacy are less likely to participate in SDM [52, 64, 65]. Although many patients would prefer to play a collaborative role, those with inadequate health literacy most often played a passive role in decision-making [52]. Recent reviews revealed the paucity of studies investigating the process of shared decision-making in dentistry [62, 66]. Small cross-sectional studies of adult patients in dental practices showed that in general patients prefer to play a more active and collaborative role in dental care decision-making [67, 68]. Other studies have addressed how to facilitate SDM by using decisional aids [69–72]. Despite the recognition by oral health experts of the importance of health literacy in SDM [73, 74], there are no studies that specifically examine this topic. On a routine basis, dental professionals will face issues related to assessment and management interventions that will demand patient involvement in the decision-making process. As we have seen throughout this chapter, older adults are a group at higher risk for demonstrating inadequate levels of health literacy. Extrapolating from the large healthcare research literature, we can anticipate that older patients with poor health literacy may not fully engage in the shared decision-making process or comprehend the benefits and risks of proposed dental interventions. In the next section, we will outline interventions designed to improve the process of shared decision-making for patients with inadequate health literacy.

Mrs. Williams undergoes the procedure as recommended by the endodontist. There are no post-procedure complications. She's a little sore afterward but glad that it's over. The endodontist sends her home with age-friendly patient education materials including images explaining post root canal care. He follows up with her by telephone the next day to discuss how she's doing.

6 Interventions

Older adults are high-risk groups for the presence of inadequate health literacy. It is therefore incumbent upon dentists to implement interventions that facilitate dentist-patient communication and improve the process of shared decision among in patients with inadequate health literacy. The American Dental Association has formulated guidelines aimed at improving communication and shared decision-making tools for patients with inadequate health literacy [75]. We complement these recommendations with those of experts in other healthcare fields [76–78].

6.1 Universal Precautions

Given the high prevalence of inadequate health literacy in older adults, it is reasonable to widely implement "lowest common denominator" approaches to address the problem of inadequate health literacy. The US Agency for Healthcare Research and Quality developed the Health Literacy Universal Precautions Toolkit to improve clinician-patient communication in patients with different levels of health literacy [79]. The implementation of universal precautions implies a dental practice commitment to make changes that improve communication and foster older patients' involvement in shared decision-making regardless of their level of health literacy. The interventions may consist of staff training on the principles of communication and SDM, as well as some of the recommendations in this section.

6.2 Teach-Back

The teach-back is a technique in which a patient is prompted to restate information previously conveyed by a clinician with the purpose of ensuring patient recall and understanding [45, 80]. This involves asking a patient to explain in their own words the diagnosis or treatment plan. The provider then can correct any errors or fill gaps in understanding. A growing body of evidence supports the use of the teach-back technique in improving patients' knowledge, self-management skills, and adherence [81]. It may not add additional time to the dental encounter.

6.3 Age-Friendly Written Materials

Age-related changes in visual and cognitive performance may impair older adults' ability to read and understand patient education materials [82, 83]. These changes may be further amplified by the effects of multimorbidity, frailty, and disability. The US the Centers for Medicare and Medicaid Services (CMS) has produced a toolkit with a set of evidence-based guidelines on how to design age-friendly reading materials (Table 2) [84]. Clinicians can use the US Centers for Disease Control (CDC) Clear Communication Index (Index), which provides evidence-based criteria to assess public communication products [85].

6.4 Image-Based Materials (Pictograms)

Pictograms are graphical, nonverbal symbols that are used to convey healtcare information [86]. Figure 1 shows an example of a pictogram explaining the use of a medication. Pictograms may overcome health literacy deficits and improve comprehension, recall, and adherence by patients with inadequate health literacy. Most of

Table 2 Guidelines for preparing age-friendly written materials [84]

Content	Organization
Use advance organizers Emphasize what patients want and need to know Create content culturally appropriate Repeat new concepts and summarize the most important points. Ensure content accurate and up to date Include information about who produced the resource and when	Pace readers by grouping content into meaningful chunks Pay attention to the orderly presentation of information Use headings and subheadings Make headings specific and informative Provide patient friendly navigational aids throughout the document (e.g., table of contents, signs, etc.)
Writing style	Motivation
Write in a conversational style Use the active voice Make sentences simple and short. Be direct, specific, and concrete Give the context first, and incorporate definitions into the text Create cohesion Use words that are familiar and culturally appropriate Use technical terms only when readers need to know them Write as simply as you can	Use a positive and friendly tone Use devices to get readers actively involved with the material Give specific instructions that are culturally appropriate Refer to trustworthy sources of information (government, healthcare organizations) Assist in reading and interpreting health statistics Offer help support or how to obtain additional information

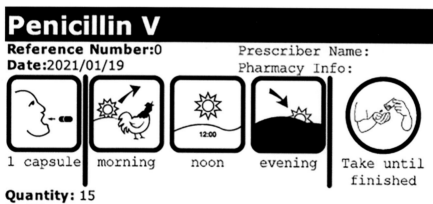

Fig. 1 Pictogram with medication instructions

the research comes from the medication adherence literature. The evidence on the effectiveness of pictograms for older adults with inadequate health is mostly positive in terms of improving patients' medication adherence [86, 87]. In conjunction with other modalities, the judicious use of pictograms may help dentists convey healthcare information to their older patients. These tools have been shown to improve patients' recall as well as their adherence to medical treatment [80].

6.5 Decision Aids

These are tools designed to assist individuals participation in the shared decision making process by fostering deliberation of healthcare options between patients, caregivers, and the healthcare professional. The goal of using decision aids is to help patients make informed decisions regarding their healthcare [88]. Dental practitioners can take advantage of decision aids to improve patients' knowledge, comprehension of risk perceptions, and participation in shared decision-making [75]. There is growing evidence of the efficacy of decision aids for improving decision-making in patients with inadequate health literacy [89].

6.6 Caregivers

Recruiting caregivers to assist older patients can go a long way in mitigating the negative effects associated with inadequate health literacy. Older patients become increasingly dependent on caregivers for assistance with their daily care and when interfacing with healthcare professionals. Caregivers' working familiarity with the oral healthcare of their loved ones may be useful in ameliorating the effect of the patient's limited health literacy. Dental professionals must be careful in ensuring that the caregivers have in fact an adequate level of health literacy [90].

7 Practical Considerations for Oral Healthcare Professionals

Time constraints are a barrier for oral healthcare professionals seeking to assess older patients for OHL. However, incorporating a practical and efficient approach may be feasible to implement in a busy dental practice. It is certainly important to be sensitive and avoid stigmatizing language when dealing with older patients who may have inadequate health literacy. Office staff may begin the screening of patients in the waiting area by asking the single question "How confident are you filling out medical/dental forms by yourself?" Staff can then document in the chart those with suspected inadequate health literacy. Thereafter, the dental professional could ask the patients for permission to include available caregivers during the encounter. Caregiver participation may occur on-site or by telephone or secure video conferencing. Keeping handy in the dental office age-appropriate written educational materials that include pictograms allows for further reinforcement of dental information. When discussing proposed diagnostic and therapeutic interventions, decisional aids that may include graphics may assist during shared decision-making

After a week, the patient returns to the dental clinic for her endodontic follow-up visit. The outcome was successful after the procedure with resolution of Mrs. Williams' severe oral discomfort. The patient was advised to receive a full coverage restoration when she returns for her 1-month follow-up visit. A follow-up radiograph after 4 months revealed no periapical changes, and Mrs. Williams is asymptomatic.

8 Future Research

There are multiple gaps in the study of oral health literacy in older adults. However, three priority areas deserve special attention: assessment, impact on dental practice access and satisfaction; and interventions. Regarding the assessment of oral health literacy, this chapter reviewed existing instruments meeting most validity and reliability criteria. However, these instruments may not be feasible in busy dental practices. The obvious advantage of the single question screener for health literacy is its rapid administration. Although validated with medical patients, it has yet to be evaluated with older adult populations in dental settings. Future studies may address the correlation of the single question with existing oral health literacy instruments. The growing diversity of the older population will also demand that investigators develop and validate culturally sensitive tools to measure oral health literacy in the persons' native language. A related research area is the evaluation of the impact that inadequate health literacy has on access to dental care services. Practicing dentists are already dealing with older adults suffering from more oral diseases and associated multimorbidity, cognitive impairment, and disability which may prolong the duration of dental encounters [91]. Inadequate health literacy may pose an additional barrier to the care of older adults. An important area of investigation will be the study of dental providers' attitudes toward older adults with inadequate health literacy. On the patient side, there are other important research gaps. More studies are needed about the experiences of older persons with inadequate health literacy and how that dynamic affects access to dental services and the shared decision-making process. We discussed several different strategies to overcome the challenges of health literacy for older persons. Unfortunately, most of the interventions are based on expert opinion lacking a solid grounding on research evidence. Health literacy is a multidimensional construct and is unlikely that single interventions will suffice. Evaluating multicomponent strategies consisting of combinations of individual approaches may represent a more efficacious and cost-effective approach to deal with the burdens associated with inadequate health literacy in older adults.

9 Conclusions

Inadequate oral health literacy is prevalent in older adults and is associated with dental complications and increased utilization. There are validated instruments that can assist dentists is the assessment of their older patients' levels of health literacy.

A single question screener may be a quick approach to identifying older patients with inadequate health literacy. Adequate levels of health literacy are a prerequisite for active participation in the decision-making process. There are many options that may facilitate the shared decision-making process in patients with inadequate levels of health literacy. An overall commitment to universal precautions, use of the teach-back technique, age-friendly materials, pictograms, and decision aids may mitigate the problems associated with inadequate health literacy. Involving caregivers to help patient during dental encounters may serve to further assist patients during the process. More research is needed into the assessment of oral health literacy, its impact on dental practice access and patient satisfaction, and in the design of multicompetent interventions targeting this important problem.

References

1. Paasche-Orlow MK, Parker RM, Gazmararian JA, Nielsen-Bohlman LT, Rudd RR. The prevalence of limited health literacy. J Gen Intern Med. 2005;20:175–84.
2. Davis TC, Arnold C, Berkel HJ, Nandy I, Jackson RH, Glass J. Knowledge and attitude on screening mammography among low-literate, low-income women. Cancer. 1996;78:1912–20.
3. Baker DW, Parker RM, Williams MV, Pitkin K, Parikh NS, Coates W, Imara M. The health care experience of patients with low literacy. Arch Fam Med. 1996;5:329–34.
4. Pleasant A, Rudd RE, O'Leary C, Paasche-Orlow MK, Allen MP, Alvarado-Little W, Myers L, Parson K, Rosen S. Considerations for a new definition of health literacy. Washington, DC: National Academy of Medicine; 2016.
5. Peters E. Beyond comprehension. Curr Dir Psychol Sci. 2012;21:31–5.
6. Rothman RL, Montori VM, Cherrington A, Pignone MP. Perspective: the role of numeracy in health care. J Health Commun. 2008;13:583–95.
7. Garcia-Retamero R, Galesic M. Who profits from visual aids: overcoming challenges in people's understanding of risks [corrected]. Soc Sci Med. 2010;70:1019–25.
8. Galesic M, Garcia-Retamero R, Gigerenzer G. Using icon arrays to communicate medical risks: overcoming low numeracy. Health Psychol. 2009;28:210–6.
9. Rudd R, Horowitz AM. The role of health literacy in achieving oral health for elders. J Dent Educ. 2005;69:1018–21.
10. Firmino RT, Martins CC, Faria LDS, Martins Paiva S, Granville-Garcia AF, Fraiz FC, Ferreira FM. Association of oral health literacy with oral health behaviors, perception, knowledge, and dental treatment related outcomes: a systematic review and meta-analysis. J Public Health Dent. 2018;78:231–45.
11. Morrow D, Clark D, Tu W, Wu J, Weiner M, Steinley D, Murray MD. Correlates of health literacy in patients with chronic heart failure. Gerontologist. 2006;46:669–76.
12. Martin LT, Ruder T, Escarce JJ, Ghosh-Dastidar B, Sherman D, Elliott M, Bird CE, Fremont A, Gasper C, Culbert A, Lurie N. Developing predictive models of health literacy. J Gen Intern Med. 2009;24:1211–6.
13. Peterson PN, Shetterly SM, Clarke CL, Bekelman DB, Chan PS, Allen LA, Matlock DD, Magid DJ, Masoudi FA. Health literacy and outcomes among patients with heart failure. JAMA. 2011;305:1695–701.
14. Garcia-Retamero R, Galesic M, Gigerenzer G. Do icon arrays help reduce denominator neglect? Med Decis Mak. 2010;30:672–84.
15. Taha J, Sharit J, Czaja SJ. The impact of numeracy ability and technology skills on older adults' performance of health management tasks using a patient portal. J Appl Gerontol. 2012;33(4):416–36.

16. Baker DW, Gazmararian JA, Sudano J, Patterson M. The association between age and health literacy among elderly persons. J Gerontol B Psychol Sci Soc Sci. 2000;55:S368–74.
17. Sentell TL, Halpin HA. Importance of adult literacy in understanding health disparities. J Gen Intern Med. 2006;21:862–6.
18. Bostock S, Steptoe A. Association between low functional health literacy and mortality in older adults: longitudinal cohort study. BMJ. 2012;344:e1602.
19. Rodríguez V, Andrade AD, García-Retamero R, Anam R, Rodríguez R, Lisigurski M, Sharit J, Ruiz JG. Health literacy, numeracy, and graphical literacy among veterans in primary care and their effect on shared decision making and trust in physicians. J Health Commun. 2013;18:273–89.
20. Osborn CY, Paasche-Orlow MK, Davis TC, Wolf MS. Health literacy: an overlooked factor in understanding HIV health disparities. Am J Prev Med. 2007;33:374–8.
21. Waldrop-Valverde D, Osborn CY, Rodriguez A, Rothman RL, Kumar M, Jones DL. Numeracy skills explain racial differences in HIV medication management. AIDS Behav. 2010;14:799–806.
22. Patel PJ, Joel S, Rovena G, Pedireddy S, Saad S, Rachmale R, Shukla M, Deol BB, Cardozo L. Testing the utility of the newest vital sign (NVS) health literacy assessment tool in older African-American patients. Patient Educ Couns. 2011;85:505–7.
23. Shea JA, Beers BB, McDonald VJ, Quistberg DA, Ravenell KL, Asch DA. Assessing health literacy in African American and Caucasian adults: disparities in rapid estimate of adult literacy in medicine (REALM) scores. Fam Med. 2004;36:575–81.
24. Chaudhry SI, Herrin J, Phillips C, Butler J, Mukerjhee S, Murillo J, Onwuanyi A, Seto TB, Spertus J, Krumholz HM. Racial disparities in health literacy and access to care among patients with heart failure. J Card Fail. 2011;17:122–7.
25. Kelly PA, Haidet P. Physician overestimation of patient literacy: a potential source of health care disparities. Patient Educ Couns. 2007;66:119–22.
26. Davis TC, Long SW, Jackson RH, Mayeaux EJ, George RB, Murphy PW, Crouch MA. Rapid estimate of adult literacy in medicine: a shortened screening instrument. Fam Med. 1993;25:391–5.
27. Murray C, Johnson W, Wolf MS, Deary IJ. The association between cognitive ability across the lifespan and health literacy in old age: the Lothian Birth Cohort 1936. Intelligence. 2011;39:178–87.
28. Chin J, Morrow DG, Stine-Morrow EA, Conner-Garcia T, Graumlich JF, Murray MD. The process-knowledge model of health literacy: evidence from a componential analysis of two commonly used measures. J Health Commun. 2011;16(Suppl 3):222–41.
29. Parker RM, Baker DW, Williams MV, Nurss JR. The test of functional health literacy in adults: a new instrument for measuring patients' literacy skills. J Gen Intern Med. 1995;10:537–41.
30. Osborn CY, Weiss BD, Davis TC, Skripkauskas S, Rodrigue C, Bass PF, Wolf MS. Measuring adult literacy in health care: performance of the newest vital sign. Am J Health Behav. 2007;31(Suppl 1):S36–46.
31. Weiss BD. Quick assessment of literacy in primary care: the newest vital sign. Ann Fam Med. 2005;3:514–22.
32. Wolf MS, Curtis LM, Wilson EA, Revelle W, Waite KR, Smith SG, Weintraub S, Borosh B, Rapp DN, Park DC, Deary IC, Baker DW. Literacy, cognitive function, and health: results of the LitCog study. J Gen Intern Med. 2012;27:1300–7.
33. Weiss BD, Mays MZ, Martz W, Castro KM, DeWalt DA, Pignone MP, Mockbee J, Hale FA. Quick assessment of literacy in primary care: the newest vital sign. Ann Fam Med. 2005;3:514–22.
34. Stucky BD, Lee JY, Lee SY, Rozier RG. Development of the two-stage rapid estimate of adult literacy in dentistry. Community Dent Oral Epidemiol. 2011;39:474–80.
35. Kaur N, Kandelman D, Nimmon L, Potvin L. Oral health literacy: findings of a scoping review. EC Dent Sci. 2015;2:293–306.
36. Lee JY, Rozier RG, Lee SY, Bender D, Ruiz RE. Development of a word recognition instrument to test health literacy in dentistry: the REALD-30–a brief communication. J Public Health Dent. 2007;67:94–8.

37. Lee JY. Lower Oral health literacy may lead to poorer oral health outcomes. J Evid Based Dent Pract. 2018;18:255–7.
38. Atchison KA, Gironda MW, Messadi D, Der-Martirosian C. Screening for oral health literacy in an urban dental clinic. J Public Health Dent. 2010;70:269–75.
39. Gironda M, Der-Martirosian C, Messadi D, Holtzman J, Atchison K. A brief 20-item dental/medical health literacy screen (REALMD-20). J Public Health Dent. 2013;73:50–5.
40. Sabbahi DA, Lawrence HP, Limeback H, Rootman I. Development and evaluation of an oral health literacy instrument for adults. Community Dent Oral Epidemiol. 2009;37:451–62.
41. Gong DA, Lee JY, Rozier RG, Pahel BT, Richman JA, Vann WF Jr. Development and testing of the Test of Functional Health Literacy in Dentistry (TOFHLiD). J Public Health Dent. 2007;67:105–12.
42. Wallace LS, Rogers ES, Roskos SE, Holiday DB, Weiss BD. Brief report: screening items to identify patients with limited health literacy skills. J Gen Intern Med. 2006;21:874–7.
43. Osborn CY, Cavanaugh K, Wallston KA, Rothman RL. Self-efficacy links health literacy and numeracy to glycemic control. J Health Commun. 2010;15(Suppl 2):146–58.
44. Williams MV, Davis T, Parker RM, Weiss BD. The role of health literacy in patient-physician communication. Fam Med. 2002;34:383–9.
45. Schillinger D, Piette J, Grumbach K, Wang F, Wilson C, Daher C, Leong-Grotz K, Castro C, Bindman AB. Closing the loop: physician communication with diabetic patients who have low health literacy. Arch Intern Med. 2003;163:83–90.
46. Kalichman SC, Ramachandran B, Catz S. Adherence to combination antiretroviral therapies in HIV patients of low health literacy. J Gen Intern Med. 1999;14:267–73.
47. Baker DW, Gazmararian JA, Williams MV, Scott T, Parker RM, Green D, Ren J, Peel J. Functional health literacy and the risk of hospital admission among Medicare managed care enrollees. Am J Public Health. 2002;92:1278–83.
48. Wolf MS, Gazmararian JA, Baker DW. Health literacy and functional health status among older adults. Arch Intern Med. 2005;165:1946–52.
49. Schillinger D, Grumbach K, Piette J, Wang F, Osmond D, Daher C, Palacios J, Sullivan GD, Bindman AB. Association of health literacy with diabetes outcomes. JAMA. 2002;288:475–82.
50. Estrada CA, Martin-Hryniewicz M, Peek BT, Collins C, Byrd JC. Literacy and numeracy skills and anticoagulation control. Am J Med Sci. 2004;328:88–93.
51. Berkman ND, Sheridan SL, Donahue KE, Halpern DJ, Crotty K. Low health literacy and health outcomes: an updated systematic review. Ann Intern Med. 2011;155:97–107.
52. Naik AD, Street RL Jr, Castillo D, Abraham NS. Health literacy and decision making styles for complex antithrombotic therapy among older multimorbid adults. Patient Educ Couns. 2011;85:499–504.
53. Hardie NA, Kyanko K, Busch S, Losasso AT, Levin RA. Health literacy and health care spending and utilization in a consumer-driven health plan. J Health Commun. 2011;16(Suppl 3):308–21.
54. Holtzman JS, Atchison KA, Macek MD, Markovic D. Oral health literacy and measures of periodontal disease. J Periodontol. 2017;88:78–88.
55. Batista MJ, Lawrence HP, Sousa M. Oral health literacy and oral health outcomes in an adult population in Brazil. BMC Public Health. 2017;18:60.
56. Baskaradoss JK. Relationship between oral health literacy and oral health status. BMC Oral Health. 2018;18:172.
57. Tenani CF, De Checchi MHR, Bado FMR, Ju X, Jamieson L, Mialhe FL. Influence of oral health literacy on dissatisfaction with oral health among older people. Gerodontology. 2020;37:46–52.
58. Makoul G, Clayman ML. An integrative model of shared decision making in medical encounters. Patient Educ Couns. 2006;60:301–12.
59. Elwyn G, Frosch D, Thomson R, Joseph-Williams N, Lloyd A, Kinnersley P, Cording E, Tomson D, Dodd C, Rollnick S, Edwards A, Barry M. Shared decision making: a model for clinical practice. J Gen Intern Med. 2012;27:1361–7.

60. Woolf SH, Chan EC, Harris R, Sheridan SL, Braddock CH 3rd, Kaplan RM, Krist A, O'Connor AM, Tunis S. Promoting informed choice: transforming health care to dispense knowledge for decision making. Ann Intern Med. 2005;143:293–300.
61. King JS, Eckman MH, Moulton BW. The potential of shared decision making to reduce health disparities. J Law Med Ethics. 2011;39(Suppl 1):30–3.
62. Alzahrani AAH, Gibson BJ. Scoping review of the role of shared decision making in dental implant consultations. JDR Clin Trans Res. 2018;3:130–40.
63. Dubow J. Adequate literacy and health literacy: prerequisites for informed health care decision making. Issue Brief (Public Policy Inst (Am Assoc Retired Pers)). 2004;(IB70):1–11.
64. DeWalt DA, Boone RS, Pignone MP. Literacy and its relationship with self-efficacy, trust, and participation in medical decision making. Am J Health Behav. 2007;31(Suppl 1):S27–35.
65. Smith SK, Dixon A, Trevena L, Nutbeam D, McCaffery KJ. Exploring patient involvement in healthcare decision making across different education and functional health literacy groups. Soc Sci Med. 2009;69:1805–12.
66. Asa'ad F. Shared decision-making (SDM) in dentistry: a concise narrative review. J Eval Clin Pract. 2019;25:1088–93.
67. Chapple H, Shah S, Caress AL, Kay EJ. Exploring dental patients' preferred roles in treatment decision-making – a novel approach. Br Dent J. 2003;194:321–7. discussion 317
68. Reissmann DR, Bellows JC, Kasper J. Patient preferred and perceived control in dental care decision making. JDR Clin Trans Res. 2019;4:151–9.
69. Bauer J, Spackman S, Chiappelli F, Prolo P. Model of evidence-based dental decision making. J Evid Based Dent Pract. 2005;5:189–97.
70. Johnson BR, Schwartz A, Goldberg J, Koerber A. A chairside aid for shared decision making in dentistry: a randomized controlled trial. J Dent Educ. 2006;70:133–41.
71. Jevsevar DS. Shared decision making tool: should I take antibiotics before my dental procedure? J Am Acad Orthop Surg. 2013;21:190–2.
72. Kupke J, Wicht MJ, Stutzer H, Derman SH, Lichtenstein NV, Noack MJ. Does the use of a visualised decision board by undergraduate students during shared decision-making enhance patients' knowledge and satisfaction? A randomised controlled trial. Eur J Dent Educ. 2013;17:19–25.
73. Barber S. Shared decision-making in orthodontics: are we there yet? J Orthod. 2019;46:21–5.
74. Rajagopal S, Kelly A. Shared decision making in endodontics. Prim Dent J. 2020;9:31–6.
75. Association AD. Health literacy in dentistry action plan: 2010–2015. ADA: Chicago IL; 2009.
76. Berkman ND, Sheridan SL, Donahue KE, Halpern DJ, Viera A, Crotty K, Holland A, Brasure M, Lohr KN, Harden E, Tant E, Wallace I, Viswanathan M. Health literacy interventions and outcomes: an updated systematic review. Evid Rep Technol Assess (Full Rep). 2011;(199):1–941.
77. Visscher BB, Steunenberg B, Heijmans M, Hofstede JM, Deville W, van der Heide I, Rademakers J. Evidence on the effectiveness of health literacy interventions in the EU: a systematic review. BMC Public Health. 2018;18:1414.
78. Walters R, Leslie SJ, Polson R, Cusack T, Gorely T. Establishing the efficacy of interventions to improve health literacy and health behaviours: a systematic review. BMC Public Health. 2020;20:1040.
79. DeWalt DA, Broucksou KA, Hawk V, Brach C, Hink A, Rudd R, Callahan L. Developing and testing the health literacy universal precautions toolkit. Nurs Outlook. 2011;59:85–94.
80. Sudore RL, Schillinger D. Interventions to improve care for patients with limited health literacy. J Clin Outcomes Manag. 2009;16:20–9.
81. Ha Dinh TT, Bonner A, Clark R, Ramsbotham J, Hines S. The effectiveness of the teach-back method on adherence and self-management in health education for people with chronic disease: a systematic review. JBI Database System Rev Implement Rep. 2016;14:210–47.
82. Span MM, Ridderinkhof KR, van der Molen MW. Age-related changes in the efficiency of cognitive processing across the life span. Acta Psychol. 2004;117:155–83.

83. Valentijn SA, van Boxtel MP, van Hooren SA, Bosma H, Beckers HJ, Ponds RW, Jolles J. Change in sensory functioning predicts change in cognitive functioning: results from a 6-year follow-up in the maastricht aging study. J Am Geriatr Soc. 2005;53:374–80.
84. US Centers for Medicare and Medicaid Services (CMS). Toolkit for making written material clear and effective. Centers for Medicare and Medicaid Services; 2020.
85. Baur C, Prue C. The CDC Clear Communication Index is a new evidence-based tool to prepare and review health information. Health Promot Pract. 2014;15:629–37.
86. Barros IM, Alcantara TS, Mesquita AR, Santos AC, Paixao FP, Lyra DP Jr. The use of pictograms in the health care: a literature review. Res Social Adm Pharm. 2014;10:704–19.
87. Sletvold H, Sagmo LAB, Torheim EA. Impact of pictograms on medication adherence: a systematic literature review. Patient Educ Couns. 2020;103:1095–103.
88. Volk RJ, Llewellyn-Thomas H, Stacey D, Elwyn G. Ten years of the International Patient Decision Aid Standards Collaboration: evolution of the core dimensions for assessing the quality of patient decision aids. BMC Med Inform Decis Mak. 2013;13(Suppl 2):S1.
89. van Weert JC, van Munster BC, Sanders R, Spijker R, Hooft L, Jansen J. Decision aids to help older people make health decisions: a systematic review and meta-analysis. BMC Med Inform Decis Mak. 2016;16:45.
90. Yuen EYN, Knight T, Ricciardelli LA, Burney S. Health literacy of caregivers of adult care recipients: a systematic scoping review. Health Soc Care Community. 2018;26:e191–206.
91. Gilliss CL. The grand challenges and nursing. Nurs Outlook. 2010;58:66–7.

Barriers to Access to Dental Care

Janet Yellowitz

1 Introduction

As a group, older adults are at increased risk for oral diseases and many are not regular users of professional dental services. While oral health is essential to one's general health and well-being, it is often neglected, increasing one's risk of a wide range of diseases. Maintaining one's dentition into later years increases ones' risk of having oral disease. Even without any natural teeth, older adults remain at increased risk for oral cancer. Quality of life can be influenced by a functional and esthetic mouth free of discomfort. Older adults with a healthy mouth are reported to have better general health, treatment outcomes, nutritional status, and quality of life [1].

Although the majority of oral diseases can be prevented or treated, older adults suffer disproportionately from oral and dental diseases and often have limited access to oral health care. Many older adults are unwilling or unable to receive routine care, which is complicated by having poor access to care. A combination of these factors can result in a high prevalence of oral health problems in older adults which increases their risk for general and oral complications. While the population of older adults is diverse and heterogeneous, many experience extensive oral disease, due to the cumulative effect of oral disease(s) throughout their lifetime. This unfortunate situation becomes more complicated when faced with multiple barriers to care.

It is not one's age that determines use of dental services, but rather utilization of care is the result of social, behavioral, health, and economic factors. Many older adults experience limited access to oral health due to a wide range of barriers, the topic of this chapter. Individually, these factors can become unique barriers to accessing care for older adults. Barriers to professional oral health care include but

---

J. Yellowitz (✉)
University of Maryland School of Dentistry, Baltimore, MD, USA
e-mail: JYellowitz@umaryland.edu

© The Author(s), under exclusive license to Springer Nature Switzerland AG 2022
C.-M. Hogue, J. G. Ruiz (eds.), *Oral Health and Aging*,
https://doi.org/10.1007/978-3-030-85993-0_16

are not limited to no perceived need, place of residence, dentition status, economic factors, education level, lack of knowledge, fear, health literacy, social isolation, professional attitudes, lack of effective oral health policies, insurance, transportation, availability, accessibility, and characteristics of dental providers. Each of these variables can impact older adults' use of dental services. Some of these factors serve as barriers while other can enable access to care. Generally, it is not a single deterrent but rather a combination of barriers that affect the receipt of care. Addressing these barriers is critical if we are to improve older adults' health and their access to and use of oral health-care services in the future.

This chapter will address key barriers that impact dental care utilization by community-dwelling older adults. Each barrier can play a role in older adults' use of dental services, and when multiple barriers are present, attempting to address them can become unsurmountable to older adults. Understanding barriers to care can help dental and dental public health communities be better prepared to address the many confounding factors impeding the use of dental services by older adults.

2 Age-Related Changes, the Presence of Pain, and Self-Perceived Needs

Many older adults do not seek professional dental care primarily because they believe that they do not have any treatment needs, and this is primarily related to them having no dental pain. Older adults with natural teeth often do not experience pain or have a reduced pain sensation in their teeth as a result of age-related physiologic changes, especially to the dental pulp. With advancing years, the pulp tissue in the teeth of older adults is often reduced or obliterated. Associated with the reduction of pulp tissue is a decreased sensitivity of the pulp to disease. This physiologic change occurs in response to the development of reparative dentin, which reduces the size, volume, and contents of the pulp. This change typically occurs following years of occlusal forces, restorations, and trauma. The decreased pulpal sensitivity occurs even in the presence of extensive dental caries and/or periodontal disease and serves as a key barrier to the dental care for older adults, especially for those who only seek care when dental pain is present. While this information is not new to dental professionals, much of the public is unaware of these changes. Dental professionals need to inform patients of all ages of the impending changes that can occur as they age and the impact of aging on their oral cavity. Having a well-informed populace will assist older adults to be better informed when making decisions about determining their need for professional dental services.

Seeking routine preventive oral care on a regular basis decreases one's risk for disease by instituting early preventive and/or treatment strategies. Rather than waiting for pain to present, older adults can reduce the risk of severe, debilitating disease from occurring by seeking preventive dental care. Unfortunately, some older adults will not seek out care even when they are having pain or discomfort, while some mistakenly believe that they will have no dental needs when they are older. In a 2017 study, over 50% of respondents had not attended a dentist in over 36 months, for the reasons that "I have no problem or need for treatment" (62%) and "I have no teeth, and therefore I have no need to go" (54%) [2].

Older adults' attitudes related to their need for care are often related to negative childhood experiences and long-standing family beliefs. While dental professionals recommend routine preventive care, some older adults believe the message to be self-serving and choose to wait for pain to occur before seeking treatment. Some older adults choose to live with dental discomfort rather than to seek care, attributing their pain and discomfort to an inevitability of dental decline with age or simply as a problem of aging, not preventable disease. Individuals seeking care typically do so with the belief that their situation will get worse without professional help.

3 The Presence and Absence of Natural Teeth

For many older adults, having natural teeth is strongly associated with having professional dental services, while having no natural teeth (edentulous) is associated with infrequent dental care. Older adults often identify dental professionals to be solely focused on caring for problems associated with their teeth, and many seem to live with the assumption that having no natural teeth means they have no need to see a dentist.

Decades ago, following the delivery of a complete set of dentures, dentists told patients that they did not have to return unless they had a problem. With advances in science, the message to new denture wearers changed to telling them they needed to return for routine checkups. Some denture patients are informed that being edentulous does not reduce their risk for oral cancer and soft tissue pathology and that they could benefit from a routine evaluation, with possible modification of their dental prosthesis. However, most new denture wearers do not return for a preventive examination until posed with a dental problem. A 2017 report of the Medical Expenditure Panel Survey found that only 16% of edentulous adults 50 years and older self-reported a dental visit during the previous 12 months, compared to 52% of those with natural teeth [3].

4 Dental Fear and Communication Between Older Adults and Providers

Communication between dentists and patients is a critical aspect of providing optimum care. Yet physical, psychological, and literacy issues of both patients and professionals can present as barriers to effective communication. For successful implementation of oral health-care services for older adults, there is a need to understand and respond to their oral health beliefs, perceived needs, and preferred type of care services, all of which are shaped by their cultural beliefs and values. This poses challenges to oral health-care providers, especially when serving a diverse older adult population with people coming from different cultural backgrounds.

Older adults who report fear as a major barrier for seeking dental care are more likely to seek care for pain than for preventive services. Dental fear originates from multiple sources including but not limited to their oral health knowledge, previous unpleasant or painful dental experience, being unfamiliar with dental disease, pain, dental procedures, dental professionals, as well as the cost of care. A fear of dentistry may occur as the result of a dental professional not clearly explaining treatment recommendations, causing discomfort, or not ensuring the patient comprehends the treatment plan. Having appropriate information about treatment options, consequences, and costs of care helps older adults make informed decisions and to address their comfort with receiving care. Both dental professionals and older adults need to address the patients' fears and concerns associated with dental care. By addressing older adults' fears of dental care, dental professionals can help to ensure older adults are able to maintain good oral health and be sufficiently comfortable in a dental office.

While dental professionals' knowledge, attitudes, and comfort can influence older adults' use of dental services, it is important to address the patient's concerns about the extent and purpose of proposed treatments. Most dental professionals recommend a minimum of semiannual preventive care visits and may explain the specific purpose of the next dental visits. In addition, dental professionals need to explain to patients their risk for oral disease as well as to explain the need for professional oral health care is lifelong. Older adults benefit from a clear understanding of the many consequences of oral disease and their role in disease management. Were the public better informed of this message, they may be able to address some of their dental fears and hesitancies about dental care.

5 Oral Health-Care Professional Perspectives

Dental professionals can be both enablers and barriers to access to oral health care for older adults. Barriers to health care include the attitudes of providers as well as being the result of experiences providing care to older adults. Oral health-care providers have reported the challenges of delivering care to older adults to include inadequate training, lack of experience, and the need for additional time and loss revenue to treat older adults in private practice. Although not unique to caring for older adults, a dental professional with a friendly, polite, respectful, and friendly demeanor is valued and endears patients, which can help them to overcome their fears so to return to the provider. Recognizing individual's fears and concerns, taking time to talk with patients, and providing a relaxed environment can help to reduce patient hesitancy.

6 Cost of Care and Dental Insurance

All health care, including oral health care is costly, especially for those on a fixed income. The cost of dental care is a major barrier to dental care for older adults and is further complicated by the limited availability of cost-effective dental insurance for older adults. Choosing to spend money on health care when on a fixed income can impact all parts of one's life – as decisions to spend money involve the consideration of many factors including need, risk, benefit, and time justification.

While adults 65 years and older are the least likely cohort to be covered by private dental insurance, those with dental insurance are 2.5 times more likely to make a regular dental visit compared to those without insurance [4]. Similarly, having supplemental medical insurance increases an older adult's chance of using dental services, possibly because the person can divert some of the savings from their medical care to their out-of-pocket dental expenses [5]. In the United States, adults without health-care insurance, without a personal health-care provider, who had delayed medical care because of cost, and who had their last medical visit longer than 12 months ago had greater odds of not having a dental visit within the last 12 months [6]. While some dental professionals choose to offer reduced fees or payment plans to older adults for their care, this is not a universal practice and has an undetermined impact on the decision to obtain care. For older adults on a fixed income as well as those without dental insurance, choosing to obtain routine preventive dental care can be cost prohibitive.

Not having private or public dental insurance can seriously impact the use of dental services. While dental insurance can be purchased while employed, it is only available to retired adults as a postretirement dental benefit, spousal coverage, or through certain Medicare Advantage plans in the United States. In general, most dental insurance plans directed to older adults contain limited benefits. An additional barrier to care for older adults with dental insurance is their limited awareness or ability to understand the insurance benefits. Without a clear understanding of their insurance benefits, many choose not to seek out dental care. In the United States, many aging adults delay routine and needed dental care because they think there is a dental benefit in the Medicare program. In a recent study of older adults' knowledge, only 34% of respondents knew that dental care is not included in Medicare [7]. A similar lack of knowledge or being unaware they are eligible for dental benefits occurs in older adults covered by the Medical Assistance or Medicaid program.

7 Geographic Residence

The location of older adults' residence is associated with their oral health status and dental service utilization, with many older adults geographically isolated from healthcare services. The location of older adult's residence becomes an important barrier to consider given that the proportion of older adults is higher in rural than urban areas and their numbers are expected to increase in the next decade [8]. Studies in several countries have documented that residence in rural areas is associated with more unmet dental needs and lower dental utilization rates than for those living in urban areas [9, 10].

In general, older adults living in rural areas are similar to those who self-report dental fear, that is, they are less likely to visit a dentist in the past year compared to those with a higher education and those who have seen the dentist in their past [11]. Older adults in rural areas are also more likely to report a functional problem and to rate their health as poor [8]. Similarly, rural older adults with lower financial resources are more likely to delay seeking care.

8 Transportation

Access to available transportation is a barrier to health care for many older adults. Transportation is a basic but a necessary step for ongoing health-care and medication access. Without transportation, delays in treatment occur, the use of home remedies increases, and disease exacerbations accumulate and worsen health outcomes [12]. In some communities, low-cost transportation services are available to those who meet eligibility criteria, such as those who have a disability that limits mobility, which can present as an important barrier for those with lower incomes or who do not meet the specific criteria [13]. In some communities, older adults have access to reduced fees for transportation. Poorer populations face more barriers to health-care access in general, and transportation barriers are no exception. Older adults with a lower socioeconomic status (SES) have greater challenges with transportation to health care than those with a higher SES.

Urban and rural locations often differ in transportation options, cost of transportation, and availability of and distance to health-care providers. People living in rural areas report more problems with transportation and travel distance to health-care providers and have a higher burden of travel for health care when measured by distance and time traveled. In general, older adults living in rural areas and those who self-report dental fear were less likely to visit a dentist in the past year compared to those with a secondary or higher education and those with filled tooth surfaces who tend to see the dentist more often [11].

9 Conclusions

Reducing barriers to dental care for older adults will improve access to oral health care. Helping older adults' access oral health services can ultimately improve their oral health status which will improve their general health. With the use of preventive dental visits, oral diseases can be addressed as well as the oral manifestations of systemic disease [6].

Older adults suffer disproportionately from oral disease and limited access to oral health care. Many older adults are either unwilling or unable to receive routine care, putting them at greater risk for general and oral complications. Some present with extensive oral disease, the cumulative effects of disease throughout their lifetime, an even more complicated situation when older adults who are frail, homebound, or in long-term care institutions. To optimally care for this aging cohort, oral health professionals need to be knowledgeable about age-related changes and the many health and cognitive conditions commonly found in older adults. For many providers, additional didactic and clinical training in delivering oral health care to older adults is needed.

While many barriers to good dental health of older adults include systemic health conditions, chronic diseases, limited resources, health literacy, and limitations in activities of daily living, more research is needed to know if alternative models of care, such as mobile dental vans or the presence of more dental professionals, would be successful.

References

1. United States & National Institute of Dental and Craniofacial Research (U.S.). Oral health in America: a report of the Surgeon General. Rockville: Department of Health and Human Services, U.S. Public Health Service; 2000.
2. Shanahan D, O'Neill D. Barriers to dental attendance in older patients. Ir Med J. 2017;110:548.
3. Foiles Sifuentes AM, Castaneda-Avila MA, Lapane KL. The relationship of aging, complete tooth loss, and having a dental visit in the last 12 months. Clin Exp Dent Res. 2020;6(5):550–7. https://doi.org/10.1002/cre2.309.
4. Manski RJ, Goodman HS, Reid BC, Macek MD. Dental insurance visits and expenditures among older adults. Am J Public Health. 2004;94:759–64.
5. Gross DJ, Alecxih L, Gibson MJ, Corea J, Caplan C, Brangan N. Out-of-pocket health spending by poor and near-poor elderly Medicare beneficiaries. Health Serv Res. 1999;34:241–54.
6. Lutfiyya MN, Gross AJ, Soffe B, et al. Dental care utilization: examining the associations between health services deficits and not having a dental visit in past 12 months. BMC Public Health. 2019;19:265. https://doi.org/10.1186/s12889-019-6590-y.
7. Macek MD, Atchison KA, Chen H, et al. Oral health conceptual knowledge and its relationships with oral health outcomes: findings from a Multi-site Health Literacy Study. Community Dent Oral Epidemiol. 2017;45:323–9. https://doi.org/10.1111/cdoe.12294.
8. Baernholdt M, Yan G, Hinton I, Rose K, Mattos M. Quality of life in rural and urban adults 65 years and older: findings from the National Health and Nutrition Examination survey. J Rural Health. 2012;28(4):339–47. https://doi.org/10.1111/j.1748-0361.2011.00403.x.
9. Vargas CM, Yellowitz JA, Hayes KL. Oral health status of older rural adults in the United States. J Am Dent Assoc. 2003;134:479–86.
10. Chalmers JM. Geriatric oral health issues in Australia. Int Dent J. 2001;51:188–99.
11. Mariño R, Giacaman RA. Patterns of use of oral health care services and barriers to dental care among ambulatory older Chilean. BMC Oral Health. 2017;17(1):38. https://doi.org/10.1186/s12903-016-0329-2.
12. Montini T, Tseng TY, Patel H, Shelley D. Barriers to dental services for older adults. Am J Health Behav. 2014;38(5):781–8. https://doi.org/10.5993/AJHB.38.5.15. PMID: 24933147.
13. Syed ST, Gerber BS, Sharp LK. Traveling towards disease: transportation barriers to health care access. J Community Health. 2013;38(5):976–93. https://doi.org/10.1007/s10900-013-9681-1.

Index

A
Active aging, 19, 20
Advance care planning (ACP), 217, 218
Affordable Care Act, 244
Ageism, 19
Age-related changes
    clinical investigation, 2
    definition, 112
    oral cavity structure and function, 2, 3
        edentulism/toothlessness, 4, 5
        masticatory function, 8, 9
        oral microbes, 7, 8
        oral mucosa membrane, 2
        salivary glands, 5, 6
        teeth, 4
        tongue-lip motor function, 6, 7
Alimentary bolus, 97
Alzheimer's disease, 162
American Dental Education Association (ADEA), 245
American Society of Anesthesiologists (ASA) physical scoring system, 147, 149
Anaphylaxis, 151
Antidepressants, 213
Antiretroviral therapies, 89
Asphyxiations, 60
Aspiration, 209
Aspiration pneumonia, 58
Atraumatic restorative treatment (ART), 138, 139
Autoimmune disease, 157, 158

B
Barriers
    age related changes, 280, 281
    cost of care, dental insurance, 283
    dental professionals, 282
    geographic residence, 283, 284
    natural teeth, 281
    older adults *vs.* providers, 281, 282
    presence of pain, 280, 281
    prevalence, 279
    quality of life, 279
    self-perceived needs, 280, 281
    social, behavioral, health and economic factors, 279
    transportation, 284
Body mass index (BMI), 31
Bone and general healing capacity, 121
Brief oral health status examination (BOHSE), 168, 206, 207

C
Cardiovascular disorders, 154
Caries and restorative dentistry
    atraumatic restorative treatment, 138, 139
    diagnosing root surface caries, 134
    exposed root surfaces, 133, 134
    global epidemiology, 131
    long term care facilities, 132, 133
    older adults, 132
    operative management, 137, 138

Caries and restorative dentistry (*cont.*)
   prevention strategies
      chlorhexidine interventions, 136
      CPP-ACP intervention, 137
      fluoride interventions, 136
      oral hygiene advice, 135, 136
      professionally administered interventions, 137
   removable partial denture, 139–141
   risk assessment, 135
Commensal flora, 213
Commission on Dental Accreditation (CODA), 245
COVID-19 pandemic, 182, 190–195, 230, 231, 247–249

D

Decayed, missing or filled teeth (DMFT) scores, 14
Decision making capacity, 217
Delirium
   communication, 170, 171
   definition, 163
   dental appointments, 170
   etiology, 164
   evidence-based behavioral approaches, 171
   future research, 172
   involvement of caregivers, 171
   key issues, 170
   management, 164
   mouth intervention, 169
   oral health and cognitive health, 167
   oral health assessments, 167, 168
   oral self care resistant behaviors, 172
   prevalence, 164
Dementia, 18
   assessment and diagnosis, 162, 163
   communication, 170, 171
   definition, 161
   dental appointments, 170
   etiology, 162
   evidence-based behavioral approaches, 171
   future research, 172
   involvement of caregivers, 171
   key issues, 170
   management, 163
   vs. mild cognitive impairment, 161, 162
   mouth intervention, 169
   neurodegenerative disorders, 162
   oral health and cognitive health, 165, 166
   oral health assessments, 167, 168
   oral self care resistant behaviors, 172
   types of, 162, 163
Dental caries, 21
Dental health registration (DHR), 206, 207
Depression
   causes, 165
   communication, 170, 171
   definition, 164
   dental appointments, 170
   evidence-based behavioral approaches, 171
   first-line treatment, 165
   future research, 172
   involvement of caregivers, 171
   key issues, 170
   mouth intervention, 169
   oral health and cognitive health, 167
   oral health assessments, 167, 168
   oral self care resistant behaviors, 172
   randomized controlled trials, 170
   screening, 165
Diabetes mellitus (DM), 88
Dietary modifications, 69
Drug-related mucocutaneous eruptions, 151
Dry mouth, 22, 23, 85
Dry mouth/xerostomia, 247
Durable power of attorney for health care (DPAHC), 217
Dynamic imaging grade of swallowing toxicity (DIGEST), 63
Dysgeusia, 211
Dysphagia, 209
   consequences of
      asphyxiation risk, 60
      aspiration pneumonia, 58
      dehydration, 60
      malnutrition, 59
      oral health- related quality of life, 60
      pneumonia, 58
   definition, 53
   esophageal phase impairments, 54, 55
   management approaches
      behavioral interventions, 69
      dietary modifications, 69
      pharmacologic interventions, 69
      postural adjustments, 69
      proactive versus reactive approaches, 70, 71
      rehabilitative interventions, 70

Index
289

surgical interventions, 68
swallowing maneuvers, 69
oral phase impairments, 54
pharyngeal phase impairments, 54
prevention of, 53
   chlorhexidine, 64
   daily mouth care, 64, 65
   mechanically ventilated critically ill patients, 67, 68
   suctioning, 66
   tooth brushing, 67
   toothpaste, 67
risk factors, 55–58
signs and symptoms, 53
Dysphagia handicap index (DHI), 62

E
Eastern cooperative oncology group (ECOG), 205
Eating assessment tool-10 (EAT-10), 62
Elder abuse, 226–228
Endocrine diseases, 88, 155
Esophageal phase impairments, 54, 55
Ethics
   changing models of care delivery, 226–228
   COVID-19 pandemic, 230, 231
   definition, 223
   elder abuse, 226–228
   embracing narrative, 231–233
   geriatric patient, 224–226, 230, 231
   history of racism, 228–230
   informed consent, 224–226
   medical mistrust, 228–230
   principles, 231–233
Expiratory muscle strength training (EMST), 70

F
Fiberoptic endoscopic evaluation of swallowing (FEES), 63
Fine-needle aspiration puncture, 101
Food frequency questionnaires (FFQ), 32
Frailty, 19
   bidirectional relationship, 257
   definition, 253
   evidence-based treatments, 255, 256
   future research, 258, 259
   health care professionals, 257–259
   oral frailty, 256, 257

recognition, 254, 255
risk factors, 254
Frailty index (FI), 254
Functional dentition, 36

G
Gastrointestinal disorders, 153
Gender longevity gap, 16
Glossitis, 155
Graft *vs.* host disease, 90
Gum (periodontal) disease, 247

H
Halitosis, 214
Health disparity, 111
   definition, 242
   dental coverage, 243, 244
   literacy, 244
   living conditions and disabilities, 245
   quality of life, 243
   tooth decay, 245, 246
   tooth loss, 246
   tooth retention, 242
Health in aging, 111
Health literacy
   definition, 264
   future research, 273
   inadequate health literacy, 267, 268
   interventions
      age-friendly written materials, 270, 271
      caregivers, 272
      decision aids, 272
      image-based materials, 270, 271
      teach back, 270
      universal precautions, 270
   oral health care professionals, 272, 273
   prevalence, 264
   recognition, 265–267
   SDM, 268, 269
Hela cells, 229
Hematologic disease, 155
Hepatitis C, 89
Hospice
   definition, 203
   ECOG, 205
   KPS, 205
Human papilloma virus (HPV), 23
Human T lymphotropic virus infection, 89

Hyposalivation
  diagnosis
    fine-needle aspiration puncture, 101
    imaging techniques, 101
    intraoral and facial examination, 100
    medical history, 99
    minor salivary gland biopsy, 101
    practical considerations, 104, 105
    questionnaires, 101
    sialometry, 100
  drugs, 92–96
  salivary disorders
    alimentary bolus, 97
    biofilm, changes in, 98
    swallowing, 97
    taste, changes in, 97
  salivary dysfunction
    age, 86
    chronic renal failure, 89
    dehydration, 89
    drugs, 90, 91, 96
    endocrine diseases, 88
    gender, 86
    genetic diseases, 89
    head and neck cancers with radio- and chemotherapy, 90
    infectious diseases, 89
    lifestyle factors, 96
    medical and psychological conditions, 87
    neurologic disorders, 88
    psychological conditions, 89
    rheumatological diseases, 88
  topical salivary substitutes and stimulators, 105
  treatment
    changes or reduction of drugs, 102
    local measures, 102, 103
    practical considerations, 104, 105
    preventive measures, 102
    Sjogren's syndrome, 103
    systemic sialagogues, 103

I
Immune system, 214
Implant-supported dentures (ISD), 35
Informed consent, 216, 217, 224–226
Instrumental swallow evaluation, 63
International Dysphagia Diet Standardization Initiative (IDDSI) framework, 60
Intraglandular lymphadenopathy, 89

K
Kaposi sarcoma, 89
Karnofsky performance scale (KPS), 204, 205

L
Lichenoid drug reaction, 153
Liquid food swallowing, 49
Living Will (LW), 217
Lobulated tongue, 158
Long-term care facilities (LTCFs), 132, 133
  aging, 177
  COVID-19 pandemic, 190–195
  dental care services, 178
  description, 178, 179
  edentulism rates, 177
  failure, 178
  integration, 191, 192
  residents, 179–182
  types, 182–190
Lower acrylic resin RPD, 140
Lupus erythematosus disease, 157

M
Malnutrition screening tool (MST), 34
Malnutrition universal screening tool (MUST), 31, 34
Managing oral hygiene using threat reduction (MOUTh), 169
Masseter muscle echo intensity (MMEI), 8
Masseter muscle thickness (MMT), 8
Masticatory function, 8, 9
Medicaid program, 244
Mild cognitive impairment (MCI), 161
Mini nutritional assessment (MNA), 30, 31
Minimally invasive dentistry (MID), 138
Minor salivary gland biopsy, 101
MNA short-form (MNA-SF), 33
Modified barium swallow impairment profile (MBSImP®), 63
Modified barium swallow study (MBS), 63
Modified functional feeding assessment (FFAm) subscale, 6
Mucositis/stomatitis, 209, 210
Multidisciplinary feeding profile (MFP), 6
Muscle quantity, 8

N
Narrative ethics, 231–233
Neurocognitive disorders, 156
Neurologic disorders, 88
Newest vital sign (NVS), 265, 266

Index   291

Non-Hodgkin lymphoma, 89
Nutrition
    adaptive and maladaptive behaviors, 36, 37
    diet and nutritional status, 35
    dietary intake, 32
    healthcare providers
        with dentures, 38, 40
        with tooth loss, 37, 38
    healthcare providers with dentures, 38, 39
    medical, surgical, and dental history, 31, 32
    oral risk factors, 32
    risk factors, 30
    screening and assessment tools, 33
        malnutrition screening tool, 34
        malnutrition universal screening tool, 34
        MNA-SF, 33
        nutritional risk screening 2002, 34
        SELF-MNA, 34
    screening tools, 30
    tooth loss, with or without replacement with dentures, 34
    weight status and change, 30, 31
Nutritional risk screening 2002 (NRS 2002), 34

O
Oral cancer, 23
Oral candidiasis, 155
Oral conditions, in older populations
    active aging, 19, 20
    ageism, 19
    chronic conditions, 17, 18
    chronological concept, 13
    dementia, 18
    dental caries, 21
    disability, 18
    DMFT scores, 14
    dry mouth, 22, 23
    ethnic differences, 17
    frailty, 19
    gender, 16
    multimorbidity, 18
    oral mucosa lesions, 23
    periodontitis, 22
    sociodemographic changes, 15, 16
    sub-groups, 14
    tooth loss, 20, 21
Oral health assessment tool (OHAT), 207
Oral health literacy (OHL), 264
Oral health- related quality of life (OHrQoL), 60
Oral healthcare
    COVID-19, 247–249
    dry mouth/xerostomia, 247
    gum disease, 247
    health disparity
        definition, 242
        dental coverage, 243, 244
        literacy, 244
        living conditions and disabilities, 245
        quality of life, 243
        tooth decay, 245, 246
        tooth loss, 246
        tooth retention, 242
    older adult population, 239–241
    oral cancer /pre-cancer, 247
    SDOH, 241, 242
Oral infections, 213, 214
Oral microbiome, 7, 8
Oral mucosa, 213
Oral mucosa lesions, 23
Oral mucosa membrane, 2
Oral performance instrument, 7
Oral phase impairments, 54
Oral praxis subtest (OPS), 6
Orofacial pain, 211–213
Oropharyngeal cancer, 23
Osseointegration process, 121
Ozar's central values of dental practice, 232

P
Palliative care
    cognitive impairment, 209
    definition, 202, 203
    dental care professional, 205, 206
    dysgeusia, 211
    end of life
        ACP and advance directives, 217, 218
        decision making capacity, 217
        informed consent, 216, 217
        SDM, 216
        withholding and withdrawal of life support, 215, 216
    functional impairment and frailty, 208
    halitosis, 214 (*see* Hospice)
    KPS, 204
    mucositis/stomatitis, 209, 210
    oral assessment, 206, 207
    oral diseases, 201
    oral infections, 213, 214
    orofacial pain, 211–213
    polypharmacy, 208
    poor oral hygiene, 207
    PPS, 204
    saliva, 210, 211
    swallowing disorders and aspiration, 209
    World Health Organization, 201

Palliative performance scale (PPS), 204, 205
Peri-implant mucositis, 122
Peri-implantitis, 122
Periodontal disease
    dental office, 123
    health in aging, 111
    health disparities, 111
    management of, 112, 116–118
    masticatory function and cognition, 114–116
    normal oral aging vs. true oral pathology, 112–116
    preserving teeth or placing implant
        bone and general healing capacity, 121
        complications, 122
        diabetes, 121–122
        maintenance protocol, 122
        plaque control, 120
        tooth replacement, 120, 121
    prevalence of, 110, 111
    proinflammatory phenotype, 114
    projections, 110
    salivary function, 113
    social support, 119
    tooth loss, 111
    tooth retention, 114
Periodontitis, 22, *see* Periodontal disease
Pharyngeal phase impairments, 54
Physician orders for life-sustaining treatment (POLST), 217
Pictograms, 270, 271
Plaque control, 120
Pneumonia, 58
Postural adjustments, 69
Presbyphagia, 55
Programs of all-inclusive care for the elders (PACE), 227, 228
Protein-energy malnutrition (PEM), 59

Q
Questionnaires, 101

R
Rapid estimate of adult literacy in medicine (REALM), 265
Rehabilitative interventions, 70
Removable partial denture. (RPD), 139–141
Renal disorders, 153, 155
Respiratory disorders, 156, 157
Rheumatological diseases, 88

S
Saliva, 85, 210, 211, 213
Salivary gland hypofunction (SGH), 22
Salivary glands, 5, 6
Sarcoidosis, 90
Sarcopenia, 253, 257
Self-administered version (Self-MNA), 33
Self-MNA, 34
Shared decision making (SDM), 268, 269
Short physical performance battery (SPPB), 254
Shortened dental arch, 141
Sialometry, 100
Sialorrhea, 210
Sjögren's syndrome (SS), 88, 157
Social determinants of health (SDOH), 5, 241, 242
Socio-economic status (SES), 284
Solid food swallowing, 50
Solid food test, 62
Spontaneous swallowing, 48
Swallowing
    anatomy
        musculature, 52
        neurophysiology, 52, 53
    definition, 48
    evaluation
        clinical, 61
        instrumental swallow evaluation, 63
    physiology
        liquid, 49, 50
        solid, 50, 51
    screening tests, 62
    spontaneous, 48
    volitional, 48
Swallowing maneuvers, 69
Sydney swallowing questionnaire (SSQ), 62
Systemic disease
    ASA classification, 147, 149
    clinical background, 145, 146
    clinical manifestation, in orofacial areas
        autoimmune disease, 157, 158
        cardiovascular disorders, 154
        endocrine disorders, 155
        gastrointestinal disorders, 153
        hematologic disease, 155
        neurocognitive disorders, 156
        renal disorders, 153, 155
        respiratory disorders, 156, 157
    geriatric assessment, 146–148
    medical risk assessment, 147
        adverse reaction, 151, 153

Index

before, during, and after dental procedure, 150, 151
bleeding, 149
drug interactions, 151
infection, 147, 149

T
Teeth, 4
Test of functional health literacy in adults (TOFHLA), 265, 266
Test of functional health literacy in dentistry (TOFHLiD), 266
Test of masticating and swallowing solids (TOMASS), 62
Tobacco use, 23
Tongue-lip motor function (TLMF), 6, 7
Tooth loss, 20, 21
    peridontal disease, 111
Tooth replacement, 120, 121
Tooth retention, 242, 243
Tuberculosis, 89
Two stage rapid estimate of adult literacy in dentistry (TS-REALD), 266

U
Unintentional weight gain, 31
Upper and lower cobalt-chromium RPDs, 140
Upper gastrointestinal tract (GI) cancers, 31

V
Vesiculobullous/ulcerative lesions, 152
Videofluoroscopic examination of swallow (VFSS), 63
Videofluoroscopic swallowing study (VFS), 63
Volitional swallowing, 48

W
Water swallow test, 62
Withdrawal and withholding of life support, 215, 216
"World Population Aging 2019", 110

X
Xerostomia, 22, 210
    diagnosis
        fine-needle aspiration puncture, 101
        imaging techniques, 101
        intraoral and facial examination, 100
        medical history, 99
        minor salivary gland biopsy, 101
        practical considerations, 104, 105
        questionnaires, 101
        sialometry, 100
    drugs, 92–96
    salivary disorders
        alimentary bolus, 97
        biofilm, changes in, 98
        swallowing, 97
        taste, changes in, 97
    salivary dysfunction
        age, 86
        chronic renal failure, 89
        dehydration, 89
        drugs, 90, 91, 96
        endocrine diseases, 88
        gender, 86
        genetic diseases, 89
        head and neck cancers with radio- and chemotherapy, 90
        infectious diseases, 89
        lifestyle factors, 96
        medical and psychological conditions, 87
        neurologic disorders, 88
        psychological conditions, 89
        rheumatological diseases, 88
    topical salivary substitutes and stimulators, 105
    treatment
        changes or reduction of drugs, 102
        local measures, 102, 103
        practical considerations, 104, 105
        preventive measures, 102
        Sjogren's syndrome, 103
        systemic sialagogues, 103

Z
Zenker's diverticulum, 54

Printed in the United States
by Baker & Taylor Publisher Services